Genetic Disorders

SOURCEBOOK

Fifth Edition

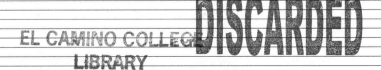

Health Reference Series

Fifth Edition

Genetic Disorders

SOURCEBOOK

Basic Consumer Health Information about Heritable Disorders, Including Disorders Resulting from Abnormalities in Specific Genes, Such as Hemophilia, Sickle Cell Disease, and Cystic Fibrosis, Chromosomal Disorders, Such as Down Syndrome, Fragile X Syndrome, and Klinefelter Syndrome, and Complex Disorders with Environmental and Genetic Components, Such as Alzheimer Disease, Cancer, Heart Disease, and Obesity

Along with Information about the Human Genome Project, Genetic Testing and Newborn Screening, Gene Therapy and Other Current Research Initiatives, the Special Needs of Children with Genetic Disorders, a Glossary of Terms, and a Directory of Resources for Further Help and Information

Edited by
Sandra J. Judd

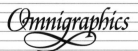

Omnigraphics

155 W. Congress, Suite 200, Detroit, MI 48226

Bibliographic Note

Because this page cannot legibly accommodate all the copyright notices, the Bibliographic Note portion of the Preface constitutes an extension of the copyright notice.

Edited by Sandra J. Judd

Health Reference Series
Karen Bellenir, *Managing Editor*
David A. Cooke, MD, FACP, *Medical Consultant*
Elizabeth Collins, *Research and Permissions Coordinator*
EdIndex, Services for Publishers, *Indexers*

* * *

Omnigraphics, Inc.
Matthew P. Barbour, *Senior Vice President*
Kevin M. Hayes, *Operations Manager*

* * *

Peter E. Ruffner, *Publisher*
Copyright © 2014 Omnigraphics, Inc.
ISBN 978-0-7808-1301-4
E-ISBN 978-0-7808-1302-1

Library of Congress Cataloging-in-Publication Data

Genetic disorders sourcebook : basic consumer health information about heritable disorders, including disorders resulting from abnormalities in specific genes, such as hemophilia, sickle cell disease, and cystic fibrosis, chromosomal disorders, such as Down syndrome, fragile x syndrome, and Klinefelter syndrome, and complex disorders with environmental and genetic components, such as Alzheimer disease, cancer, heart disease, and obesity; along with information about the human genome project, genetic testing and newborn screening, gene therapy and other current research initiatives, the special needs of children with genetic disorders, a glossary of terms, and a directory of resources for further help and information / edited by Sandra J. Judd. -- Fifth edition.
    pages cm
  Includes bibliographical references and index.
  Summary: "Provides basic consumer health information about disorders caused by gene and chromosome abnormalities and those with genetic and environmental components, along with facts about genetic testing and treatment research, and guidance for parents of children with special needs. Includes index, glossary of related terms, and other resources"-- Provided by publisher.
  ISBN 978-0-7808-1301-4 (hardcover : alk. paper) 1. Human chromosome abnormalities--Popular works. I. Judd, Sandra J.
  RB155.5.G455 2013
  616'.042--dc23
                                                                    2013026642

Table of Contents

Visit www.healthreferenceseries.com to view *A Contents Guide to the Health Reference Series*, a listing of more than 16,000 topics and the volumes in which they are covered.

Part III: Chromosome Abnormalities

Part IV: Complex Disorders with Genetic and Environmental Components

Part VI: Information for Parents of Children with Genetic Disorders

Preface

About This Book

Genes provide the information that directs the human body's basic cellular activities. Research on the human genome has shown that the DNA sequences of any two individuals are 99.9 percent identical. That 0.1 percent variation, however, is profoundly important. It contributes to visible differences, like height and hair color, and also to invisible differences, such as increased risk for—or protection from—a myriad of diseases and disorders.

As medical researchers unlock the secrets of the human genome, they are learning that nearly all diseases have a genetic component. Some are caused by a mutation in a gene or group of genes. Such mutations can occur randomly or as the result of exposure to hazardous conditions or substances. Other disorders are hereditary. These can be passed down from generation to generation within a family. Finally, many—perhaps most—genetic disorders are caused by a combination of small variations in genes operating in concert with environmental factors.

Genetic Disorders Sourcebook, Fifth Edition offers updated information on how genes work and how genetic mutations affect health. It provides facts about the most common genetic disorders, including those that arise from mutations in specific genes—for example, muscular dystrophy, sickle cell anemia, and cystic fibrosis—as well as those arising from chromosomal abnormalities—such as Down syndrome and fragile X syndrome. A section on disorders with genetic and environmental components explains the hereditary components of Alzheimer disease, cancer, diabetes, mental illness, obesity, addiction, and others. Reports on current research initiatives provide detailed information on the newest breakthroughs in the causes and treatments of genetic disorders, including strategies, like gene therapy, nutrigenomics, and pharmacogenetics that could radically change how we treat these disorders in the future. A section for parents of children with genetic disorders offers information about assistive technologies, educational options, transition to adulthood, and estate planning. Information about genetic counseling, prenatal testing, newborn screening, and preventing genetic discrimination is also provided. The book concludes with a glossary of genetic terms and a list of resources for additional help and information.

How to Use This Book

This book is divided into parts and chapters. Parts focus on broad areas of interest. Chapters are devoted to single topics within a part.

Part I: Introduction to Genetics describes how genes work and explains what is known about how genetic mutations affect health. It details how genetic inheritance works, explains when genetic counseling might be advisable, and describes how genetic testing works and the type of information it can provide. The part concludes with a discussion of the legal framework currently in place to prevent discrimination on the basis of genetic background.

Part II: Disorders Resulting from Abnormalities in Specific Genes provides basic information about the types of disorders that are caused by changes in one or more genes. These include blood and clotting disorders, connective tissue disorders, heart rhythm disorders, muscular dystrophy and other neuromuscular disorders, cystic fibrosis, and hearing and vision disorders. Individual chapters include information about the inheritance, symptoms, diagnosis, and treatment of each disorder.

Part III: Chromosome Abnormalities offers detailed information about the types of disorders caused by changes in chromosomes. It explains how Down syndrome, fragile X syndrome, Turner syndrome, and other chromosomal disorders are inherited and describes the diagnostic tests and treatment techniques used.

Part IV: Complex Disorders with Genetic and Environmental Components explains what is known about the causes of addiction, obesity, mental health disorders, heart disease, diabetes, cancer, and other disorders with both genetic and environmental components. It describes the genetic associations related to each disorder and discusses the research advances that may lead to improved prevention efforts and treatment outcomes.

Part V: Genetic Research describes recent advances in the field of genetics as doctors seek ways to use knowledge of an individual's genetic background to target disease prevention and treatment techniques. It includes a discussion of what has been discovered during the course of the Human Genome Project and describes promising new avenues of research, including nutrigenomics, pharmacogenomics, and gene therapy.

Part VI: Information for Parents of Children with Genetic Disorders addresses the challenges of raising special needs children. It discusses early interventions, assistive technologies, educational concerns, and the transition into adulthood. The part also explains government benefits available to children and adults with disabilities and offers estate planning information for families of children with special needs.

Part VII: Additional Help and Information includes a glossary of terms related to human genetics and a directory of resources offering additional help and support.

Bibliographic Note

This volume contains documents and excerpts from publications issued by the following U.S. government agencies: Centers for Disease Control and Prevention (CDC); Genetics Home Reference; National Cancer Institute; National Dissemination Center for Children with Disabilities; National Heart, Lung, and Blood Institute; National Human Genome Research Institute; National Institute of Arthritis and Musculoskeletal and Skin Diseases; National Institute of Child Health and Human Development; National Institute of Diabetes and Digestive and Kidney Diseases; National Institute of Neurological Disorders and Stroke; National Institute on Alcohol Abuse and Alcoholism; National Institute on Deafness and Other Communication Disorders; National Institutes of Health; Oak Ridge National Laboratory; Office on Women's Health; Rare Diseases Clinical Research Network; U.S. Department of Education; U.S. Department of Health and Human Services; and the U.S. Social Security Administration.

In addition, this volume contains copyrighted documents from the following organizations: About.com; A.D.A.M., Inc.; American Association for Pediatric Ophthalmology and Strabismus; Australian

Mitochondrial Disease Foundation; Children's Hospital of Philadelphia; Duke Institute for Genome Sciences and Policy; Emory University School of Medicine—Department of Human Genetics; Genetic Science Learning Center; HealthDay/ScoutNews LLC; Hormone Health Network; Kansas State University News Services; Magic Foundation; Massachusetts General Hospital; Massachusetts Institute of Technology News Office; Minnesota Department of Health—Newborn Screening Program; Miriam Hospital; National Collaborative on Workforce and Disability for Youth; National Marfan Foundation; Nemours Foundation; Pacer Center; Parkinson's Disease Foundation; PsychCentral; Queensland University of Technology; Sainte-Justine University Hospital Research Center; Spastic Paraplegia Foundation; Texas Heart Institute; United Leukodystrophy Foundation; University of Chicago Medical Center; University of Illinois at Chicago; University of Leicester Press Office; University of Michigan Health System; University of Michigan Health System—YourChild: Development and Behavior Resources; University of North Carolina Medical Center News Office; University of Ottawa Heart Institute; University of Virginia School of Medicine—Department of Psychiatry and Neurobehavioral Sciences; University of Washington Medical Center—Patient and Family Education Services; Utah Department of Health Asthma Program; Washington University in St. Louis School of Medicine—Office of Medical Public Affairs; and the World Institute on Disability.

Full citation information is provided on the first page of each chapter or section. Every effort has been made to secure all necessary rights to reprint the copyrighted material. If any omissions have been made, please contact Omnigraphics to make corrections for future editions.

Acknowledgements

Thanks go to the many organizations, agencies, and individuals who have contributed materials for this *Sourcebook* and to medical consultant Dr. David Cooke and prepress services provider WhimsyInk. Special thanks go to managing editor Karen Bellenir and permissions coordinator Liz Collins for their help and support.

About the Health Reference Series

The *Health Reference Series* is designed to provide basic medical information for patients, families, caregivers, and the general public. Each volume takes a particular topic and provides comprehensive coverage. This is especially important for people who may be dealing with a newly diagnosed disease or a chronic disorder in themselves or in a family member. People looking for preventive guidance, information about disease warning signs, medical statistics, and risk factors for health problems will also find answers to their questions in the *Health Reference Series*. The *Series*, however, is not intended to serve as a tool for diagnosing illness, in prescribing treatments, or as a substitute for the physician/patient relationship. All people concerned about medical symptoms or the possibility of disease are encouraged to seek professional care from an appropriate healthcare provider.

A Note about Spelling and Style

Health Reference Series editors use *Stedman's Medical Dictionary* as an authority for questions related to the spelling of medical terms and the *Chicago Manual of Style* for questions related to grammatical structures, punctuation, and other editorial concerns. Consistent adherence is not always possible, however, because the individual volumes within the *Series* include many documents from a wide variety of different producers and copyright holders, and the editor's primary goal is to present material from each source as accurately as is possible following the terms specified by each document's producer. This sometimes means that information in different chapters or sections may follow other guidelines and alternate spelling authorities. For example, occasionally a copyright holder may require that eponymous terms be shown in possessive forms (Crohn's disease *vs.* Crohn disease) or that British spelling norms be retained (leukaemia *vs.* leukemia).

Locating Information within the Health Reference Series

The *Health Reference Series* contains a wealth of information about a wide variety of medical topics. Ensuring easy access to all the fact sheets, research reports, in-depth discussions, and other material contained within the individual books of the series remains one of our highest priorities. As the *Series* continues to grow in size and scope, however, locating the precise information needed by a reader may become more challenging.

A Contents Guide to the Health Reference Series was developed to direct readers to the specific volumes that address their concerns. It presents an extensive list of diseases, treatments, and other topics of general interest compiled from the Tables of Contents and major index headings. To access *A Contents Guide to the Health Reference Series*, visit www.healthreferenceseries.com.

Medical Consultant

Medical consultation services are provided to the *Health Reference Series* editors by David A. Cooke, MD, FACP. Dr. Cooke is a graduate of Brandeis University, and he received his M.D. degree from the University of Michigan. He completed residency training at the University of Wisconsin Hospital and Clinics. He is board-certified in Internal Medicine. Dr. Cooke currently works as part of the University of Michigan Health System and practices in Ann Arbor, MI. In his free time, he enjoys writing, science fiction, and spending time with his family.

Our Advisory Board

We would like to thank the following board members for providing guidance to the development of this series:

Dr. Lynda Baker, Associate Professor of Library and Information Science, Wayne State University, Detroit, MI

Nancy Bulgarelli, William Beaumont Hospital Library, Royal Oak, MI

Karen Imarisio, Bloomfield Township Public Library, Bloomfield Township, MI

Karen Morgan, Mardigian Library, University of Michigan-Dearborn, Dearborn, MI

Rosemary Orlando, St. Clair Shores Public Library, St. Clair Shores, MI

Health Reference Series *Update Policy*

The inaugural book in the *Health Reference Series* was the first edition of *Cancer Sourcebook* published in 1989. Since then, the *Series* has been enthusiastically received by librarians and in the medical community. In order to maintain the standard of providing high-quality health information for the layperson the editorial staff at Omnigraphics felt it was necessary to implement a policy of updating volumes when warranted.

Medical researchers have been making tremendous strides, and it is the purpose of the *Health Reference Series* to stay current with the most recent advances. Each decision to update a volume is made on an individual basis. Some of the considerations include how much new information is available and the feedback we receive from people who use the books. If there is a topic you would like to see added to the update list, or an area of medical concern you feel has not been adequately addressed, please write to:

Editor
Health Reference Series
Omnigraphics, Inc.
155 W. Congress, Suite 200
Detroit, MI 48226
E-mail: editorial@omnigraphics.com

Part One

Introduction to Genetics

Chapter 1

Cells and DNA: The Basics

What is a cell?

Cells are the basic building blocks of all living things. The human body is composed of trillions of cells. They provide structure for the body, take in nutrients from food, convert those nutrients into energy, and carry out specialized functions. Cells also contain the body's hereditary material and can make copies of themselves.

Cells have many parts, each with a different function. Human cells contain the following major parts, listed in alphabetical order:

- **Cytoplasm:** Within cells, the cytoplasm is made up of a jelly-like fluid (called the cytosol) and other structures that surround the nucleus.

- **Cytoskeleton:** The cytoskeleton is a network of long fibers that make up the cell's structural framework. The cytoskeleton has several critical functions, including determining cell shape, participating in cell division, and allowing cells to move. It also provides a track-like system that directs the movement of organelles and other substances within cells.

- **Endoplasmic reticulum (ER):** This organelle helps process molecules created by the cell. The endoplasmic reticulum also transports these molecules to their specific destinations either inside or outside the cell.

Excerpted from "Cells and DNA," Genetics Home Reference (http://ghr.nlm
.nih.gov), May 13, 2013.

- **Golgi apparatus:** The Golgi apparatus packages molecules processed by the endoplasmic reticulum to be transported out of the cell.

- **Lysosomes and peroxisomes:** These organelles are the recycling center of the cell. They digest foreign bacteria that invade the cell, rid the cell of toxic substances, and recycle worn-out cell components.

- **Mitochondria:** Mitochondria are complex organelles that convert energy from food into a form that the cell can use. They have their own genetic material, separate from the DNA (deoxyribonucleic acid) in the nucleus, and can make copies of themselves.

- **Nucleus:** The nucleus serves as the cell's command center, sending directions to the cell to grow, mature, divide, or die. It also houses DNA, the cell's hereditary material. The nucleus is surrounded by a membrane called the nuclear envelope, which protects the DNA and separates the nucleus from the rest of the cell.

- **Plasma membrane:** The plasma membrane is the outer lining of the cell. It separates the cell from its environment and allows materials to enter and leave the cell.

- **Ribosomes:** Ribosomes are organelles that process the cell's genetic instructions to create proteins. These organelles can float freely in the cytoplasm or be connected to the endoplasmic reticulum (see above).

What is DNA?

DNA, or deoxyribonucleic acid, is the hereditary material in humans and almost all other organisms. Nearly every cell in a person's body has the same DNA. Most DNA is located in the cell nucleus (where it is called nuclear DNA), but a small amount of DNA can also be found in the mitochondria (where it is called mitochondrial DNA or mtDNA).

The information in DNA is stored as a code made up of four chemical bases: adenine (A), guanine (G), cytosine (C), and thymine (T). Human DNA consists of about three billion bases, and more than 99 percent of those bases are the same in all people. The order, or sequence, of these bases determines the information available for building and maintaining an organism, similar to the way in which letters of the alphabet appear in a certain order to form words and sentences.

DNA bases pair up with each other, A with T and C with G, to form units called base pairs. Each base is also attached to a sugar molecule and a phosphate molecule. Together, a base, sugar, and phosphate are called a nucleotide. Nucleotides are arranged in two long strands that form a spiral called a double helix. The structure of the double helix is somewhat like a ladder, with the base pairs forming the ladder's rungs and the sugar and phosphate molecules forming the vertical sidepieces of the ladder.

An important property of DNA is that it can replicate, or make copies of itself. Each strand of DNA in the double helix can serve as a pattern for duplicating the sequence of bases. This is critical when cells divide because each new cell needs to have an exact copy of the DNA present in the old cell.

What is mitochondrial DNA?

Although most DNA is packaged in chromosomes within the nucleus, mitochondria also have a small amount of their own DNA. This genetic material is known as mitochondrial DNA or mtDNA.

Mitochondria are structures within cells that convert the energy from food into a form that cells can use. Each cell contains hundreds to thousands of mitochondria, which are located in the fluid that surrounds the nucleus (the cytoplasm).

Mitochondria produce energy through a process called oxidative phosphorylation. This process uses oxygen and simple sugars to create adenosine triphosphate (ATP), the cell's main energy source. A set of enzyme complexes, designated as complexes I–V, carry out oxidative phosphorylation within mitochondria.

In addition to energy production, mitochondria play a role in several other cellular activities. For example, mitochondria help regulate the self-destruction of cells (apoptosis). They are also necessary for the production of substances such as cholesterol and heme (a component of hemoglobin, the molecule that carries oxygen in the blood).

Mitochondrial DNA contains thirty-seven genes, all of which are essential for normal mitochondrial function. Thirteen of these genes provide instructions for making enzymes involved in oxidative phosphorylation. The remaining genes provide instructions for making molecules called transfer RNAs (tRNAs) and ribosomal RNAs (rRNAs), which are chemical cousins of DNA. These types of RNA help assemble protein building blocks (amino acids) into functioning proteins.

What is a gene?

A gene is the basic physical and functional unit of heredity. Genes, which are made up of DNA, act as instructions to make molecules called proteins. In humans, genes vary in size from a few hundred DNA bases to more than two million bases. The Human Genome Project has estimated that humans have between twenty thousand and twenty-five thousand genes.

Every person has two copies of each gene, one inherited from each parent. Most genes are the same in all people, but a small number of genes (less than 1 percent of the total) are slightly different between people. Alleles are forms of the same gene with small differences in their sequence of DNA bases. These small differences contribute to each person's unique physical features.

What is a chromosome?

In the nucleus of each cell, the DNA molecule is packaged into thread-like structures called chromosomes. Each chromosome is made up of DNA tightly coiled many times around proteins called histones that support its structure.

Chromosomes are not visible in the cell's nucleus—not even under a microscope—when the cell is not dividing. However, the DNA that makes up chromosomes becomes more tightly packed during cell division and is then visible under a microscope. Most of what researchers know about chromosomes was learned by observing chromosomes during cell division.

Each chromosome has a constriction point called the centromere, which divides the chromosome into two sections, or "arms." The short arm of the chromosome is labeled the "p arm." The long arm of the chromosome is labeled the "q arm." The location of the centromere on each chromosome gives the chromosome its characteristic shape, and can be used to help describe the location of specific genes.

How many chromosomes do people have?

In humans, each cell normally contains twenty-three pairs of chromosomes, for a total of forty-six. Twenty-two of these pairs, called autosomes, look the same in both males and females. The twenty-third pair, the sex chromosomes, differ between males and females. Females have two copies of the X chromosome, while males have one X and one Y chromosome.

Chapter 2

How Genes Work

What are proteins and what do they do?

Proteins are large, complex molecules that play many critical roles in the body. They do most of the work in cells and are required for the structure, function, and regulation of the body's tissues and organs.

Proteins are made up of hundreds or thousands of smaller units called amino acids, which are attached to one another in long chains. There are twenty different types of amino acids that can be combined to make a protein. The sequence of amino acids determines each protein's unique three-dimensional structure and its specific function.

Proteins can be described according to their large range of functions in the body, as shown in Table 2.1.

How do genes direct the production of proteins?

Most genes contain the information needed to make functional molecules called proteins. (A few genes produce other molecules that help the cell assemble proteins.) The journey from gene to protein is complex and tightly controlled within each cell. It consists of two major steps: transcription and translation. Together, transcription and translation are known as gene expression.

Excerpted from "How Genes Work," Genetics Home Reference (http://ghr.nlm.nih.gov), May 13, 2013.

During the process of transcription, the information stored in a gene's deoxyribonucleic acid (DNA) is transferred to a similar molecule called RNA (ribonucleic acid) in the cell nucleus. Both RNA and DNA are made up of a chain of nucleotide bases, but they have slightly different chemical properties. The type of RNA that contains the information for making a protein is called messenger RNA (mRNA) because it carries the information, or message, from the DNA out of the nucleus into the cytoplasm.

Translation, the second step in getting from a gene to a protein, takes place in the cytoplasm. The mRNA interacts with a specialized complex called a ribosome, which "reads" the sequence of mRNA bases. Each sequence of three bases, called a codon, usually codes for one particular amino acid. (Amino acids are the building blocks of proteins.) A type of RNA called transfer RNA (tRNA) assembles the protein, one amino acid at a time. Protein assembly continues until the ribosome encounters a "stop" codon (a sequence of three bases that does not code for an amino acid).

The flow of information from DNA to RNA to proteins is one of the fundamental principles of molecular biology. It is so important that it is sometimes called the "central dogma."

Table 2.1. Examples of protein functions

Function	Description	Example
Antibody	Antibodies bind to specific foreign particles, such as viruses and bacteria, to help protect the body.	Immunoglobulin G (IgG)
Enzyme	Enzymes carry out almost all of the thousands of chemical reactions that take place in cells. They also assist with the formation of new molecules by reading the genetic information stored in deoxyribonucleic acid (DNA).	Phenylalanine hydroxylase
Messenger	Messenger proteins, such as some types of hormones, transmit signals to coordinate biological processes between different cells, tissues, and organs.	Growth hormone
Structural component	These proteins provide structure and support for cells. On a larger scale, they also allow the body to move.	Actin
Transport/ storage	These proteins bind and carry atoms and small molecules within cells and throughout the body.	Ferritin

Can genes be turned on and off in cells?

Each cell expresses, or turns on, only a fraction of its genes. The rest of the genes are repressed, or turned off. The process of turning genes on and off is known as gene regulation. Gene regulation is an important part of normal development. Genes are turned on and off in different patterns during development to make a brain cell look and act different from a liver cell or a muscle cell, for example. Gene regulation also allows cells to react quickly to changes in their environments. Although we know that the regulation of genes is critical for life, this complex process is not yet fully understood.

Gene regulation can occur at any point during gene expression, but most commonly occurs at the level of transcription (when the information in a gene's DNA is transferred to mRNA). Signals from the environment or from other cells activate proteins called transcription factors. These proteins bind to regulatory regions of a gene and increase or decrease the level of transcription. By controlling the level of transcription, this process can determine the amount of protein product that is made by a gene at any given time.

What is the epigenome?

DNA modifications that do not change the DNA sequence can affect gene activity. Chemical compounds that are added to single genes can regulate their activity; these modifications are known as epigenetic changes. The epigenome comprises all of the chemical compounds that have been added to the entirety of one's DNA (genome) as a way to regulate the activity (expression) of all the genes within the genome. The chemical compounds of the epigenome are not part of the DNA sequence, but are on or attached to DNA ("epi-" means above in Greek). Epigenomic modifications remain as cells divide and in some cases can be inherited through the generations. Environmental influences, such as a person's diet and exposure to pollutants, can also impact the epigenome.

Epigenetic changes can help determine whether genes are turned on or off and can influence the production of proteins in certain cells, ensuring that only necessary proteins are produced. For example, proteins that promote bone growth are not produced in muscle cells. Patterns of epigenome modification vary among individuals, different tissues within an individual, and even different cells.

A common type of epigenomic modification is called methylation. Methylation involves attaching small molecules called methyl groups, each consisting of one carbon atom and three hydrogen atoms, to segments of DNA. When methyl groups are added to a particular gene, that gene is turned off or silenced, and no protein is produced from that gene.

Because errors in the epigenetic process, such as modifying the wrong gene or failing to add a compound to a gene, can lead to abnormal gene activity or inactivity, they can cause genetic disorders. Conditions including cancers, metabolic disorders, and degenerative disorders have all been found to be related to epigenetic errors.

Scientists continue to explore the relationship between the genome and the chemical compounds that modify it. In particular, they are studying what effect the modifications have on gene function, protein production, and human health.

How do cells divide?

There are two types of cell division: mitosis and meiosis. Most of the time when people refer to "cell division," they mean mitosis, the process of making new body cells. Meiosis is the type of cell division that creates egg and sperm cells.

Mitosis is a fundamental process for life. During mitosis, a cell duplicates all of its contents, including its chromosomes, and splits to form two identical daughter cells. Because this process is so critical, the steps of mitosis are carefully controlled by a number of genes. When mitosis is not regulated correctly, health problems such as cancer can result.

The other type of cell division, meiosis, ensures that humans have the same number of chromosomes in each generation. It is a two-step process that reduces the chromosome number by half—from forty-six to twenty-three—to form sperm and egg cells. When the sperm and egg cells unite at conception, each contributes twenty-three chromosomes so the resulting embryo will have the usual forty-six. Meiosis also allows genetic variation through a process of DNA shuffling while the cells are dividing.

How do genes control the growth and division of cells?

A variety of genes are involved in the control of cell growth and division. The cell cycle is the cell's way of replicating itself in an organized, step-by-step fashion. Tight regulation of this process ensures that a dividing cell's DNA is copied properly, any errors in the DNA are repaired, and each daughter cell receives a full set of chromosomes. The cycle has checkpoints (also called restriction points), which allow certain genes to check for mistakes and halt the cycle for repairs if something goes wrong.

If a cell has an error in its DNA that cannot be repaired, it may undergo programmed cell death (apoptosis). Apoptosis is a common process throughout life that helps the body get rid of cells it doesn't need. Cells that undergo apoptosis break apart and are recycled by a type of white blood cell called a macrophage. Apoptosis protects the body by removing genetically damaged cells that could lead to cancer, and it plays an important role in the development of the embryo and the maintenance of adult tissues.

Cancer results from a disruption of the normal regulation of the cell cycle. When the cycle proceeds without control, cells can divide without order and accumulate genetic defects that can lead to a cancerous tumor.

How do geneticists indicate the location of a gene?

Geneticists use maps to describe the location of a particular gene on a chromosome. One type of map uses the cytogenetic location to describe a gene's position. The cytogenetic location is based on a distinctive pattern of bands created when chromosomes are stained with certain chemicals. Another type of map uses the molecular location, a precise description of a gene's position on a chromosome. The molecular location is based on the sequence of DNA building blocks (base pairs) that make up the chromosome.

Cytogenetic location: Geneticists use a standardized way of describing a gene's cytogenetic location. In most cases, the location describes the position of a particular band on a stained chromosome: 17q12.

It can also be written as a range of bands, if less is known about the exact location: 17q12-q21

The combination of numbers and letters provide a gene's "address" on a chromosome. This address is made up of several parts:

- The chromosome on which the gene can be found. The first number or letter used to describe a gene's location represents the chromosome. Chromosomes 1 through 22 (the autosomes) are designated by their chromosome number. The sex chromosomes are designated by X or Y.

- The arm of the chromosome. Each chromosome is divided into two sections (arms) based on the location of a narrowing (constriction) called the centromere. By convention, the shorter arm is called p, and the longer arm is called q. The chromosome arm is the second part of the gene's address. For example, 5q is the long arm of chromosome 5, and Xp is the short arm of the X chromosome.

11

- The position of the gene on the p or q arm. The position of a gene is based on a distinctive pattern of light and dark bands that appear when the chromosome is stained in a certain way. The position is usually designated by two digits (representing a region and a band), which are sometimes followed by a decimal point and one or more additional digits (representing sub-bands within a light or dark area). The number indicating the gene position increases with distance from the centromere. For example: 14q21 represents position 21 on the long arm of chromosome 14. 14q21 is closer to the centromere than 14q22.

Sometimes, the abbreviations "cen" or "ter" are also used to describe a gene's cytogenetic location. "Cen" indicates that the gene is very close to the centromere. For example, 16pcen refers to the short arm of chromosome 16 near the centromere. "Ter" stands for terminus, which indicates that the gene is very close to the end of the p or q arm. For example, 14qter refers to the tip of the long arm of chromosome 14. ("Tel" is also sometimes used to describe a gene's location. "Tel" stands for telomeres, which are at the ends of each chromosome. The abbreviations "tel" and "ter" refer to the same location.)

Molecular location: The Human Genome Project, an international research effort completed in 2003, determined the sequence of base pairs for each human chromosome. This sequence information allows researchers to provide a more specific address than the cytogenetic location for many genes. A gene's molecular address pinpoints the location of that gene in terms of base pairs. It describes the gene's precise position on a chromosome and indicates the size of the gene. Knowing the molecular location also allows researchers to determine exactly how far a gene is from other genes on the same chromosome.

Different groups of researchers often present slightly different values for a gene's molecular location. Researchers interpret the sequence of the human genome using a variety of methods, which can result in small differences in a gene's molecular address.

What are gene families?

A gene family is a group of genes that share important characteristics. In many cases, genes in a family share a similar sequence of DNA building blocks (nucleotides). These genes provide instructions for making products (such as proteins) that have a similar structure or function. In other cases, dissimilar genes are grouped together in a family because proteins produced from these genes work together as a unit or participate in the same process.

Classifying individual genes into families helps researchers describe how genes are related to each other. Researchers can use gene families to predict the function of newly identified genes based on their similarity to known genes. Similarities among genes in a family can also be used to predict where and when a specific gene is active (expressed). Additionally, gene families may provide clues for identifying genes that are involved in particular diseases.

Sometimes not enough is known about a gene to assign it to an established family. In other cases, genes may fit into more than one family. No formal guidelines define the criteria for grouping genes together. Classification systems for genes continue to evolve as scientists learn more about the structure and function of genes and the relationships between them.

Chapter 3

Genetic Mutations and Health

What is a gene mutation and how do mutations occur?

A gene mutation is a permanent change in the deoxyribonucleic acid (DNA) sequence that makes up a gene. Mutations range in size from a single DNA building block (DNA base) to a large segment of a chromosome.

Gene mutations occur in two ways: they can be inherited from a parent or acquired during a person's lifetime. Mutations that are passed from parent to child are called hereditary mutations or germline mutations (because they are present in the egg and sperm cells, which are also called germ cells). This type of mutation is present throughout a person's life in virtually every cell in the body.

Mutations that occur only in an egg or sperm cell, or those that occur just after fertilization, are called new (de novo) mutations. De novo mutations may explain genetic disorders in which an affected child has a mutation in every cell, but has no family history of the disorder.

Acquired (or somatic) mutations occur in the DNA of individual cells at some time during a person's life. These changes can be caused by environmental factors such as ultraviolet radiation from the sun, or can occur if a mistake is made as DNA copies itself during cell division. Acquired mutations in somatic cells (cells other than sperm and egg cells) cannot be passed on to the next generation.

Excerpted from "Mutations and Health," Genetics Home Reference (http://ghr.nlm.nih.gov), May 13, 2013.

Mutations may also occur in a single cell within an early embryo. As all the cells divide during growth and development, the individual will have some cells with the mutation and some cells without the genetic change. This situation is called mosaicism.

Some genetic changes are very rare; others are common in the population. Genetic changes that occur in more than 1 percent of the population are called polymorphisms. They are common enough to be considered a normal variation in the DNA. Polymorphisms are responsible for many of the normal differences between people, such as eye color, hair color, and blood type. Although many polymorphisms have no negative effects on a person's health, some of these variations may influence the risk of developing certain disorders.

How can gene mutations affect health and development?

To function correctly, each cell depends on thousands of proteins to do their jobs in the right places at the right times. Sometimes, gene mutations prevent one or more of these proteins from working properly. By changing a gene's instructions for making a protein, a mutation can cause the protein to malfunction or to be missing entirely. When a mutation alters a protein that plays a critical role in the body, it can disrupt normal development or cause a medical condition. A condition caused by mutations in one or more genes is called a genetic disorder.

In some cases, gene mutations are so severe that they prevent an embryo from surviving until birth. These changes occur in genes that are essential for development, and often disrupt the development of an embryo in its earliest stages. Because these mutations have very serious effects, they are incompatible with life.

It is important to note that genes themselves do not cause disease—genetic disorders are caused by mutations that make a gene function improperly. For example, when people say that someone has "the cystic fibrosis gene," they are usually referring to a mutated version of the CFTR gene, which causes the disease. All people, including those without cystic fibrosis, have a version of the CFTR gene.

Do all gene mutations affect health and development?

No, only a small percentage of mutations cause genetic disorders—most have no impact on health or development. For example, some mutations alter a gene's DNA sequence but do not change the function of the protein made by the gene.

Often, gene mutations that could cause a genetic disorder are repaired by certain enzymes before the gene is expressed and an altered protein is produced. Each cell has a number of pathways through which enzymes recognize and repair mistakes in DNA. Because DNA can be damaged or mutated in many ways, DNA repair is an important process by which the body protects itself from disease.

A very small percentage of all mutations actually have a positive effect. These mutations lead to new versions of proteins that help an individual better adapt to changes in his or her environment. For example, a beneficial mutation could result in a protein that protects an individual and future generations from a new strain of bacteria.

Because a person's genetic code can have a large number of mutations with no effect on health, diagnosing genetic conditions can be difficult. Sometimes, genes thought to be related to a particular genetic condition have mutations, but whether these changes are involved in development of the condition has not been determined; these genetic changes are known as variants of unknown significance (VOUS). Sometimes, no mutations are found in suspected disease-related genes, but mutations are found in other genes whose relationship to a particular genetic condition is unknown. It is difficult to know whether these variants are involved in the disease.

What kinds of gene mutations are possible?

The DNA sequence of a gene can be altered in a number of ways. Gene mutations have varying effects on health, depending on where they occur and whether they alter the function of essential proteins. The types of mutations include the following:

- **Missense mutation:** This type of mutation is a change in one DNA base pair that results in the substitution of one amino acid for another in the protein made by a gene.

- **Nonsense mutation:** A nonsense mutation is also a change in one DNA base pair. Instead of substituting one amino acid for another, however, the altered DNA sequence prematurely signals the cell to stop building a protein. This type of mutation results in a shortened protein that may function improperly or not at all.

- **Insertion:** An insertion changes the number of DNA bases in a gene by adding a piece of DNA. As a result, the protein made by the gene may not function properly.

- **Deletion:** A deletion changes the number of DNA bases by removing a piece of DNA. Small deletions may remove one or a few base pairs within a gene, while larger deletions can remove an entire gene or several neighboring genes. The deleted DNA may alter the function of the resulting protein(s).

- **Duplication:** A duplication consists of a piece of DNA that is abnormally copied one or more times. This type of mutation may alter the function of the resulting protein.

- **Frameshift mutation:** This type of mutation occurs when the addition or loss of DNA bases changes a gene's reading frame. A reading frame consists of groups of three bases that each code for one amino acid. A frameshift mutation shifts the grouping of these bases and changes the code for amino acids. The resulting protein is usually nonfunctional. Insertions, deletions, and duplications can all be frameshift mutations.

- **Repeat expansion:** Nucleotide repeats are short DNA sequences that are repeated a number of times in a row. For example, a trinucleotide repeat is made up of three-base-pair sequences, and a tetranucleotide repeat is made up of four-base-pair sequences. A repeat expansion is a mutation that increases the number of times that the short DNA sequence is repeated. This type of mutation can cause the resulting protein to function improperly.

Can a change in the number of genes affect health and development?

People have two copies of most genes, one copy inherited from each parent. In some cases, however, the number of copies varies—meaning that a person can be born with one, three, or more copies of particular genes. Less commonly, one or more genes may be entirely missing. This type of genetic difference is known as copy number variation (CNV).

Copy number variation results from insertions, deletions, and duplications of large segments of DNA. These segments are big enough to include whole genes. Variation in gene copy number can influence the activity of genes and ultimately affect many body functions.

Researchers were surprised to learn that copy number variation accounts for a significant amount of genetic difference between people. More than 10 percent of human DNA appears to contain these differences in gene copy number. While much of this variation does not affect health or development, some differences likely influence a person's risk of disease and response to certain drugs. Future research will focus on the consequences of copy number variation in different parts of the genome and study the contribution of these variations to many types of disease.

Can changes in the number of chromosomes affect health and development?

Human cells normally contain twenty-three pairs of chromosomes, for a total of forty-six chromosomes in each cell. A change in the number of chromosomes can cause problems with growth, development, and function of the body's systems. These changes can occur during the formation of reproductive cells (eggs and sperm), in early fetal development, or in any cell after birth. A gain or loss of chromosomes from the normal forty-six is called aneuploidy.

A common form of aneuploidy is trisomy, or the presence of an extra chromosome in cells. "Tri-" is Greek for "three"; people with trisomy have three copies of a particular chromosome in cells instead of the normal two copies. Down syndrome is an example of a condition caused by trisomy. People with Down syndrome typically have three copies of chromosome 21 in each cell, for a total of forty-seven chromosomes per cell.

Monosomy, or the loss of one chromosome in cells, is another kind of aneuploidy. "Mono-" is Greek for "one"; people with monosomy have one copy of a particular chromosome in cells instead of the normal two copies. Turner syndrome is a condition caused by monosomy. Women with Turner syndrome usually have only one copy of the X chromosome in every cell, for a total of forty-five chromosomes per cell.

Rarely, some cells end up with complete extra sets of chromosomes. Cells with one additional set of chromosomes, for a total of sixty-nine chromosomes, are called triploid. Cells with two additional sets of chromosomes, for a total of ninety-two chromosomes, are called tetraploid. A condition in which every cell in the body has an extra set of chromosomes is not compatible with life.

In some cases, a change in the number of chromosomes occurs only in certain cells. When an individual has two or more cell populations with a different chromosomal makeup, this situation is called chromosomal mosaicism. Chromosomal mosaicism occurs from an error in cell division in cells other than eggs and sperm. Most commonly, some cells end up with one extra or missing chromosome (for a total of forty-five or forty-seven chromosomes per cell), while other cells have the usual forty-six chromosomes. Mosaic Turner syndrome is one example of chromosomal mosaicism. In females with this condition, some cells have forty-five chromosomes because they are missing one copy of the X chromosome, while other cells have the usual number of chromosomes.

Many cancer cells also have changes in their number of chromosomes. These changes are not inherited; they occur in somatic cells

(cells other than eggs or sperm) during the formation or progression of a cancerous tumor.

Can changes in the structure of chromosomes affect health and development?

Changes that affect the structure of chromosomes can cause problems with growth, development, and function of the body's systems. These changes can affect many genes along the chromosome and disrupt the proteins made from those genes.

Structural changes can occur during the formation of egg or sperm cells, in early fetal development, or in any cell after birth. Pieces of DNA can be rearranged within one chromosome or transferred between two or more chromosomes. The effects of structural changes depend on their size and location, and whether any genetic material is gained or lost. Some changes cause medical problems, while others may have no effect on a person's health.

Changes in chromosome structure include the following:

- **Translocations:** A translocation occurs when a piece of one chromosome breaks off and attaches to another chromosome. This type of rearrangement is described as balanced if no genetic material is gained or lost in the cell. If there is a gain or loss of genetic material, the translocation is described as unbalanced.

- **Deletions:** Deletions occur when a chromosome breaks and some genetic material is lost. Deletions can be large or small, and can occur anywhere along a chromosome.

- **Duplications:** Duplications occur when part of a chromosome is copied (duplicated) too many times. This type of chromosomal change results in extra copies of genetic material from the duplicated segment.

- **Inversions:** An inversion involves the breakage of a chromosome in two places; the resulting piece of DNA is reversed and reinserted into the chromosome. Genetic material may or may not be lost as a result of the chromosome breaks. An inversion that involves the chromosome's constriction point (centromere) is called a pericentric inversion. An inversion that occurs in the long (q) arm or short (p) arm and does not involve the centromere is called a paracentric inversion.

- **Isochromosomes:** An isochromosome is a chromosome with two identical arms. Instead of one long (q) arm and one short (p) arm, an isochromosome has two long arms or two short arms. As a result, these abnormal chromosomes have an extra copy of some genes and are missing copies of other genes.

- **Dicentric chromosomes:** Unlike normal chromosomes, which have a single constriction point (centromere), a dicentric chromosome contains two centromeres. Dicentric chromosomes result from the abnormal fusion of two chromosome pieces, each of which includes a centromere. These structures are unstable and often involve a loss of some genetic material.

- **Ring chromosomes:** Ring chromosomes usually occur when a chromosome breaks in two places and the ends of the chromosome arms fuse together to form a circular structure. The ring may or may not include the chromosome's constriction point (centromere). In many cases, genetic material near the ends of the chromosome is lost.

Many cancer cells also have changes in their chromosome structure. These changes are not inherited; they occur in somatic cells (cells other than eggs or sperm) during the formation or progression of a cancerous tumor.

Can changes in mitochondrial DNA affect health and development?

Mitochondria are structures within cells that convert the energy from food into a form that cells can use. Although most DNA is packaged in chromosomes within the nucleus, mitochondria also have a small amount of their own DNA (known as mitochondrial DNA or mtDNA). In some cases, inherited changes in mitochondrial DNA can cause problems with growth, development, and function of the body's systems. These mutations disrupt the mitochondria's ability to generate energy efficiently for the cell.

Conditions caused by mutations in mitochondrial DNA often involve multiple organ systems. The effects of these conditions are most pronounced in organs and tissues that require a lot of energy (such as the heart, brain, and muscles). Although the health consequences of inherited mitochondrial DNA mutations vary widely, frequently observed features include muscle weakness and wasting, problems with movement, diabetes, kidney failure, heart disease, loss of intellectual functions (dementia), hearing loss, and abnormalities involving the eyes and vision.

Mitochondrial DNA is also prone to somatic mutations, which are not inherited. Somatic mutations occur in the DNA of certain cells during a person's lifetime and typically are not passed to future generations. Because mitochondrial DNA has a limited ability to repair itself when it is damaged, these mutations tend to build up over time. A buildup of somatic mutations in mitochondrial DNA has been associated with some forms of cancer and an increased risk of certain age-related disorders such as heart disease, Alzheimer disease, and Parkinson disease. Additionally, research suggests that the progressive accumulation of these mutations over a person's lifetime may play a role in the normal process of aging.

What are complex or multifactorial disorders?

Researchers are learning that nearly all conditions and diseases have a genetic component. Some disorders, such as sickle cell anemia and cystic fibrosis, are caused by mutations in a single gene. The causes of many other disorders, however, are much more complex. Common medical problems such as heart disease, diabetes, and obesity do not have a single genetic cause—they are likely associated with the effects of multiple genes in combination with lifestyle and environmental factors. Conditions caused by many contributing factors are called complex or multifactorial disorders.

Although complex disorders often cluster in families, they do not have a clear-cut pattern of inheritance. This makes it difficult to determine a person's risk of inheriting or passing on these disorders. Complex disorders are also difficult to study and treat because the specific factors that cause most of these disorders have not yet been identified. By 2010, however, researchers predict they will have found the major contributing genes for many common complex disorders.

What does it mean to have a genetic predisposition to a disease?

A genetic predisposition (sometimes also called genetic susceptibility) is an increased likelihood of developing a particular disease based on a person's genetic makeup. A genetic predisposition results from specific genetic variations that are often inherited from a parent. These genetic changes contribute to the development of a disease but do not directly cause it. Some people with a predisposing genetic variation will never get the disease while others will, even within the same family.

Genetic variations can have large or small effects on the likelihood of developing a particular disease. For example, certain mutations in the BRCA1 or BRCA2 genes greatly increase a person's risk of developing breast cancer and ovarian cancer. Variations in other genes, such as BARD1 and BRIP1, also increase breast cancer risk, but the contribution of these genetic changes to a person's overall risk appears to be much smaller.

Current research is focused on identifying genetic changes that have a small effect on disease risk but are common in the general population. Although each of these variations only slightly increases a person's risk, having changes in several different genes may combine to increase disease risk significantly. Changes in many genes, each with a small effect, may underlie susceptibility to many common diseases, including cancer, obesity, diabetes, heart disease, and mental illness.

In people with a genetic predisposition, the risk of disease can depend on multiple factors in addition to an identified genetic change. These include other genetic factors (sometimes called modifiers) as well as lifestyle and environmental factors. Diseases that are caused by a combination of factors are described as multifactorial. Although a person's genetic makeup cannot be altered, some lifestyle and environmental modifications (such as having more frequent disease screenings and maintaining a healthy weight) may be able to reduce disease risk in people with a genetic predisposition.

What information about a genetic condition can statistics provide?

Statistical data can provide general information about how common a condition is, how many people have the condition, or how likely it is that a person will develop the condition. Statistics are not personalized, however—they offer estimates based on groups of people. By taking into account a person's family history, medical history, and other factors, a genetics professional can help interpret what statistics mean for a particular patient.

Some statistical terms are commonly used when describing genetic conditions and other disorders. Some of these terms are presented in Table 3.1.

How are genetic conditions and genes named?

Naming genetic conditions: Genetic conditions are not named in one standard way (unlike genes, which are given an official name and symbol by a formal committee). Doctors who treat families with a particular disorder are often the first to propose a name for the condition. Expert working groups may later revise the name to improve its usefulness. Naming is important because it allows accurate and effective communication about particular conditions, which will ultimately help researchers find new approaches to treatment.

Table 3.1. Common statistical terms

Statistical term	Description	Examples
Incidence	The incidence of a gene mutation or a genetic disorder is the number of people who are born with the mutation or disorder in a specified group per year. Incidence is often written in the form "1 in [a number]" or as a total number of live births.	About 1 in 200,000 people in the United States are born with syndrome A each year. An estimated 15,000 infants with syndrome B were born last year worldwide.
Prevalence	The prevalence of a gene mutation or a genetic disorder is the total number of people in a specified group at a given time who have the mutation or disorder. This term includes both newly diagnosed and preexisting cases in people of any age. Prevalence is often written in the form "1 in [a number]" or as a total number of people who have a condition.	Approximately 1 in 100,000 people in the United States have syndrome A at the present time. About 100,000 children worldwide currently have syndrome B.
Mortality	Mortality is the number of deaths from a particular disorder occurring in a specified group per year. Mortality is usually expressed as a total number of deaths.	An estimated 12,000 people worldwide died from syndrome C in 2002.
Lifetime risk	Lifetime risk is the average risk of developing a particular disorder at some point during a lifetime. Lifetime risk is often written as a percentage or as "1 in [a number]." It is important to remember that the risk per year or per decade is much lower than the lifetime risk. In addition, other factors may increase or decrease a person's risk as compared with the average.	Approximately 1 percent of people in the United States develop disorder D during their lifetimes. The lifetime risk of developing disorder D is 1 in 100.

Disorder names are often derived from one or a combination of sources:

- The basic genetic or biochemical defect that causes the condition (for example, alpha-1 antitrypsin deficiency);

- One or more major signs or symptoms of the disorder (for example, hypermanganesemia with dystonia, polycythemia, and cirrhosis);

- The parts of the body affected by the condition (for example, craniofacial-deafness-hand syndrome);

- The name of a physician or researcher, often the first person to describe the disorder (for example, Marfan syndrome, which was named after Dr. Antoine Bernard-Jean Marfan);

- A geographic area (for example, familial Mediterranean fever, which occurs mainly in populations bordering the Mediterranean Sea); or

- The name of a patient or family with the condition (for example, amyotrophic lateral sclerosis, which is also called Lou Gehrig disease after the famous baseball player who had the condition).

Disorders named after a specific person or place are called eponyms. There is debate as to whether the possessive form (e.g., Alzheimer's disease) or the nonpossessive form (Alzheimer disease) of eponyms is preferred. As a rule, medical geneticists use the nonpossessive form, and this form may become the standard for doctors in all fields of medicine.

Naming genes: The HUGO Gene Nomenclature Committee (HGNC) designates an official name and symbol (an abbreviation of the name) for each known human gene. Some official gene names include additional information in parentheses, such as related genetic conditions, subtypes of a condition, or inheritance pattern. The HGNC is a nonprofit organization funded by the U.K. Medical Research Council and the U.S. National Institutes of Health. The Committee has named more than thirteen thousand of the estimated twenty thousand to twenty-five thousand genes in the human genome.

During the research process, genes often acquire several alternate names and symbols. Different researchers investigating the same gene may each give the gene a different name, which can cause confusion. The HGNC assigns a unique name and symbol to each human gene, which allows effective organization of genes in large databanks, aiding the advancement of research.

Chapter 4

Genetic Inheritance

What does it mean if a disorder seems to run in my family?

A particular disorder might be described as "running in a family" if more than one person in the family has the condition. Some disorders that affect multiple family members are caused by gene mutations, which can be inherited (passed down from parent to child). Other conditions that appear to run in families are not caused by mutations in single genes. Instead, environmental factors such as dietary habits or a combination of genetic and environmental factors are responsible for these disorders.

It is not always easy to determine whether a condition in a family is inherited. A genetics professional can use a person's family history (a record of health information about a person's immediate and extended family) to help determine whether a disorder has a genetic component. He or she will ask about the health of people from several generations of the family, usually first-, second-, and third-degree relatives. First-degree relatives are your parents, children, brothers, and sisters. Second-degree relatives are your grandparents, aunts and uncles, nieces and nephews, and grandchildren. Third-degree relatives are your first cousins.

Excerpted from "Inheriting Genetic Conditions," Genetics Home Reference (http://ghr.nlm.nih.gov), May 13, 2013.

Why is it important to know my family medical history?

A family medical history is a record of health information about a person and his or her close relatives. A complete record includes information from three generations of relatives, including children, brothers and sisters, parents, aunts and uncles, nieces and nephews, grandparents, and cousins.

Families have many factors in common, including their genes, environment, and lifestyle. Together, these factors can give clues to medical conditions that may run in a family. By noticing patterns of disorders among relatives, healthcare professionals can determine whether an individual, other family members, or future generations may be at an increased risk of developing a particular condition.

A family medical history can identify people with a higher-than-usual chance of having common disorders, such as heart disease, high blood pressure, stroke, certain cancers, and diabetes. These complex disorders are influenced by a combination of genetic factors, environmental conditions, and lifestyle choices. A family history also can provide information about the risk of rarer conditions caused by mutations in a single gene, such as cystic fibrosis and sickle cell anemia.

While a family medical history provides information about the risk of specific health concerns, having relatives with a medical condition does not mean that an individual will definitely develop that condition. On the other hand, a person with no family history of a disorder may still be at risk of developing that disorder.

Knowing one's family medical history allows a person to take steps to reduce his or her risk. For people at an increased risk of certain cancers, health care professionals may recommend more frequent screening (such as mammography or colonoscopy) starting at an earlier age. Healthcare providers may also encourage regular checkups or testing for people with a medical condition that runs in their family. Additionally, lifestyle changes such as adopting a healthier diet, getting regular exercise, and quitting smoking help many people lower their chances of developing heart disease and other common illnesses.

The easiest way to get information about family medical history is to talk to relatives about their health. Have they had any medical problems, and when did they occur? A family gathering could be a good time to discuss these issues. Additionally, obtaining medical records and other documents (such as obituaries and death certificates) can help complete a family medical history. It is important to keep this information up-to-date and to share it with a healthcare professional regularly.

What are the different ways in which a genetic condition can be inherited?

Some genetic conditions are caused by mutations in a single gene. These conditions are usually inherited in one of several straightforward patterns, depending on the gene involved:

- **Autosomal dominant:** One mutated copy of the gene in each cell is sufficient for a person to be affected by an autosomal dominant disorder. Each affected person usually has one affected parent. Autosomal dominant disorders tend to occur in every generation of an affected family. Huntington disease and neurofibromatosis type 1 are autosomal dominant disorders.

- **Autosomal recessive:** Two mutated copies of the gene are present in each cell when a person has an autosomal recessive disorder. An affected person usually has unaffected parents who each carry a single copy of the mutated gene (and are referred to as carriers). Autosomal recessive disorders are typically not seen in every generation of an affected family. Cystic fibrosis and sickle cell anemia are autosomal recessive disorders.

- **X-linked dominant:** X-linked dominant disorders are caused by mutations in genes on the X chromosome. Females are more frequently affected than males, and the chance of passing on an X-linked dominant disorder differs between men and women. Families with an X-linked dominant disorder often have both affected males and affected females in each generation. A characteristic of X-linked inheritance is that fathers cannot pass X-linked traits to their sons (no male-to-male transmission). Fragile X syndrome is an X-linked dominant disorder.

- **X-linked recessive:** X-linked recessive disorders are also caused by mutations in genes on the X chromosome. Males are more frequently affected than females, and the chance of passing on the disorder differs between men and women. Families with an X-linked recessive disorder often have affected males, but rarely affected females, in each generation. A characteristic of X-linked inheritance is that fathers cannot pass X-linked traits to their sons (no male-to-male transmission). Hemophilia and Fabry disease are X-linked recessive disorders.

- **Codominant:** In codominant inheritance, two different versions (alleles) of a gene can be expressed, and each version makes a slightly different protein. Both alleles influence the genetic trait or determine the characteristics of the genetic condition. ABO blood group and alpha-1 antitrypsin deficiency are codominant conditions.

- **Mitochondrial:** This type of inheritance, also known as maternal inheritance, applies to genes in mitochondrial DNA. Mitochondria, which are structures in each cell that convert molecules into energy, each contain a small amount of DNA. Because only egg cells contribute mitochondria to the developing embryo, only females can pass on mitochondrial mutations to their children. Disorders resulting from mutations in mitochondrial DNA can appear in every generation of a family and can affect both males and females, but fathers do not pass these disorders to their children. Leber hereditary optic neuropathy (LHON) is a mitochondrial disorder.

Many other disorders are caused by a combination of the effects of multiple genes or by interactions between genes and the environment. Such disorders are more difficult to analyze because their genetic causes are often unclear, and they do not follow the patterns of inheritance described above. Examples of conditions caused by multiple genes or gene/environment interactions include heart disease, diabetes, schizophrenia, and certain types of cancer.

If a genetic disorder runs in my family, what are the chances that my children will have the condition?

When a genetic disorder is diagnosed in a family, family members often want to know the likelihood that they or their children will develop the condition. This can be difficult to predict in some cases because many factors influence a person's chances of developing a genetic condition. One important factor is how the condition is inherited:

- **Autosomal dominant inheritance:** A person affected by an autosomal dominant disorder has a 50 percent chance of passing the mutated gene to each child. The chance that a child will not inherit the mutated gene is also 50 percent.

- **Autosomal recessive inheritance:** Two unaffected people who each carry one copy of the mutated gene for an autosomal recessive disorder (carriers) have a 25 percent chance with each pregnancy of having a child affected by the disorder. The chance with each pregnancy of having an unaffected child who is a carrier of the disorder is 50 percent, and the chance that a child will not have the disorder and will not be a carrier is 25 percent.

- **X-linked dominant inheritance:** The chance of passing on an X-linked dominant condition differs between men and women because men have one X chromosome and one Y chromosome, while women have two X chromosomes. A man passes on his Y chromosome to all of his sons and his X chromosome to all of his daughters. Therefore, the sons of a man with an X-linked dominant disorder will not be affected, but all of his daughters will inherit the condition. A woman passes on one or the other of her X chromosomes to each child. Therefore, a woman with an X-linked dominant disorder has a 50 percent chance of having an affected daughter or son with each pregnancy.

- **X-linked recessive inheritance:** Because of the difference in sex chromosomes, the probability of passing on an X-linked recessive disorder also differs between men and women. The sons of a man with an X-linked recessive disorder will not be affected, and his daughters will carry one copy of the mutated gene. With each pregnancy, a woman who carries an X-linked recessive disorder has a 50 percent chance of having sons who are affected and a 50 percent chance of having daughters who carry one copy of the mutated gene.

- **Codominant inheritance:** In codominant inheritance, each parent contributes a different version of a particular gene, and both versions influence the resulting genetic trait. The chance of developing a genetic condition with codominant inheritance, and the characteristic features of that condition, depend on which versions of the gene are passed from parents to their child.

- **Mitochondrial inheritance:** Mitochondria, which are the energy-producing centers inside cells, each contain a small amount of DNA. Disorders with mitochondrial inheritance result from mutations in mitochondrial DNA. Although these disorders can affect both males and females, only females can pass mutations in mitochondrial DNA to their children. A woman with a disorder caused by changes in mitochondrial DNA will pass the mutation to all of her daughters and sons, but the children of a man with such a disorder will not inherit the mutation.

It is important to note that the chance of passing on a genetic condition applies equally to each pregnancy. For example, if a couple has a child with an autosomal recessive disorder, the chance of having another child with the disorder is still 25 percent (or one in four). Having one child with a disorder does not "protect" future children from inheriting the condition. Conversely, having a child without the condition does not mean that future children will definitely be affected.

Although the chances of inheriting a genetic condition appear straightforward, factors such as a person's family history and the results of genetic testing can sometimes modify those chances. In addition, some people with a disease-causing mutation never develop any health problems or may experience only mild symptoms of the disorder. If a disease that runs in a family does not have a clear-cut inheritance pattern, predicting the likelihood that a person will develop the condition can be particularly difficult.

Estimating the chance of developing or passing on a genetic disorder can be complex. Genetics professionals can help people understand these chances and help them make informed decisions about their health.

What are reduced penetrance and variable expressivity?

Reduced penetrance and variable expressivity are factors that influence the effects of particular genetic changes. These factors usually affect disorders that have an autosomal dominant pattern of inheritance, although they are occasionally seen in disorders with an autosomal recessive inheritance pattern.

Reduced penetrance: Penetrance refers to the proportion of people with a particular genetic change (such as a mutation in a specific gene) who exhibit signs and symptoms of a genetic disorder. If some people with the mutation do not develop features of the disorder, the condition is said to have reduced (or incomplete) penetrance. Reduced penetrance often occurs with familial cancer syndromes. For example, many people with a mutation in the BRCA1 or BRCA2 gene will develop cancer during their lifetime, but some people will not. Doctors cannot predict which people with these mutations will develop cancer or when the tumors will develop.

Reduced penetrance probably results from a combination of genetic, environmental, and lifestyle factors, many of which are unknown. This phenomenon can make it challenging for genetics professionals to interpret a person's family medical history and predict the risk of passing a genetic condition to future generations.

Variable expressivity: Although some genetic disorders exhibit little variation, most have signs and symptoms that differ among affected individuals. Variable expressivity refers to the range of signs and symptoms that can occur in different people with the same genetic condition. For example, the features of Marfan syndrome vary widely—some people have only mild symptoms (such as being tall and thin with long, slender fingers), while others also experience life-threatening complications involving the heart and blood vessels. Although the features are highly variable, most people with this disorder have a mutation in the same gene (FBN1).

As with reduced penetrance, variable expressivity is probably caused by a combination of genetic, environmental, and lifestyle factors, most of which have not been identified. If a genetic condition has highly variable signs and symptoms, it may be challenging to diagnose.

What do geneticists mean by anticipation?

The signs and symptoms of some genetic conditions tend to become more severe and appear at an earlier age as the disorder is passed from one generation to the next. This phenomenon is called anticipation. Anticipation is most often seen with certain genetic disorders of the nervous system, such as Huntington disease, myotonic dystrophy, and fragile X syndrome.

Anticipation typically occurs with disorders that are caused by an unusual type of mutation called a trinucleotide repeat expansion. A trinucleotide repeat is a sequence of three DNA building blocks (nucleotides) that is repeated a number of times in a row. DNA segments with an abnormal number of these repeats are unstable and prone to errors during cell division. The number of repeats can change as the gene is passed from parent to child. If the number of repeats increases, it is known as a trinucleotide repeat expansion. In some cases, the trinucleotide repeat may expand until the gene stops functioning normally. This expansion causes the features of some disorders to become more severe with each successive generation.

Most genetic disorders have signs and symptoms that differ among affected individuals, including affected people in the same family. Not all of these differences can be explained by anticipation. A combination of genetic, environmental, and lifestyle factors is probably responsible for the variability, although many of these factors have not been identified. Researchers study multiple generations of affected family members and consider the genetic cause of a disorder before determining that it shows anticipation.

What are genomic imprinting and uniparental disomy?

Genomic imprinting and uniparental disomy are factors that influence how some genetic conditions are inherited.

Genomic imprinting: People inherit two copies of their genes—one from their mother and one from their father. Usually both copies of each gene are active, or "turned on," in cells. In some cases, however, only one of the two copies is normally turned on. Which copy is active depends on the parent of origin: some genes are normally active only when they are inherited from a person's father; others are active only when inherited from a person's mother. This phenomenon is known as genomic imprinting.

In genes that undergo genomic imprinting, the parent of origin is often marked, or "stamped," on the gene during the formation of egg and sperm cells. This stamping process, called methylation, is a chemical reaction that attaches small molecules called methyl groups to certain segments of DNA. These molecules identify which copy of a gene was inherited from the mother and which was inherited from the father. The addition and removal of methyl groups can be used to control the activity of genes.

Only a small percentage of all human genes undergo genomic imprinting. Researchers are not yet certain why some genes are imprinted and others are not. They do know that imprinted genes tend to cluster together in the same regions of chromosomes. Two major clusters of imprinted genes have been identified in humans, one on the short (p) arm of chromosome 11 (at position 11p15) and another on the long (q) arm of chromosome 15 (in the region 15q11 to 15q13).

Uniparental disomy: Uniparental disomy (UPD) occurs when a person receives two copies of a chromosome, or part of a chromosome, from one parent and no copies from the other parent. UPD can occur as a random event during the formation of egg or sperm cells or may happen in early fetal development.

In many cases, UPD likely has no effect on health or development. Because most genes are not imprinted, it doesn't matter if a person inherits both copies from one parent instead of one copy from each parent. In some cases, however, it does make a difference whether a gene is inherited from a person's mother or father. A person with UPD may lack any active copies of essential genes that undergo genomic imprinting. This loss of gene function can lead to delayed development, mental retardation, or other medical problems.

Several genetic disorders can result from UPD or a disruption of normal genomic imprinting. The most well-known conditions include Prader-Willi syndrome, which is characterized by uncontrolled eating and obesity, and Angelman syndrome, which causes mental retardation and impaired speech. Both of these disorders can be caused by UPD or other errors in imprinting involving genes on the long arm of chromosome 15. Other conditions, such as Beckwith-Wiedemann syndrome (a disorder characterized by accelerated growth and an increased risk of cancerous tumors), are associated with abnormalities of imprinted genes on the short arm of chromosome 11.

Are chromosomal disorders inherited?

Although it is possible to inherit some types of chromosomal abnormalities, most chromosomal disorders (such as Down syndrome and Turner syndrome) are not passed from one generation to the next.

Some chromosomal conditions are caused by changes in the number of chromosomes. These changes are not inherited, but occur as random events during the formation of reproductive cells (eggs and sperm). An error in cell division called nondisjunction results in reproductive cells with an abnormal number of chromosomes. For example, a reproductive cell may accidentally gain or lose one copy of a chromosome. If one of these atypical reproductive cells contributes to the genetic makeup of a child, the child will have an extra or missing chromosome in each of the body's cells.

Changes in chromosome structure can also cause chromosomal disorders. Some changes in chromosome structure can be inherited, while others occur as random accidents during the formation of reproductive cells or in early fetal development. Because the inheritance of these changes can be complex, people concerned about this type of chromosomal abnormality may want to talk with a genetics professional.

Some cancer cells also have changes in the number or structure of their chromosomes. Because these changes occur in somatic cells (cells other than eggs and sperm), they cannot be passed from one generation to the next.

Why are some genetic conditions more common in particular ethnic groups?

Some genetic disorders are more likely to occur among people who trace their ancestry to a particular geographic area. People in an ethnic group often share certain versions of their genes, which have been passed down from common ancestors. If one of these shared genes contains a disease-causing mutation, a particular genetic disorder may be more frequently seen in the group.

Examples of genetic conditions that are more common in particular ethnic groups are sickle cell anemia, which is more common in people of African, African-American, or Mediterranean heritage; and Tay-Sachs disease, which is more likely to occur among people of Ashkenazi (eastern and central European) Jewish or French Canadian ancestry. It is important to note, however, that these disorders can occur in any ethnic group.

Chapter 5

Genetic Counseling

What is a genetic consultation?

A genetic consultation is a health service that provides information and support to people who have, or may be at risk for, genetic disorders. During a consultation, a genetics professional meets with an individual or family to discuss genetic risks or to diagnose, confirm, or rule out a genetic condition.

Genetics professionals include medical geneticists (doctors who specialize in genetics) and genetic counselors (certified healthcare workers with experience in medical genetics and counseling). Other healthcare professionals such as nurses, psychologists, and social workers trained in genetics can also provide genetic consultations.

Consultations usually take place in a doctor's office, hospital, genetics center, or other type of medical center. These meetings are most often in-person visits with individuals or families, but they are occasionally conducted in a group or over the telephone.

Why might someone have a genetic consultation?

Individuals or families who are concerned about an inherited condition may benefit from a genetic consultation. The reasons that a person might be referred to a genetic counselor, medical geneticist, or other genetics professional include the following:

Excerpted from "Genetic Consultation," Genetics Home Reference (http://ghr.nlm.nih.gov), May 13, 2013.

- A personal or family history of a genetic condition, birth defect, chromosomal disorder, or hereditary cancer.

- Two or more pregnancy losses (miscarriages), a stillbirth, or a baby who died.

- A child with a known inherited disorder, a birth defect, mental retardation, or developmental delay.

- A woman who is pregnant or plans to become pregnant at or after age thirty-five. (Some chromosomal disorders occur more frequently in children born to older women.)

- Abnormal test results that suggest a genetic or chromosomal condition.

- An increased risk of developing or passing on a particular genetic disorder on the basis of a person's ethnic background.

- People related by blood (for example, cousins) who plan to have children together. (A child whose parents are related may be at an increased risk of inheriting certain genetic disorders.)

A genetic consultation is also an important part of the decision-making process for genetic testing. A visit with a genetics professional may be helpful even if testing is not available for a specific condition, however.

What happens during a genetic consultation?

A genetic consultation provides information, offers support, and addresses a patient's specific questions and concerns. To help determine whether a condition has a genetic component, a genetics professional asks about a person's medical history and takes a detailed family history (a record of health information about a person's immediate and extended family). The genetics professional may also perform a physical examination and recommend appropriate tests.

If a person is diagnosed with a genetic condition, the genetics professional provides information about the diagnosis, how the condition is inherited, the chance of passing the condition to future generations, and the options for testing and treatment.

During a consultation, a genetics professional will do the following things:

- Interpret and communicate complex medical information.

- Help each person make informed, independent decisions about his or her health care and reproductive options.

- Respect each person's individual beliefs, traditions, and feelings.

A genetics professional will *not* do the following things:

- Tell a person which decision to make.

- Advise a couple not to have children.

- Recommend that a woman continue or end a pregnancy.

- Tell someone whether to undergo testing for a genetic disorder.

How can I find a genetics professional in my area?

To find a genetics professional in your community, you may wish to ask your doctor for a referral. If you have health insurance, you can also contact your insurance company to find a medical geneticist or genetic counselor in your area who participates in your plan.

Several resources for locating a genetics professional in your community are available online:

- The American College of Medical Genetics (ACMG) has a searchable directory of genetics centers in the United States. You can view a list of all clinics or search by clinic name, services provided, city, state, or zip code.

- The National Society of Genetic Counselors offers a searchable directory of genetic counselors in the United States. You can search by location, name, area of practice or specialization, or zip code.

- The National Cancer Institute provides a Cancer Genetics Services Directory, which lists professionals who provide services related to cancer genetics. You can search by type of cancer or syndrome, location, and/or provider name.

Chapter 6

Testing for Genetic Disorders

Chapter Contents

Section 6.1

What You Need to Know about Genetic Testing

Excerpted from "Frequently Asked Questions about
Genetic Testing," National Human Genome Research
Institute (www.genome.gov), April 30, 2013.

Genetic research is leading to the development of more genetic
tests that can be used for the diagnosis of genetic conditions. Genetic
testing is available for infants, children, and adults. Genetic tests can
be used to diagnose a disease in an individual with symptoms and to
help measure risk of developing a disease. Adults can undergo pre-
conception testing before deciding to become pregnant, and prenatal
testing can be performed during a pregnancy. Results of genetic tests
can help physicians select appropriate treatments for their patients.

What is genetic testing?

Genetic tests look for alterations in a person's genes or changes
in the level or structure of key proteins coded for by specific genes.
Genetic tests can also be used to look at levels of ribonucleic acid
(RNA) that play a role in certain conditions. Abnormal results on
these tests could mean that someone has a genetic disorder.

Types of genetic tests include the following:

- **Gene tests:** Individual genes or relatively short lengths of deoxyribonucleic acid (DNA) or RNA are tested.

- **Chromosomal tests:** Whole chromosomes or very long lengths
  of DNA are tested.

- **Biochemical tests:** Protein levels or enzyme activities are
  tested.

What is a gene test?

Gene tests look for signs of a disease or disorder in DNA or
RNA taken from a person's blood, other body fluids like saliva, or

tissues. These tests can look for large changes, such as a gene that has a section missing or added, or small changes, such as a missing, added, or altered chemical base (subunit) within the DNA strand. Gene tests may also detect genes with too many copies, individual genes that are too active, genes that are turned off, or genes that are lost entirely.

Gene tests examine a person's DNA in a variety of ways. Some tests use DNA probes. A probe is a short string of DNA with base sequence complementary to (able to bind with) the sequence of an altered gene. These probes usually have fluorescent tags attached to them. During the test, a probe looks for its complement within a person's genome. If the altered gene is found, the complementary probe binds to it, and the fluorescent label can be used to identify the presence of the alteration.

Another type of gene test relies on DNA or RNA sequencing. This test directly compares the base-by-base sequence of DNA or RNA in a patient's sample to a normal version of the DNA or RNA sequence.

What is a chromosomal test?

Chromosomes are the large DNA-containing structures in the nucleus of a cell. Humans normally have twenty-three pairs of chromosomes: twenty-two pairs of autosomes (numbered 1 through 22) and one pair of sex chromosomes (either XX for females or XY for males). Chromosomal tests look at features of a person's chromosomes, including their structure, number, and arrangement. These tests look for changes, such as pieces of a chromosome being deleted, expanded, or being switched to a different chromosomal location.

Types of chromosomal tests include the following:

- **Karyotype:** This test gives a picture of all of a person's chromosomes from the largest to the smallest. This type of testing can identify changes in chromosome number and large changes in DNA structure. A karyotype would, for instance, identify Down syndrome caused by the presence of an extra copy of chromosome 21.

- **FISH analysis (fluorescent in situ hybridization):** This test identifies certain regions on chromosomes using fluorescent DNA probes. FISH analysis can find small pieces of chromosomes that are missing or have extra copies. These small changes can be missed by the overall karyotype test. FISH analysis can, for instance, be used to reveal the missing fragments of DNA on chromosome 22 that are characteristic of velocardiofacial syndrome.

What is a biochemical test?

Biochemical tests look at the amounts or activities of key proteins. Since genes contain the DNA code for making proteins, abnormal amounts or activities of proteins can signal genes that are not working normally. These types of tests are often used for newborn screening. For example, biochemical screening can detect infants who have metabolic conditions such as phenylketonuria (PKU).

What information can genetic testing give?

Genetic testing can do the following things:

1. Give a diagnosis if someone has symptoms.

2. Show whether a person is a carrier for a genetic disease. Carriers have an altered gene, but will not get the disease. However, they can pass the altered gene on to their children.

3. Help expectant parents know whether an unborn child will have a genetic condition. This is called prenatal testing.

4. Screen newborn infants for abnormal or missing proteins that can cause disease. This is called newborn screening.

5. Show whether a person has an inherited disposition to a certain disease before symptoms start.

6. Determine the type or dose of a medicine that is best for a certain person. This is called pharmacogenetics.

People in families at high risk for a genetic disease have to live with uncertainty about their future and their children's future. A genetic test result that can show that a known alteration causing disease is not present in a person can provide a sense of relief.

A genetic test result showing that a person has a disease-causing gene alteration can also provide benefits. Such a test result might lead a person to take steps to lower his or her chance of developing a disease. For example, as the result of such a finding, someone could be screened earlier and more frequently for the disease and/or could make changes to health habits like diet and exercise. Such a genetic test result can lower a person's feelings of uncertainty, and this information can also help people to make informed choices about their future, such as whether to have a baby.

What are reasons to get different types of genetic tests?

Diagnostic testing: This type of testing is used to confirm a diagnosis when a person has signs or symptoms that suggest a genetic disease. The particular genetic test used depends on the disease for which a person is tested. For example, if a patient has physical features that suggest Down syndrome, a chromosomal test is used to see if the patient has an extra copy of chromosome 21. To test for Duchenne muscular dystrophy, a gene test is done to look for missing sections in the dystrophin gene.

Predictive testing: Predictive testing can show which people have a higher chance of getting a disease before symptoms appear. For example, one type of predictive test screens for inherited genetic risk factors that make it more likely for someone to develop certain cancers, such as colon or breast cancer, or diseases that usually develop later in life, such as adult-onset (Type 2) diabetes. Someone with an inherited genetic risk factor may have an increased chance of getting a disease, although this does not mean that the person will certainly get the disease.

Presymptomatic: This is a type of predictive testing that can indicate which family members are at risk for a certain genetic condition already known to be present in their family. This type of testing is done with people who do not yet show symptoms of that disease. This can be done for Huntington disease, for example. For some diseases, this type of testing can lead to prevention or treatment options. For example, when a disease-causing alteration for Graves disease is found in a family, testing is recommended for all close blood relatives (such as parents and siblings). Graves disease is an autoimmune disease that leads to overactivity of the thyroid gland (hyperthyroidism). Family members with the genetic alteration can be offered treatment, including surgery to remove the thyroid. With other types of diseases, there are no prevention or treatment options. For example, there is no treatment for family members who have a gene alteration causing Huntington disease. People with this alteration are certain to get the disease.

Preconception/carrier testing: This type of testing can tell individuals if they have (carry) a gene alteration for a type of inherited disorder called an autosomal recessive disorder. Autosomal means that the altered gene is on one of the twenty-two chromosomes other than the sex chromosomes (X or Y chromosomes). Recessive means that the person with only one altered copy of the disease gene will not get the disease, but might pass the alteration to their children. If both parents are carriers, their children might inherit an alteration from each parent and get the disease. Examples of autosomal recessive disorders are cystic fibrosis and Tay-Sachs disease.

Prenatal testing: This is available to pregnant women during pregnancy. Some reasons to have genetic testing include the following:

- Age of the mother. Women age thirty-five or older are at a higher risk for having a child with chromosomal abnormalities or other birth defects. However, some tests are recommended for all pregnant women, regardless of age.

- A family history of an inherited condition such as Duchenne muscular dystrophy.

- Ancestry or ethnic background indicating that the parents might have a higher chance of carrying an inherited disorder such as sickle cell anemia, common in people of African descent; thalassemia, common in people of Italian, Greek, Middle Eastern, Southern Asian, or African descent; or Tay-Sachs disease, common in people of eastern European (Ashkenazi) Jewish descent.

- To screen for common genetic disorders that may occur during pregnancy, such as Down syndrome or spina bifida.

Three diagnostic procedures are common in prenatal testing: ultrasound, amniocentesis, and chorionic villus sampling (CVS). Ultrasound uses the reflection of sound waves to create an overall picture of the developing fetus. Amniocentesis involves testing a sample of amniotic fluid from the womb surrounding the fetus. CVS involves taking a tiny sample of tissue from a region of the placenta that carries fetal cells rather than maternal cells.

Newborn screening: This is the most widespread type of genetic testing. It is an important public health program that can find disorders in newborns that might have long-term health effects. Newborn screening analyzes infant blood samples for abnormal or missing gene products (proteins). For example, infants are often screened for phenylketonuria (PKU), a metabolic disease in which an enzyme deficiency can cause severe mental retardation if the child is not treated. Metabolic disorders are diseases in which gene alterations lead to an inability to break down (metabolize) food and other substances. In the past, newborn screening focused on only a few disorders that lead to mental retardation. Regulations vary from state to state, but all states are now required by law to test for at least twenty-one disorders, although some states test for thirty or more disorders. These programs now test for disorders that can lead to increased risk of infectious disease, premature death, hearing loss, and heart problems.

Pharmacogenetic testing: This type of testing examines a person's genes to understand how drugs may move through the body and be broken down. The goal of pharmacogenetic testing is to help select drug treatments that are best for each person. For example, a test used in patients who have chronic myelogenous leukemia (CML) can show which of these patients would benefit from a medicine called imatinib. Another test looks at the liver enzyme cytochrome P450 (CYP450). This enzyme breaks down certain types of drugs, such as warfarin, which is used to prevent blood clots. Alterations in the CYP450 gene can affect how well people's bodies break down certain drugs. By taking a single dose of a drug, people with a less active form of the enzyme might get too much of the drug in their body, while people with a more active form of the enzyme might get too little of the drug. Too much warfarin, for example, can lead to internal bleeding, while too little warfarin may still allow blood clots to form. Pharmacogenetic testing can help make sure that people get the right amount of a medicine based on their particular genetic makeup.

How do I decide whether to be tested?

People have many different reasons for being tested or not being tested. For many, it is important to know whether a disease can be prevented if a gene alteration causing a disease is found. For example, those who have inherited predispositions to breast or colon cancer have options such as earlier and more frequent disease screening or early treatment. Pharmacogenetic testing can indicate the best medicine or dose of a medicine for a certain person.

In other cases, there may be no treatment for the disease. For example are no preventive steps or cures for Huntington's disease, but test results might help a person make life decisions, such as career choice, family planning, or insurance coverage.

People can seek advice about genetic testing from a genetic counselor. Genetic counselors help individuals and families understand the scientific, emotional, and ethical factors surrounding the decision to have genetic testing and how to deal with the results of those tests.

What about direct-to-consumer genetic tests available on the internet?

A variety of genetic tests are being offered directly to consumers, often over the internet. Such direct-to-consumer (DTC) genetic testing usually involves the individual scraping a few cells from inside the cheek and mailing the sample to a laboratory that performs the test. If you are considering such genetic tests, it is a good idea to first discuss the issue with your health care provider or a genetic counselor.

Your test results may show that you are at increased risk for a condition, such as Alzheimer disease, for which there is currently no effective prevention or cure. Such knowledge may help you plan your life, but it may also make you and your loved ones anxious or depressed.

Finally, ask yourself if you are prepared to make changes in your lifestyle based on the test results. If you are not willing to take actions like stopping smoking or exercising more, such tests may not be of much benefit to you.

Here are some major types of direct-to-consumer genetic tests:

- **Health-related:** These tests can detect changes in all or selected parts of your genome for variants that may influence your risk of developing certain diseases. Be aware that current tests provide just a partial picture of your disease risk. For most diseases, many pieces of the genetic puzzle remain to be discovered, along with how those pieces interact with lifestyle and environmental factors. This means that today's tests may falsely reassure people with undiscovered risk factors, or needlessly alarm people with undiscovered protective factors.

- **Nutrigenetic:** These tests are offered by companies that claim they can use information about your genetic makeup to develop an individualized diet plan. A government report published in 2006 found that such tests may be misleading or even harmful because they make claims that cannot be scientifically proven.

- **Nonmedical/other:** Other nonmedical types of tests may scan your genome for genetic variants related to various aspects of your life. These may include genetic markers that might be related to your physical traits, your ancestry, or your personality. These tests often do not claim to provide specific information about disease risk, but some of the results may have implications for your health. As with other DTC tests, there are concerns that the validity and reliability of these tests are not adequate.

Section 6.2

Prenatal Genetic Testing

Adapted with permission from
"A Guide to Prenatal Genetics Testing," © 2012 University of
Washington Medical Center, Seattle, Washington. All rights reserved.

This section describes prenatal tests that give information about your baby's health. It is your choice whether or not to have these tests done. Talk with your health care provider to learn more and to help you decide if any of these tests are right for you.

If you have any of these tests done, you will be asked to read more about each one. You will also be asked to read and sign a consent form for each test.

There is a lot you can do during your pregnancy to keep you and your baby healthy. Taking prenatal vitamins, eating healthy foods, exercising, and getting enough sleep are all important.

The human body is complicated. Even if you do everything "right" during your pregnancy, babies do not always develop normally. Between 3 percent and 5 percent of babies (between 3 and 5 out of 100) have some kind of health problem when they are born.

This section gives some basic information about these tests to help you make the best decision for you.

What Are the Tests?

There are two basic kinds of tests:

- Screening tests predict the chance, or odds, that your baby has a certain birth defect.

- Diagnostic tests tell you if your baby does or does not have a certain birth defect.

Table 6.1 lists the tests and when they are done. It also gives a brief description of each test and what it will tell you. The rest of this section gives more details about these tests, if you would like to read about them before you talk with your health care provider.

Table 6.1. Prenatal Tests

Screening Tests

Name of Test	When	Description	What It Tells You
Nuchal translucency (NT) ultrasound	11 to 14 weeks	Abdominal ultrasound to measure small space behind baby's neck	Chances your baby has a chromosome problem
Integrated screen	11 to 14 weeks and 15 to 22 weeks	NT ultrasound plus two separate blood samples	Chances your baby has Down syndrome, trisomy 18, or spina bifida
Quad screen	15 to 22 weeks	One blood sample	Chances your baby has Down syndrome, trisomy 18, or spina bifida

Diagnostic Tests

Name of Test	When	Description	What It Tells You
Chorionic villus sampling (CVS)	11 to 14 weeks	Sample of placenta, taken through the vagina or abdomen	Whether or not your baby has chromosome problems and sometimes other inherited diseases
Amniocentesis (with ultrasound)	16 to 22 weeks	Sample of fluid from around your baby, taken through your abdomen	Whether or not your baby has chromosome problems, spina bifida, and sometimes other inherited diseases

Other Tests

Name of Test	When	Description	What It Tells You
Anatomy ultrasound	18 to 22 weeks	Abdominal ultrasound to check baby's growth and development	Whether or not abnormalities are suspected and if further testing is needed

Screening Tests

Nuchal Translucency (NOO-kul trans-LOO-sun-see) or NT Ultrasound

This screening test is done between eleven and fourteen weeks of pregnancy. Using ultrasound, your baby's length is measured to confirm your due date. Ultrasound is also used to measure the small space under the skin behind your baby's neck. This space is called the nuchal translucency (NT). The larger this space of fluid is, the greater the chance your baby has a chromosome problem. An NT ultrasound can be done only by specially trained staff.

Integrated (IN-tuh-grey-tud) Screen

This test uses the results of the NT ultrasound and two blood tests. The first blood sample is taken between eleven and fourteen weeks, usually the same day as the NT ultrasound. The second blood sample is taken between fifteen and twenty-two weeks. The blood tests look for patterns of proteins and hormones that are linked to certain birth defects.

An integrated screen tells you the chances that your baby has Down syndrome, trisomy 18, or spina bifida. It does not diagnose these conditions. Most women who get an abnormal integrated screen result still have a healthy baby.

The integrated screen can detect:

- Ninety out of one hundred cases (90 percent) of Down syndrome;

- Ninety out of one hundred cases (90 percent) of trisomy 18;

- Eighty out of one hundred cases (80 percent) of spina bifida.

But, it will not detect all cases of these birth defects. And, it does not test for any other health problems.

Quad Screen

This screening test involves one blood sample that is taken between fifteen and twenty-two weeks. It's like the integrated screen, because it also looks for patterns of proteins and hormones that are linked to certain birth defects.

A quad screen tells you the chances that your baby has Down syndrome, trisomy 18, or spina bifida. It does not diagnose these conditions. Most women who get an abnormal quad screen result still have a healthy baby.

The quad screen can detect:

- Eighty-five out of one hundred cases (85 percent) of Down syndrome;

- Seventy-five out of one hundred cases (75 percent) of trisomy 18;

- Eighty out of one hundred cases (80 percent) of spina bifida.

But, it will not detect all cases of these birth defects. And, it does not test for any other health problems.

A quad screen may be a good test to have if you do not start prenatal care until your fourth month or if an NT ultrasound is not available.

Advanced Aneuploidy Screening with Cell-Free DNA

You may have heard in the news or seen articles on the Internet about a new blood test that can screen for Down syndrome. This test is called advanced aneuploidy screening with cell-free deoxyribonucleic acid (DNA). It uses a blood sample from the mother, and it is done starting at ten weeks of pregnancy. It screens for specific chromosome disorders in the baby.

Everyone has some free (not contained within a cell) DNA in their blood. When you are pregnant, most of that cell-free DNA is from you, but some is from your pregnancy. In this test, the total amount of cell-free DNA from chromosomes 21, 18, and 13 is measured in your blood.

Like the other screening tests, this test does not tell you if the baby has, or does not have, a chromosome problem. But if there is an increased amount of DNA from one of these chromosomes in your blood, there is a high chance that the baby has trisomy for that chromosome.

Currently, only women who have a high risk of having a baby with Down syndrome, trisomy 18, or trisomy 13 can have this test. If you have already had a child with one of these trisomies, or if you have another type of screen and the results are abnormal, you may be offered advanced aneuploidy screening with cell-free DNA.

Diagnostic Tests

Anatomy (uh-NAT-uh-mee) Ultrasound

This test is done between eighteen and twenty-two weeks. An ultrasound is used to look at your baby, the amount of fluid around him, your placenta, and your uterus. It checks to see that the baby is growing and that all major organs are formed.

Your baby is developed enough at this age that an ultrasound may find problems such as a severe heart defect, spina bifida, a missing kidney, and severe cleft lip. Although this test will not diagnose chromosome problems, it may show signs of them or other conditions.

Chorionic Villus Sampling (kor-ee-ON-ic VILL-us sampling) or CVS

This diagnostic test is usually done between eleven and fourteen weeks. The doctor uses either a thin, flexible needle or a thin plastic tube to remove a small sample of the placenta. An ultrasound is done at the same time, so your baby can be seen during the procedure.

The placenta sample is used to diagnose chromosome problems. If an inherited condition such as muscular dystrophy or hemophilia runs in your family, the sample can be used to test your baby for that condition.

The chance of miscarriage after CVS is one to two women in one hundred (1 percent to 2 percent).

Amniocentesis (AM-nee-oh-sen-TEE-sis) or Amnio

This diagnostic test is usually done between sixteen and twenty-two weeks. The doctor uses a thin, flexible needle to take two tablespoons of fluid from around your baby. An ultrasound is done at the same time, so your baby can be seen during the procedure.

Table 6.2. Ancestry Based Carrier Screening

Ancestral Group	Hereditary Condition	Chance of Being a Carrier
African-American	Beta Thalassemia	10% (10 out of 100)
	Sickle Cell Disease	11% (11 out of 100)
Eastern European (Ashkenazi) Jewish	Canavan Disease	2.5% (2 to 3 out of 100)
	Cystic Fibrosis	3% to 4% (3 to 4 out of 100)
	Familial Dysautonomia	3% (3 out of 100)
	Tay-Sachs Disease	3% (3 out of 100)
European Caucasian	Cystic Fibrosis	3% (3 out of 100)
Mediterranean	Beta Thalassemia	3% to 5% (3 to 5 out of 100)
	Sickle Cell Disease	2% to 30% (2 to 30 out of 100)
East and Southeast Asian[a]	Alpha Thalassemia	5% (5 out of 100)
	Beta Thalassemia	2% to 4% (2 to 4 out of 100)
Hispanic[a]	Beta Thalassemia	0.25% to 8% (fewer than 1 to 8 out of 100)
	Sickle Cell Disease	0.6% to 14% (fewer than 1 to 14 out of 100)
Middle Eastern and South Central Asian[a]	Beta Thalassemia	0.5% to 5.5% (fewer than 1 to 6 out of 100)
	Sickle Cell Disease	5% to 25% (5 to 25 out of 100)

[a] Numbers for this group are estimates and may vary depending on exact ethnicity.

The fluid is used to diagnose chromosome problems and spina bifida. If an inherited condition like muscular dystrophy or hemophilia runs in your family, the fluid can be used to test your baby for that condition.

The chance that having an amniocentesis will cause a miscarriage is one in four hundred women (0.25 percent).

Ancestry Based Carrier Screening

Your ancestry, or ethnicity, is one clue to help learn if your baby could have a rare genetic disease. Each ancestral group has conditions that can be inherited that are more common in that group compared to other ethnic groups. The conditions that are linked with each ancestral group are listed in Table 6.2.

Most times, a couple can have a child with one of these disorders only when both parents are "carriers" for the same disorder. Carriers usually have no symptoms of the disease. Also, most carriers have no family history of the disease. If someone in your family has one of these conditions, tell your health care provider.

If you and your partner are both carriers for the same genetic condition, then your baby could inherit that condition. If you want to know for sure before birth, an amniocentesis or a CVS can be done. The integrated screen, quad screen, and ultrasound will not diagnose these disorders.

To see if you are a carrier for these hereditary conditions, you will need to give a small blood sample. It is your choice whether or not to have any or all of these tests.

Table 6.2 is adapted from "Ancestry Based Carrier Screening" published by the National Society of Genetic Counselors, Inc., 2005.

Deciding Whether to Do These Tests

Choosing whether to have any of these tests, or deciding which ones are best for you, can be hard. There is no "right" choice. Some women choose only an anatomy ultrasound and no other tests. Others may choose an integrated screen and anatomy ultrasound. And, if one of these tests is abnormal, they may have amniocentesis. Some women prefer a CVS or amniocentesis without any of the screening tests.

Making an Informed Decision

These are some questions you may want to ask yourself as you think about having genetic testing:

- Do I want to have any of this information?

- How would learning about these birth defects before my baby is born help me and my health care provider prepare and plan?

- How would this information help me make choices about my pregnancy if a birth defect is found?

- Will taking these tests help me feel more reassured?

Your health care provider can talk more with you about your choices.

Section 6.3

Newborn Screening

About Newborn Screening

Newborn screening is the practice of testing every newborn for certain harmful or potentially fatal disorders that aren't otherwise apparent at birth.

Many of these are metabolic disorders (often called "inborn errors of metabolism") that interfere with the body's use of nutrients to maintain healthy tissues and produce energy. Other disorders that screening can detect include problems with hormones or the blood.

In general, metabolic and other inherited disorders can hinder an infant's normal physical and mental development in a variety of ways. And parents can pass along the gene for a certain disorder without even knowing that they're carriers.

With a simple blood test, doctors often can tell whether newborns have certain conditions that eventually could cause problems. Although these conditions are considered rare and most babies are given a clean bill of health, early diagnosis and proper treatment can make the difference between lifelong impairment and healthy development.

Screening: Past, Present, and Future

In the early 1960s, scientist Robert Guthrie, PhD, developed a blood test that could determine whether newborns had the metabolic disorder phenylketonuria (PKU). People with PKU lack an enzyme needed to process the amino acid phenylalanine, which is necessary for normal growth in kids and for normal protein use throughout life. However, if too much phenylalanine builds up, it damages brain tissue and eventually can cause substantial developmental delay.

If kids born with PKU are put on a special diet right away, they can avoid the developmental delay the condition caused in past generations and lead normal lives.

Since the development of the PKU test, researchers have developed additional blood tests that can screen newborns for other disorders that, unless detected and treated early, can cause physical problems, developmental delay, and in some cases, death.

The federal government has set no national standards, so screening requirements vary from state to state and are determined by individual state public health departments. Many states have mandatory newborn screening programs, but parents can refuse the testing for their infant if they choose.

Almost all states now screen for more than thirty disorders. One screening technique, the tandem mass spectrometry (or MS/MS), can screen for more than twenty inherited metabolic disorders with a single drop of blood.

Which Tests Are Offered?

Traditionally, state decisions about what to screen for have been based on weighing the costs against the benefits. "Cost" considerations include:

- the risk of false positive results (and the worry they cause);
- the availability of treatments known to help the condition;
- financial costs.

So what can you do? Your best strategy is to stay informed. Discuss this issue with both your obstetrician or health care provider and your future baby's doctor before you give birth. Know what tests are routinely done in your state and in the hospital where you'll deliver (some hospitals go beyond what's required by state law).

If your state isn't offering screening for the expanded panel of disorders, you may want to ask your doctors about supplemental screening, though you'll probably have to pay for additional tests yourself.

If you're concerned about whether your infant was screened for certain conditions, ask your child's doctor for information about which tests were done and whether further tests are recommended.

Newborn screening varies by state and is subject to change, especially given advancements in technology. However, the disorders listed here are the ones typically included in newborn screening programs.

PKU

When this disorder is detected early, feeding an infant a special formula low in phenylalanine can prevent mental retardation. A low-phenylalanine diet will need to be followed throughout childhood and adolescence and perhaps into adult life. This diet cuts out all high-protein foods, so people with PKU often need to take a special artificial formula as a nutritional substitute. Incidence: 1 in 10,000 to 25,000.

Congenital Hypothyroidism

This is the disorder most commonly identified by routine screening. Affected babies don't have enough thyroid hormone and so develop retarded growth and brain development. (The thyroid, a gland at the front of the neck, releases chemical substances that control metabolism and growth.)

If the disorder is detected early, a baby can be treated with oral doses of thyroid hormone to permit normal development. Incidence: 1 in 4,000.

Galactosemia

Babies with galactosemia lack the enzyme that converts galactose (one of two sugars found in lactose) into glucose, a sugar the body is able to use. As a result, milk (including breast milk) and other dairy products must be eliminated from the diet. Otherwise, galactose can build up in the system and damage the body's cells and organs, leading to blindness, severe mental retardation, growth deficiency, and even death.

Incidence: 1 in 60,000 to 80,000. Several less severe forms of galactosemia that may be detected by newborn screening may not require any intervention.

Sickle Cell Disease

Sickle cell disease is an inherited blood disease in which red blood cells mutate into abnormal "sickle" shapes and can cause episodes of pain, damage to vital organs such as the lungs and kidneys, and even death. Young children with sickle cell disease are especially prone to certain dangerous bacterial infections, such as pneumonia (inflammation of the lungs) and meningitis (inflammation of the brain and spinal cord).

Studies suggest that newborn screening can alert doctors to begin antibiotic treatment before infections occur and to monitor symptoms of possible worsening more closely. The screening test can also detect other disorders affecting hemoglobin (the oxygen-carrying substance in the blood).

Incidence: about 1 in every 500 African-American births and 1 in every 1,000 to 1,400 Hispanic-American births; also occurs with some frequency among people of Mediterranean, Middle Eastern, and South Asian descent.

Biotinidase Deficiency

Babies with this condition don't have enough biotinidase, an enzyme that recycles biotin (a B vitamin) in the body. The deficiency may cause seizures, poor muscle control, immune system impairment, hearing loss, mental retardation, coma, and even death. If the deficiency is detected in time, however, problems can be prevented by giving the baby extra biotin. Incidence: 1 in 72,000 to 126,000.

Congenital Adrenal Hyperplasia

This is actually a group of disorders involving a deficiency of certain hormones produced by the adrenal gland. It can affect the development of the genitals and may cause death due to loss of salt from the kidneys. Lifelong treatment through supplementation of the missing hormones manages the condition. Incidence: 1 in 12,000.

Maple Syrup Urine Disease (MSUD)

Babies with MSUD are missing an enzyme needed to process three amino acids that are essential for the body's normal growth. When not processed properly, these can build up in the body, causing urine to smell like maple syrup or sweet, burnt sugar. These babies usually have little appetite and are extremely irritable.

If not detected and treated early, MSUD can cause mental retardation, physical disability, and even death. A carefully controlled diet that cuts out certain high-protein foods containing those amino acids can prevent this. Like people with PKU, those with MSUD are often given a formula that supplies the necessary nutrients missed in the special diet they must follow. Incidence: 1 in 250,000.

Tyrosinemia

Babies with this amino acid metabolism disorder have trouble processing the amino acid tyrosine. If it accumulates in the body, it can cause mild retardation, language skill difficulties, liver problems, and even death from liver failure. Treatment requires a special diet and sometimes a liver transplant. Early diagnosis and treatment seem to offset long-term problems, although more information is needed. Incidence: not yet determined. Some babies have a mild self-limited form of tyrosinemia.

Cystic Fibrosis

Cystic fibrosis (CF) is a genetic disorder that particularly affects the lungs and digestive system and makes kids who have it more vulnerable to repeated lung infections. There is no known cure—treatment involves trying to prevent serious lung infections (sometimes with antibiotics) and providing adequate nutrition. Early detection may help doctors reduce the problems associated with CF, but the real impact of newborn screening has yet to be determined. Incidence: 1 in 2,000 Caucasian babies; less common in African Americans, Hispanics, and Asians.

Medium Chain Acyl CoA Dehydrogenase (MCAD) Deficiency

MCAD (medium chain acyl CoA dehydrogenase) deficiency is a fatty acid metabolism disorder. Kids who have it are prone to repeated episodes of low blood sugar (hypoglycemia), which can cause seizures and interfere with normal growth and development. Treatment involves making sure kids don't fast (skip meals) and supplies extra nutrition (usually by intravenous nutrients) when they're ill. Early detection and treatment can help affected children live normal lives.

Toxoplasmosis

Toxoplasmosis is a parasitic infection that can be transmitted through the mother's placenta to an unborn child. The disease-causing organism can invade the brain, eye, and muscles, possibly resulting in blindness and mental retardation. The benefit of early detection and treatment is uncertain. Incidence: 1 in 1,000. But only one or two states screen for toxoplasmosis.

Hearing Screening

Most but not all states require newborns' hearing to be screened before they're discharged from the hospital. If your baby isn't examined then, be sure that he or she does get screened within the first three weeks of life.

Kids develop critical speaking and language skills in their first few years. A hearing loss that's caught early can be treated to help prevent interference with that development.

Should I Request Additional Tests?

If you answer "yes" to any of these questions, talk to your doctor and perhaps a genetic counselor about additional tests:

- Do you have a family history of an inherited disorder?

- Have you previously given birth to a child who's affected by a disorder?

- Did an infant in your family die because of a suspected metabolic disorder?

- Do you have another reason to believe that your child may be at risk for a certain condition?

How Screening Is Done

In the first two or three days of life, your baby's heel will be pricked to obtain a small blood sample for testing. Most states have a state or regional laboratory perform the analyses, although some use a private lab.

It's generally recommended that the sample be taken after the first twenty-four hours of life. Some tests, such as the one for PKU, may not be as sensitive if they're done too soon after birth. However, because mothers and newborns are often discharged within a day, some babies may be tested within the first twenty-four hours. If this happens, experts recommend that a repeat sample be taken no more than one to two weeks later. It's especially important that the PKU screening test be run again for accurate results. Some states routinely do two tests on all infants.

Getting the Results

Different labs have different procedures for notifying families and pediatricians of the results. Some may send the results to the hospital where your child was born and not directly to your child's doctor, which may mean a delay in getting the results to you.

And although some states have a system that allows doctors to access the results via phone or computer, others may not. Ask your doctor how you'll get the results and when you should expect them.

If a test result comes back abnormal, try not to panic. This does not necessarily mean that your child has the disorder in question. A screening test is not the same as diagnostic test. The initial screening provides only preliminary information that must be followed up with more specific diagnostic testing.

If testing confirms that your child does have a disorder, your doctor may refer you to a specialist for further evaluation and treatment. Keep in mind that dietary restrictions and supplements, along with proper medical supervision, often can prevent most of the serious physical and mental problems that were associated with metabolic disorders in the past.

You also may wonder whether the disorder can be passed on to any future children. You'll want to discuss this with your doctor and perhaps a genetic counselor. Also, if you have other children who weren't screened for the disorder, consider having testing done. Again, speak with your doctor.

Know Your Options

Because state programs are subject to change, you'll want to find up-to-date information about your state's (and individual hospital's) program. Talk to your doctor or contact your state's department of health for more information.

Section 6.4

Screening for Critical Congenital Heart Defects

Excerpted from "Screening for Critical Congenital Heart Defects,"
Centers for Disease Control and Prevention (www.cdc.gov), May 13, 2013.

Congenital heart defects (CHDs) account for nearly 30 percent of infant deaths due to birth defects.[1] In the United States, about 7,200 (or 18 per 10,000) babies born every year have critical congenital heart defects (CCHDs, which also are known as critical congenital heart disease).[2] These CCHDs are coarctation of the aorta, double-outlet right ventricle, D-transposition of the great arteries, Ebstein anomaly, hypoplastic left heart syndrome, interrupted aortic arch, pulmonary atresia (intact septum), single ventricle, total anomalous pulmonary venous connection, tetralogy of Fallot, tricuspid atresia, and truncus arteriosus. Babies with CCHDs usually require surgery or catheter intervention in the first year of life. CCHDs can potentially be detected using pulse oximetry screening, which is a test to determine the amount of oxygen in the blood and pulse rate. Pulse oximetry screening is most likely to detect seven of the CCHDs. These seven main screening targets are hypoplastic left heart syndrome, pulmonary atresia (with intact septum), tetralogy of Fallot, total anomalous pulmonary venous return, transposition of the great arteries, tricuspid atresia, and truncus arteriosus. Other heart defects can be just as severe as the main screening targets and also require treatment soon after birth. However, pulse oximetry screening may not detect these heart defects as consistently as the seven disorders listed as the main screening targets.

The Importance of Screening for Critical Congenital Heart Defects

Some babies born with a heart defect appear healthy at first and can be sent home with their families before their heart defect is detected. It is estimated that about three hundred infants with an unrecognized CCHD are discharged each year from newborn nurseries in the United States.[3] These babies are at risk of having serious complications within the first few days or weeks of life and often require emergency care.

Newborn screening using pulse oximetry can identify some infants with a CCHD before they show signs of a CCHD. Once identified, babies with a CCHD can be seen by cardiologists and can receive specialized care and treatment that can prevent disability and death early in life. Treatment can include medications and surgery.

When and How Babies Are Screened

Pulse oximetry is a simple bedside test to determine the amount of oxygen in a baby's blood and the baby's pulse rate. Low levels of oxygen in the blood can be a sign of a CCHD. The test is done using a machine called a pulse oximeter, with sensors placed on the baby's skin. The test is painless and takes only a few minutes. Screening is done when a baby is twenty-four to forty-eight hours of age, or as late as possible if the baby is to be discharged from the hospital before he or she is twenty-four hours of age.

Pulse oximetry screening does not replace a complete history and physical examination, which sometimes can detect a CCHD before the development of low levels of oxygen in the blood. Pulse oximetry screening, therefore, should be used along with the physical examination.

CCHD Screening Results

If the results are "negative" ("pass" or in-range result), it means that the baby's test results did not show signs of a CCHD. This type of screening test does not detect all CCHDs, so it is possible for a baby with a negative screening result to still have a CCHD or other congenital heart defect. If the results are "positive" ("fail" or out-of-range result), it means that the baby's test results showed low levels of oxygen in the blood, which can be a sign of a CCHD. This does not always mean that the baby has a CCHD. It just means that more testing is needed.

The baby's doctor might recommend that the infant get screened again or have more specific tests, like an echocardiogram (an ultrasound picture of the heart), to diagnose a CCHD. Babies who are found to have a CCHD also might be evaluated by a clinical geneticist. This could help identify genetic syndromes associated with CCHDs and inform families about future risks.

References

1. Broussard CS, Gilboa SM, Lee KA, Oster M, Petrini JR, Honein MA. Racial/Ethnic Differences in Infant Mortality Attributable to Birth Defects by Gestational Age. *Pediatrics.* 2012; 130:e518–27.

2. Adapted from Reller, MD, Strickland, MJ, Riehle-Colarusso, TJ, Mahle, WT, Correa, A. Prevalence of congenital heart defects in metropolitan Atlanta, 1998–2005. *J Pediatr.* 2008;153:807–13.

3. Adapted from Aamir T, Kruse L, Ezeakudo O. Delayed diagnosis of critical congenital cardiovascular malformations (CCVM) and pulse oximetry screening of newborns. *Acta Paediatr.* 2007;96:1146–49.

Chapter 7

Preventing Genetic Discrimination

In 2008, President George W. Bush signed the Genetic Information Nondiscrimination Act (GINA) into law. Under GINA, employers and health insurers can no longer discriminate against individuals based upon their genetic information. GINA protects Americans from genetic discrimination while encouraging each patient to seek out medical care that is specifically tailored to his or her genetic makeup.

Yesterday

Health insurers and employers could discriminate against individuals based upon their genetic information. For example, a health insurer might refuse coverage to a woman whose deoxyribonucleic acid (DNA) increases her risk of breast cancer.

Because every person has dozens of DNA differences that could affect his or her chance of getting a disease, everyone needs to be concerned about genetic discrimination. DNA differences that increase a person's risk don't mean that he or she will develop a disease, but individuals might be targeted for discrimination based on the specific differences in their DNA.

The development of genetic tests promised to give patients new power to create personalized ways of detecting, treating, and preventing disease. But without protection from discrimination, patients were reluctant to undergo genetic testing.

"The Genetic Information Nondiscrimination Act (GINA)," U.S. Department of Health and Human Services, February 14, 2011.

While some states had passed laws against genetic discrimination, the degree of protection from these laws varied widely among the different states. Many states had no law preventing genetic discrimination.

Today

GINA protects individuals from discrimination by health insurers or employers based on genetic information.

Health Insurance

- Insurers may not discriminate against individuals based on family medical history or individuals' and family members' genetic tests and services.

- Health insurers may not use genetic information to make eligibility, coverage, underwriting, or premium-setting decisions.

- Health insurers may not request or require individuals or their family members to undergo genetic testing or to provide genetic information.

- Insurers cannot use genetic information obtained intentionally or unintentionally in decisions about enrollment or coverage.

- The use of genetic information as a preexisting condition is prohibited in both the Medicare supplemental policy and individual health insurance markets.

Employment

- GINA makes it illegal to discriminate against employees or applicants because of genetic information.

- Employers may not discriminate on the basis of genetic information when it comes to any aspect of employment.

- Whether by a supervisor, co-worker, client, or customer, harassment because of someone's genetic information is illegal.

- It is illegal for an employer to fire, demote, harass, or otherwise "retaliate" against an applicant or employee who has filed a charge of discrimination, participates in a discrimination proceeding, or opposes genetic discrimination.

- GINA makes it illegal for an employer to obtain genetic information, including family medical history, except under certain exceptions.

- Employers are forbidden from disclosing genetic information about applicants or employees.

GINA sets a minimum standard of protection that must be met across the country. It does not weaken the protections provided by any state law.

The law does not cover life insurance, disability insurance, or long-term care insurance.

Tomorrow

As genomic medicine is poised to revolutionize medicine, patients will be able to utilize advances in genetic testing to create highly personalized care and treatment plans without fear of discrimination.

Patients may be more likely to participate in medical research that involves genetic testing because they no longer need to fear genetic discrimination.

With more participants for vital medical research, doctors and scientists will be able to create new lifesaving treatments and cures based upon the underlying genetic causes of their patients' diseases.

Part Two

Disorders Resulting from Abnormalities in Specific Genes

Chapter 8

Albinism

Humans, animals, and even plants can have albinism, a condition that gives people a kind of pale appearance. But what is albinism and what causes it?

Albinism is a genetic condition where people are born without the usual pigment (color) in their bodies. Their bodies aren't able to make a normal amount of melanin, the chemical that is responsible for eye, skin, and hair color. So most people with albinism have very pale skin, hair, and eyes. Albinism can affect people of all races, and there are different kinds of albinism.

Some people with a condition called oculocutaneous albinism have extremely pale skin and eyes, and white hair. Others with this same type of albinism might have slightly more color in their hair, eyes, or skin.

For some people, albinism affects only their eyes. This is known as ocular albinism. People with ocular albinism usually have blue eyes. In some cases, the iris (the colored part of the eye) has very little color so a person's eyes might look pink or reddish. This is caused by the blood vessels inside the eye showing through the iris. In some forms of ocular albinism, the hearing nerves may be affected and the person may develop hearing problems or deafness over time.

Excerpted from "Albinism," July 2010, with permission from www.kidshealth.org. This information was provided by KidsHealth®, one of the largest resources online for medically reviewed health information for parents, kids, and teens. For more articles like this, visit www.KidsHealth.org, or www.TeensHealth.org. Copyright © 1995 –2012 The Nemours Foundation. All rights reserved.

Except for eye problems, most people with albinism are just as healthy as anyone else. In very rare cases a person's albinism is part of another condition that involves other health problems in addition to albinism. People with these types of albinism can have such health complications as bleeding, lung, bowel, and immune system problems.

Eyesight and Albinism

People with albinism often have trouble with their eyesight. They may wear glasses or contact lenses to help correct problems like near-sightedness, farsightedness, or astigmatism. Others might need eye surgery. Just as there are different degrees of albinism there are also different levels of eye problems for a person who has the condition.

Albinism does not make a person completely blind. Although some people with albinism are "legally blind," that doesn't mean they have lost their vision completely. They can still read and study—they just may need larger print or magnifiers to help them.

People with albinism can be very sensitive to light because the iris doesn't have enough color to shield the retina properly. Wearing sunglasses or tinted contact lenses can help make them more comfortable out in the sun.

Skin Precautions

Besides giving skin, eyes, and hair their color, melanin helps protect our skin from the sun. It does this by causing skin to tan instead of burn—which is why people with darker skin (more melanin) are less likely to burn than people with lighter skin. So people with albinism can sunburn very easily.

People with light skin are also particularly at risk for skin cancer. So it's important for people with albinism to use a sunscreen with a high sun protection factor (SPF) at all times and to wear clothing that offers protection from the sun, such as hats, dark-colored clothing, or long pants and long-sleeved shirts.

What Causes Albinism?

Albinism is inherited. It's not contagious—you can't "catch" it from someone else. People are born with albinism because they inherit an albinism gene or genes from their parents.

In the most common forms of oculocutaneous albinism, both parents must carry the albinism gene for a child to be born with the condition.

Even if both parents carry the gene, the chance of each of their children being born with albinism is one in four.

If just one parent has the gene and the other parent has a normal pigment gene, their children won't have oculocutaneous albinism. But each child will have a one in two chance of being a "carrier" of an albinism gene. If a child who carries the gene grows up to have a baby with someone who also does, there's a one in four chance that their baby may have albinism. Since most people who carry an albinism gene don't show any signs of the condition, a baby with albinism can be born to parents whose coloring is typical for people of their ethnic group.

The most common form of ocular albinism affects only males who have inherited an albinism gene from their mothers. Some females can have a milder form of the condition if they have inherited this gene.

How Is It Treated?

Because most people with albinism don't have health problems, treatment—apart from vision care—isn't usually necessary. But they do need to take certain precautions, such as wearing sunglasses and sunscreen when outdoors.

Albinism can't be "cured." But it only rarely leads to serious health problems. When health problems are serious, doctors usually can treat the symptoms.

Chapter 9

Alpha-1 Antitrypsin Deficiency

What is alpha-1 antitrypsin deficiency?

Alpha-1 antitrypsin deficiency (AATD) is an inherited condition that causes low levels of, or no, alpha-1 antitrypsin (AAT) in the blood. AATD occurs in approximately 1 in 2,500 individuals. This condition is found in all ethnic groups; however, it occurs most often in whites of European ancestry.

Alpha-1 antitrypsin (AAT) is a protein that is made in the liver. The liver releases this protein into the bloodstream. AAT protects the lungs so they can work normally. Without enough AAT, the lungs can be damaged, and this damage may make breathing difficult.

Everyone has two copies of the gene for AAT and receives one copy of the gene from each parent. Most people have two normal copies of the alpha-1 antitrypsin gene. Individuals with AATD have one normal copy and one damaged copy, or they have two damaged copies. Most individuals who have one normal gene can produce enough alpha-1 antitrypsin to live healthy lives, especially if they do not smoke.

People who have two damaged copies of the gene are not able to produce enough alpha-1 antitrypsin, which leads them to have more severe symptoms.

Reprinted from "Learning about Alpha-1 Antitrypsin Deficiency," National Human Genome Research Institute (www.genome.gov), January 4, 2012.

What are the symptoms of alpha-1 antitrypsin deficiency (AATD)?

AATD can present as lung disease in adults and can be associated with liver disease in a small portion of affected children. In affected adults, the first symptoms of AATD are shortness of breath with mild activity, reduced ability to exercise, and wheezing. These symptoms usually appear between the ages of twenty and forty. Other signs and symptoms can include repeated respiratory infections, fatigue, rapid heartbeat upon standing, vision problems, and unintentional weight loss.

Some individuals with AATD have advanced lung disease and have emphysema, in which the small air sacs (alveoli) in the lungs are damaged. Symptoms of emphysema include difficulty breathing, a hacking cough, and a barrel-shaped chest. Smoking or exposure to tobacco smoke increases the appearance of symptoms and damage to the lungs. Other common diagnoses include COPD (chronic obstructive pulmonary disease), asthma, chronic bronchitis, and bronchiectasis—a chronic inflammatory or degenerative condition of one or more bronchi or bronchioles.

Liver disease, called cirrhosis of the liver, is another symptom of AATD. It can be present in some affected children, about 10 percent, and has also been reported in 15 percent of adults with AATD. In its late stages signs and symptoms of liver disease can include a swollen abdomen, coughing up blood, swollen feet or legs, and yellowing of the skin and the whites of the eyes (jaundice).

Rarely, AATD can cause a skin condition known as panniculitis, which is characterized by hardened skin with painful lumps or patches. Panniculitis varies in severity and can occur at any age.

How is alpha-1 antitrypsin deficiency diagnosed?

Alpha-1 antitrypsin deficiency (AATD) is diagnosed through testing of a blood sample, when a person is suspected of having AATD. For example, AATD may be suspected when a physical examination reveals a barrel-shaped chest, or, when listening to the chest with a stethoscope, wheezing, crackles, or decreased breath sounds are heard.

Testing for AATD, using a blood sample from the individual, is simple, quick, and highly accurate. Three types of tests are usually done on the blood sample:

- Alpha-1 genotyping, which examines a person's genes and determines their genotype

- Alpha-1 antitrypsin proteinase inhibitor (PI) type of phenotype test, which determines the type of AAT protein that a person has.

- Alpha-1 antitrypsin level test, which determines the amount of AAT in a person's blood.

Individuals who have symptoms that suggest AATD or who have a family history of AATD should consider being tested.

What is the treatment for alpha-1 antitrypsin deficiency?

Treatment of alpha-1 antitrypsin deficiency (AATD) is based on a person's symptoms. There is currently no cure. The major goal of AATD management is preventing or slowing the progression of lung disease.

Treatments include bronchodilators and prompt treatment with antibiotics for upper respiratory tract infections. Lung transplantation may be an option for those who develop end-stage lung disease. Quitting smoking, if a person with AATD smokes, is essential.

Replacement (augmentation) therapy with the missing AAT protein is available, although it is used only under special circumstances. It is not known how effective this is once disease has developed or which people would benefit most.

Is alpha-1 antitrypsin deficiency inherited?

Alpha-1 antitrypsin deficiency is inherited in families in an autosomal codominant pattern. Codominant inheritance means that two different variants of the gene (alleles) may be expressed, and both versions contribute to the genetic trait.

The M gene is the most common allele of the alpha-1 gene. It produces normal levels of the alpha-1 antitrypsin protein.

The Z gene is the most common variant of the gene. It causes alpha-1 antitrypsin deficiency. The S allele is another, less common variant that causes ATTD.

If a person inherits one M gene and one Z gene or one S gene ("type PiMZ" or "type PiMS"), that person is a carrier of the disorder. While such a person may not have normal levels of alpha-1 antitrypsin, there should be enough to protect the lungs. However, carriers with the MZ alleles have an increased risk for lung disease, particularly if they smoke.

A person who inherits the Z gene from each parent is called "type PiZZ." This person has very low alpha-1 antitrypsin levels, allowing elastase—an enzyme especially of pancreatic juice that digests elastin—to damage the lungs. A person who inherits an altered version called S and Z is also likely to develop AATD.

Chapter 10

Blood Clotting Deficiency Disorders

Chapter Contents

Section 10.1

Factor V Leiden Thrombophilia

Reprinted from "Learning about Factor V Leiden Thrombophilia,"
National Human Genome Research Institute (www.genome.gov),
December 13, 2011.

What is factor V Leiden thrombophilia?

Factor V Leiden thrombophilia is an inherited disorder of blood clotting. Factor V Leiden is the name of a specific mutation (genetic alteration) that results in thrombophilia, or an increased tendency to form abnormal blood clots in blood vessels. People who have the factor V Leiden mutation are at somewhat higher than average risk for a type of clot that forms in large veins in the legs (deep venous thrombosis, or DVT) or a clot that travels through the bloodstream and lodges in the lungs (pulmonary embolism, or PE).

Factor V Leiden is the most common inherited form of thrombophilia. Between 3 and 8 percent of the Caucasian (white) U.S. and European populations carry one copy of the factor V Leiden mutation, and about one in five thousand people have two copies of the mutation. The mutation is less common in other populations.

A mutation in the factor V gene (F5) increases the risk of developing factor V Leiden thrombophilia. The protein made by F5 called factor V plays a critical role in the formation of blood clots in response to injury. The Factor V protein is involved in a series of chemical reactions that hold blood clots together. A molecule called activated protein C (APC) prevents blood clots from growing too large by inactivating factor V. In people with the factor V Leiden mutation, APC is unable to inactivate factor V normally. As a result, the clotting process continues longer than usual, increasing the chance of developing abnormal blood clots.

What are the symptoms of factor V Leiden thrombophilia?

The symptoms of factor V Leiden vary among individuals. There are some individuals who have the F5 gene and who never develop thrombosis, while others have recurring thrombosis before the age of thirty years. This variability is influenced by the number of F5 gene mutations a person has, the presence of other gene alterations related to blood clotting, and circumstantial risk factors, such as surgery, use of oral contraceptives, and pregnancy.

Symptoms of Factor V Leiden include the following:

- Having a first DVT or PE before fifty years of age

- Having recurring DVT or PE

- Having venous thrombosis in unusual sites in the body such as the brain or the liver

- Having a DVT or PE during or right after pregnancy

- Having a history of unexplained pregnancy loss in the second or third trimester

- Having a DVT or PE and a strong family history of venous thromboembolism

The use of hormones, such as oral contraceptive pills (OCPs) and hormone replacement therapy (HRT), including estrogen and estrogen-like drugs taken after menopause, increases the risk of developing DVT and PE. Healthy women taking OCPs have a three- to fourfold increased risk of developing a DVT or PE compared with women who do not take OCP. Women with factor V Leiden who take OCPs have about a thirty-five-fold increased risk of developing a DVT or PE compared with women without factor V Leiden and those who do not take OCPs. Likewise, postmenopausal women taking HRT have a two- to threefold higher risk of developing a DVT or PE than women who do not take HRT, and women with factor V Leiden who take HRT have a fifteen-fold higher risk. Women with heterozygous factor V Leiden who are making decisions about OCP or HRT use should take these statistics into consideration when weighing the risks and benefits of treatment.

How is factor V Leiden thrombophilia diagnosed?

Your doctor would suspect a diagnosis of thrombophilia if you have a history of venous thrombosis and/or a family history of venous thrombosis. The diagnosis is made using a screening test called a coagulation screening test or by genetic testing (DNA analysis) of the F5 gene.

How is factor V Leiden thrombophilia treated?

The management of individuals with factor V Leiden depends on the clinical circumstances. People with factor V Leiden who have had a DVT or PE are usually treated with blood thinners or anti-coagulants. Anticoagulants such as heparin are given for varying amounts of time depending on the person's situation. It is not usually recommended that people with factor V Leiden be treated lifelong with anticoagulants if they have had only one DVT or PE, unless there are additional risk factors present. Having had a DVT or PE in the past increases a person's risk for developing another one in the future, but having factor V Leiden does not seem to add to the risk of having a second clot. In general, individuals who have factor V Leiden but have never had a blood clot are not routinely treated with an anticoagulant. Rather, these individuals are counseled about reducing or eliminating other factors that may add to one's risk of developing a clot in the future. In addition, these individuals may require temporary treatment with an anticoagulant during periods of particularly high risk, such as major surgery.

Factor V Leiden increases the risk of developing a DVT during pregnancy by about sevenfold. Women with factor V Leiden who are planning pregnancy should discuss this with their obstetrician and/or hematologist. Most women with factor V Leiden have normal pregnancies and only require close follow-up during pregnancy. For those with a history of DVT or PE, treatment with an anticoagulant during a subsequent pregnancy can prevent recurrent problems.

What do we know about heredity and factor V Leiden thrombophilia?

Factor V Leiden is the most common inherited form of thrombophilia. The risk of developing a clot in a blood vessel depends on whether a person inherits one or two copies of the factor V Leiden mutation. Inheriting one copy of the mutation from a parent increases by fourfold to eightfold the chance of developing a clot. People who inherit two copies of the mutation, one from each parent, may have up to eighty times the usual risk of developing this type of blood clot. Considering that the risk of developing an abnormal blood clot averages about 1 in 1,000 per year in the general population, the presence of one copy of the factor V Leiden mutation increases that risk to 1 in 125 to 1 in 250. Having two copies of the mutation may raise the risk as high as 1 in 12.

Section 10.2

Hemophilia

"Hemophilia," January 2011, reprinted with permission from www .kidshealth.org. This information was provided by KidsHealth®, one of the largest resources online for medically reviewed health information written for parents, kids, and teens. For more articles like this, visit www.KidsHealth.org, or www.TeensHealth.org. Copyright © 1995–2012 The Nemours Foundation. All rights reserved.

Bumps and scrapes are a part of every child's life. For most kids, a tumble off a bike or a stray kick in a soccer game means a temporary bruise or a healing scab. However, for kids with hemophilia, these normal traumas of childhood are reason for extra concern.

Hemophilia is a rare bleeding disorder that prevents the blood from clotting properly, so a person who has it bleeds more than someone without hemophilia does. It's a genetic disorder, which means it's the result of a change in genes that was either inherited (passed on from parent to child) or occurred during development in the womb.

Currently, about seventeen thousand people in the United States have hemophilia. Hemophilia affects mostly boys—about one in every five thousand to ten thousand is born with it. Girls are more rarely affected. A male can't pass the gene for hemophilia to his sons, though all his daughters will be carriers of the disease gene. Each male child of a female carrier has a 50 percent chance of having hemophilia.

About Hemophilia

When most people get a cut, the body naturally protects itself. Sticky blood cells called platelets go to where the bleeding is and plug up the hole. This is the first step in the clotting process. When the platelets plug the hole, they release chemicals that attract more sticky platelets and also activate various proteins in the blood known as clotting factors. These proteins mix with the platelets to form fibers, and these fibers make the clot stronger and stop the bleeding.

Our bodies have twelve clotting factors that work together in this process (numbered using Roman numerals from I through XII). Having too little of factors VIII (8) or IX (9) is what causes hemophilia. A

83

person with hemophilia will lack only one factor, either factor VIII or factor IX, but not both.

There are two major kinds of hemophilia, hemophilia A and hemophilia B. About 80 percent of cases are hemophilia A, which is a factor VIII deficiency. Hemophilia B is when factor IX is lacking.

Hemophilia is classified as mild, moderate, or severe, based on the amount of the clotting factor in the person's blood. If someone produces only 1 percent or less of the affected factor, the case is called severe. Someone that produces 2 percent to 5 percent has a moderate case, and someone that produces 6 percent to 50 percent of the affected factor level is considered to have a mild case of hemophilia.

In general, a person with milder hemophilia may only bleed excessively once in a while, whereas severe hemophilia puts someone at risk for having bleeding problems much more often.

Signs and Symptoms

Signs and symptoms of hemophilia vary, depending on severity of the factor deficiency and the location of the bleeding. Few babies are diagnosed with hemophilia within the first six months of life because they're unlikely to sustain an injury that would lead to bleeding. For example, only about 50 percent of males with hemophilia bleed excessively when circumcised and only 3 percent to 5 percent of newborns with hemophilia have bleeding within the skull (called an intracranial hemorrhage).

Once babies with hemophilia begin crawling and cruising, parents may notice raised bruises on the stomach, chest, buttocks, and back. Sometimes, because bruises appear in unlikely places, parents may be suspected of child abuse before their child is diagnosed with hemophilia.

The baby may also be fussy and may not want to reach for a cup, walk, or crawl. Other symptoms include:

- prolonged nosebleeds;
- excessive bleeding from biting down on the lips or tongue;
- excessive bleeding following a tooth extraction or loss of a tooth;
- excessive bleeding following surgery;
- blood in the urine (called hematuria).

The most common type of bleeding in hemophilia involves muscles and joints. A child with hemophilia will usually refuse to move the affected joint or muscle because of pain and swelling. Recurrent joint bleeding can also lead to chronic damage.

Diagnosis

Your doctor may suspect your child has hemophilia if there's a pattern of bruising and bleeding, particularly if this includes bleeding into the joint. Diagnosing the condition requires a set of blood tests, including a complete blood count (CBC), prothrombin time (PT), activated partial thromboplastin time (PTT), factor VIII level, and factor IX level.

Treatment

Although hemophilia is a lifelong condition with no cure (other than liver transplantation, a procedure that can sometimes cause health problems more serious than hemophilia itself), it can be successfully managed with clotting factor replacement therapy—periodic infusions of the deficient clotting factor into the child's bloodstream.

Factor replacement may be given through an intravenous (IV) line either at the hematology clinic or at home by a visiting nurse or by parents (and patients themselves) who have undergone special training. Your child's hemophilia team (doctors called hematologists who specialize in treating blood disorders, nurse practitioners, nurses, and social workers) will teach you how to prepare the concentrated clotting factor and when and how to inject it into your child's vein.

Once the clotting factor is "infused," it begins to work quickly and helps prevent joint damage.

Although these treatments are effective, they are also expensive. According to the National Heart, Lung, and Blood Institute, most kids in the United States who begin receiving regular infusions early in life will incur more than $1,000,000 in health care costs by their second decade (although most health insurance plans will cover much of this).

Between 14 percent and 25 percent of children with severe hemophilia A develop inhibitors (antibodies to the clotting factor). Their bodies view the clotting factor as a foreign substance and develop antibodies that block its clotting action. This can make the hemophilia difficult to treat.

One method for overcoming the inhibitors is to increase the body's tolerance to the clotting factor by carefully infusing increasing amounts of the clotting factor over time. Inhibitors to factor IX (hemophilia B) are less common but are more difficult to treat.

Also, a new medication called recombinant factor VII has helped many patients with inhibitors. It activates another part of the coagulation process directly and bypasses the deficiencies.

Preventing Problems

Parents can help kids with hemophilia prevent problems by encouraging healthy behaviors. For example, exercise can strengthen muscles and help decrease bleeding from injuries. Swimming is strongly encouraged because it exercises all the muscle groups without putting stress on the joints.

The child's weight should also be managed properly, because excess weight can cause strain in regions of the body and increase bleeding risks. If your child is overweight, speak to your doctor for advice on weight management.

Medications can also help prevent problems in kids within hemophilia. Many patients with severe disease prevent "bleeds" by infusing clotting factors on a regular basis (usually two or three times per week). Some young children have a surgical procedure to implant a central venous catheter (a hollow, soft tube) into a vein. The catheter can be used to give concentrates of clotting factors without pain.

Your Child's Needs

Although each stage of development comes with its own set of issues, experts say the toddler and teenage years can be the most challenging for kids with hemophilia. Both phases naturally involve a child's quest for independence. For example, a toddler may not tell his or her parents about an injury that resulted from doing something that wasn't allowed (riding a bike without a helmet, jumping on the furniture, running in the house, etc.). Most kids, though, will discover that seeking prompt treatment is better than waiting until pain and swelling become severe.

Ask your family members, caregivers, and your child's teachers if they would like to learn more about hemophilia by meeting with your doctor or other members of the hemophilia team.

Kids with hemophilia can still participate in activities, though they might have to take on a different role. For example, hemophilia might prevent kids from participating in contact sports but they can still be a part of the team as the scorekeeper or assistant manager.

Another excellent option is to send them to an appropriate summer camp where they can meet other kids with hemophilia and work toward being able to give themselves clotting factor replacement therapy for a sense of control over the condition. Ask your doctor for information about finding a camp near you.

Caring for Kids with Hemophilia

When your child is an infant, you should put bumper pads in the crib, cushion furniture with sharp edges, and put gates across stairs to prevent falls.

As your baby begins to crawl and walk, special knee and elbow pads can offer protection against joint bleeds. Some parents sew a pocket in the seat of their child's pants and pad it with a piece of diaper. If your house has ceramic tile or hardwood floors, consider installing carpet or buying rugs to soften the floor surface.

Depending on how rambunctious and adventurous your toddler is, you might want to have him or her wear a helmet to protect against head injuries.

Dental care is just as important for kids with hemophilia, but routine cleanings can sometimes cause bleeding. So it's important that the dentist have experience with patients who have hemophilia and know how to handle any bleeding that may occur.

Kids with hemophilia can generally sense when a bleed has occurred. They often describe a tingly or bubbly sensation in a joint. It may also feel warm to the touch. Encourage your child to tell you when he or she senses a bleed—a quick infusion is the key to preventing long-term damage.

Doctors also recommend splinting an affected joint for a short period of time and then applying ice to decrease inflammation, promote clotting, and relieve pain. Acetaminophen (such as Tylenol) is the preferred pain reliever because many other over-the-counter pain medications contain aspirin or NSAIDs (nonsteroidal anti-inflammatory drugs, such as ibuprofen or naproxen sodium), which can affect blood platelets and lead to increased bleeding.

Bleeds must be treated promptly because prolonged bleeding can cause joint problems. The accumulation of blood in the joint spaces can erode the smooth surfaces that allow limbs to bend easily. As the surfaces roughen, inflammation and the number of bleeds can increase. This cycle can lead to chronic joint damage that may require surgery to remove the damaged joint tissue (called a synovectomy).

When to Call the Doctor

Certain bleeds require medical attention, including those injuries affecting:

- the central nervous system—any suspected trauma to the head, neck, or back;

- the face, including the eyes and ears;
- the throat or another portion of the airway;
- the gastrointestinal tract (which might produce signs such as bright red or black blood in the stool);
- the kidneys and urinary tract (if you find blood in the urine, this may require treatment and bed rest);
- the iliopsoas muscle in the trunk (which might produce signs that mimic a hip or abdominal bleed, including lower abdominal/groin or upper thigh pain, an inability to raise the leg on the affected side);
- the genital area;
- the hips or shoulders (these can be complicated bleeds because they involve the rotator joints);
- large muscle compartments, such as the thighs.

If the bleed requires going to the emergency room, make sure your child is treated at a hospital that has experience treating hemophilia. Any injury affecting the brain or any part of the central nervous system or a vital organ should be treated as an emergency and you should get medical assistance immediately.

Looking to the Future

Tremendous advances have been made in the treatment of hemophilia, and most patients can now lead full, healthy lives with careful management of their condition.

The development of clotting factors made in the laboratory has virtually eliminated the danger of transfusion-related infection with human immunodeficiency virus (HIV) or hepatitis viruses from clotting factor replacement therapy. And regular home-based infusions have helped reduce chronic joint problems.

In the future, people with hemophilia may have access to continuous infusion of clotting factors under the skin or in pill form. Some doctors are also encouraged by research involving gene therapy.

Thanks to advances like these, kids with hemophilia can now participate in a wide range of sports and have the freedom to lead more active lives.

Section 10.3

Von Willebrand Disease

Excerpted from "What Is Von Willebrand Disease?" National Heart, Lung, and Blood Institute, National Institutes of Health, June 1, 2011.

What Is von Willebrand Disease?

Von Willebrand disease (VWD) is a bleeding disorder. It affects your blood's ability to clot. If your blood doesn't clot, you can have heavy, hard-to-stop bleeding after an injury. The bleeding can damage your internal organs. Rarely, the bleeding may even cause death.

In VWD, you either have low levels of a certain protein in your blood or the protein doesn't work well. The protein is called von Willebrand factor, and it helps your blood clot.

Normally, when one of your blood vessels is injured, you start to bleed. Small blood cell fragments called platelets clump together to plug the hole in the blood vessel and stop the bleeding. Von Willebrand factor acts like glue to help the platelets stick together and form a blood clot.

Von Willebrand factor also carries clotting factor VIII (8), another important protein that helps your blood clot. Factor VIII is the protein that's missing or doesn't work well in people who have hemophilia, another bleeding disorder.

VWD is more common and usually milder than hemophilia. In fact, VWD is the most common inherited bleeding disorder. It occurs in about one out of every one hundred to one thousand people. VWD affects both males and females, while hemophilia mainly affects males.

Types of von Willebrand Disease

The three major types of VWD are called type 1, type 2, and type 3.

Type 1: People who have type 1 VWD have low levels of von Willebrand factor and may have low levels of factor VIII. Type 1 is the mildest and most common form of VWD. About three out of four people who have VWD have type 1.

Type 2: In type 2 VWD, the von Willebrand factor doesn't work well. Type 2 is divided into subtypes: 2A, 2B, 2M, and 2N. Different gene mutations (changes) cause each type, and each is treated differently. Thus, it's important to know the exact type of VWD that you have.

Type 3: People who have type 3 VWD usually have no von Willebrand factor and low levels of factor VIII. Type 3 is the most serious form of VWD, but it's very rare.

Overview

Most people who have VWD have type 1, a mild form. This type usually doesn't cause life-threatening bleeding. You may need treatment only if you have surgery, tooth extraction, or trauma. Treatment includes medicines and medical therapies.

Some people who have severe forms of VWD need emergency treatment to stop bleeding before it becomes life threatening.

Early diagnosis is important. With the proper treatment plan, even people who have type 3 VWD can live normal, active lives.

What Causes von Willebrand Disease?

Von Willebrand disease (VWD) is almost always inherited. "Inherited" means that the disorder is passed from parents to children though genes.

You can inherit type 1 or type 2 VWD if only one of your parents passes the gene on to you. You usually inherit type 3 VWD only if both of your parents pass the gene on to you. Your symptoms may be different from your parents' symptoms.

Some people have the genes for the disorder but don't have symptoms. However, they still can pass the genes on to their children.

Some people get VWD later in life as a result of other medical conditions. This type of VWD is called acquired von Willebrand syndrome.

What Are the Signs and Symptoms of von Willebrand Disease?

The signs and symptoms of von Willebrand disease (VWD) depend on which type of the disorder you have. They also depend on how serious the disorder is. Many people have such mild symptoms that they don't know they have VWD.

If you have type 1 or type 2 VWD, you may have the following mild-to-moderate bleeding symptoms:

- Frequent, large bruises from minor bumps or injuries

- Frequent or hard-to-stop nosebleeds

- Prolonged bleeding from the gums after a dental procedure
- Heavy or prolonged menstrual bleeding in women
- Blood in your stools from bleeding in your intestines or stomach
- Blood in your urine from bleeding in your kidneys or bladder
- Heavy bleeding after a cut or other accident
- Heavy bleeding after surgery

People who have type 3 VWD may have all of the symptoms listed above and severe bleeding episodes for no reason. These bleeding episodes can be fatal if not treated right away. People who have type 3 VWD also may have bleeding into soft tissues or joints, causing severe pain and swelling.

Heavy menstrual bleeding often is the main symptom of VWD in women. Doctors call this menorrhagia. They define it as follows:

- Bleeding with clots larger than about one inch in diameter
- Anemia (low red blood cell count) or low blood iron
- The need to change pads or tampons more than every hour

However, just because a woman has heavy menstrual bleeding doesn't mean she has VWD.

How Is von Willebrand Disease Diagnosed?

Early diagnosis of von Willebrand disease (VWD) is important to make sure that you're treated and can live a normal, active life.

Sometimes VWD is hard to diagnose. People who have type 1 or type 2 VWD may not have major bleeding problems. Thus, they may not be diagnosed unless they have heavy bleeding after surgery or some other trauma.

On the other hand, type 3 VWD can cause major bleeding problems during infancy and childhood. So, children who have type 3 VWD usually are diagnosed during their first year of life.

To find out whether you have VWD, your doctor will review your medical history and the results from a physical exam and tests.

Medical History

Your doctor will likely ask questions about your medical history and your family's medical history. He or she may ask about the following things:

- Any bleeding from a small wound that lasted more than fifteen minutes or started up again within the first seven days following the injury.

- Any prolonged, heavy, or repeated bleeding that required medical care after surgery or dental extractions.

- Any bruising with little or no apparent trauma, especially if you could feel a lump under the bruise.

- Any nosebleeds that occurred for no known reason and lasted more than ten minutes despite pressure on the nose, or any nosebleeds that needed medical attention.

- Any blood in your stools for no known reason.

- Any heavy menstrual bleeding (for women). This bleeding usually involves clots or lasts longer than seven to ten days.

- Any history of muscle or joint bleeding.

- Any medicines you've taken that might cause bleeding or increase the risk of bleeding. Examples include aspirin and other nonsteroidal anti-inflammatory drugs (NSAIDs), clopidogrel, warfarin, or heparin.

- Any history of liver or kidney disease, blood or bone marrow disease, or high or low blood platelet counts.

Physical Exam

Your doctor will do a physical exam to look for unusual bruising or other signs of recent bleeding. He or she also will look for signs of liver disease or anemia (a low red blood cell count).

Diagnostic Tests

No single test can diagnose VWD. Your doctor may recommend one or more blood tests to diagnose the disorder. These tests may include the following:

- **Von Willebrand factor antigen:** This test measures the amount of von Willebrand factor in your blood.

- **Von Willebrand factor ristocetin (ris-to-SEE-tin) cofactor activity:** This test shows how well your von Willebrand factor works.

- **Factor VIII clotting activity:** This test checks the clotting activity of factor VIII. Some people who have VWD have low levels of factor VIII activity, while others have normal levels.

- **Von Willebrand factor multimers:** This test is done if one or more of the first three tests are abnormal. It shows the structure of your von Willebrand factor. The test helps your doctor diagnose what type of VWD you have.

- **Platelet function test:** This test measures how well your platelets are working.

You may have these tests more than once to confirm a diagnosis. Your doctor also may refer you to a hematologist to confirm the diagnosis and for follow-up care. A hematologist is a doctor who specializes in diagnosing and treating blood disorders.

How Is von Willebrand Disease Treated?

Treatment for von Willebrand disease (VWD) is based on the type of VWD you have and how severe it is. Most cases of VWD are mild, and you may need treatment only if you have surgery, tooth extraction, or an accident.

Medicines are used to do the following things:

- Increase the amount of von Willebrand factor and factor VIII released into the bloodstream

- Replace von Willebrand factor

- Prevent the breakdown of blood clots

- Control heavy menstrual bleeding in women

Specific Treatments

One treatment for VWD is a man-made hormone called desmopressin. You usually take this hormone by injection or nasal spray. It makes your body release more von Willebrand factor and factor VIII into your bloodstream. Desmopressin works for most people who have type 1 VWD and for some people who have type 2 VWD.

Another type of treatment is von Willebrand factor replacement therapy. This involves an infusion of concentrated von Willebrand factor and factor VIII into a vein in your arm. This treatment may be used if any of the following are true:

- You can't take desmopressin or need extended treatment

- You have type 1 VWD that doesn't respond to desmopressin

- You have type 2 or type 3 VWD

Antifibrinolytic (AN-te-fi-BRIN-o-LIT-ik) medicines also are used to treat VWD. These medicines help prevent the breakdown of blood clots. They're mostly used to stop bleeding after minor surgery, tooth extraction, or an injury. These medicines may be used alone or with desmopressin and replacement therapy.

Fibrin glue is medicine that's placed directly on a wound to stop bleeding.

Treatments for Women

Treatments for women who have VWD with heavy menstrual bleeding include the following:

- **Birth control pills:** The hormones in these pills can increase the amount of von Willebrand factor and factor VIII in your blood. The hormones also can reduce menstrual blood loss. Birth control pills are the most recommended birth control method for women who have VWD.

- **A levonorgestrel intrauterine device:** This is a birth control device that contains the hormone progestin. The device is placed in the uterus (womb).

- **Aminocaproic acid or tranexamic acid:** These antifibrinolytic medicines can reduce bleeding by slowing the breakdown of blood clots.

- **Desmopressin.**

For some women who are done having children or don't want children, endometrial ablation (EN-do-ME-tre-al ab-LA-shun) is done. This procedure destroys the lining of the uterus. It has been shown to reduce menstrual blood loss in women who have VWD.

If you need a hysterectomy (HIS-ter-EK-to-me; surgical removal of the uterus) for another reason, this procedure will stop menstrual bleeding and possibly improve your quality of life. However, hysterectomy has its own risk of bleeding complications.

Living with von Willebrand Disease

If you have von Willebrand disease (VWD), you can take steps to prevent bleeding and stay healthy.

For example, avoid over-the-counter medicines that can affect blood clotting, such as aspirin, ibuprofen, and other nonsteroidal anti-inflammatory drugs (NSAIDs). Always check with your doctor before taking any medicines.

Tell your doctor, dentist, and pharmacist that you have VWD. Your dentist can ask your doctor whether you need medicine before dental work to reduce bleeding.

You also may want to tell other people about your condition, like your employee health nurse, gym trainer, and sports coach. Making them aware will allow them to act quickly if you have an injury.

Consider wearing a medical ID bracelet or necklace if you have a serious form of VWD (for example, type 3). In case of a serious accident or injury, the health care team treating you will know that you have VWD.

Be physically active and maintain a healthy weight. Physical activity helps keep muscles flexible. It also helps prevent damage to muscles and joints. Always stretch before exercising.

Some safe physical activities are swimming, biking, and walking. Football, hockey, wrestling, and lifting heavy weights are not safe activities if you have bleeding problems. Always check with your doctor before starting any exercise program.

Your parents, brothers and sisters, and children also may have VWD. Talk with them about your diagnosis and suggest that they get tested too.

Pregnancy and von Willebrand Disease

Pregnancy can be a challenge for women who have VWD. Blood levels of von Willebrand factor and factor VIII tend to increase during pregnancy. However, women who have VWD can have bleeding problems during delivery. They also are likely to have heavy bleeding for an extended time after delivery.

You can take steps to lower the risk of complications during pregnancy. If possible, talk with a hematologist and an obstetrician who specializes in high-risk pregnancies before you become pregnant.

A hematologist is a doctor who specializes in diagnosing and treating blood disorders. An obstetrician is a doctor who provides treatment and care for pregnant women.

Consider using a medical center that specializes in high-risk obstetrics and has a hematologist on staff for prenatal care and delivery.

Before you have any invasive procedure, such as amniocentesis, discuss with your doctor whether you need to take steps to prevent serious blood loss.

During your third trimester, you should have blood tests to measure von Willebrand factor and factor VIII to help plan for delivery.

You also should meet with an anesthesiologist to review your choices for anesthesia and to discuss taking medicine to reduce your bleeding risk. The term "anesthesia" refers to a loss of feeling and awareness.

Some types of anesthesia temporarily put you to sleep, while others only numb certain areas of your body.

With these steps for safety, most women who have VWD can have successful pregnancies.

Children and von Willebrand Disease

If your child has VWD that's severe enough to cause bleeding, anyone who cares for him or her should be told about the condition.

For example, the school nurse, teacher, daycare provider, coach, or any leader of after school activities should know, especially if your child has severe VWD. This information will help them handle the situation if your child has an injury.

Clinical Trials

Clinical trials test new ways to prevent, diagnose, or treat various diseases and conditions. For example, new treatments for a disease or condition (such as medicines, medical devices, surgeries, or procedures) are tested in volunteers who have the illness. Testing shows whether a treatment is safe and effective in humans before it is made available for widespread use.

By taking part in a clinical trial, you can gain access to new treatments before they're widely available. You also will have the support of a team of health care providers, who will likely monitor your health closely. Even if you don't directly benefit from the results of a clinical trial, the information gathered can help others and add to scientific knowledge.

Chapter 11

Blood Disorders (Hemoglobinopathies)

Chapter Contents

Section 11.1

Fanconi Anemia

"What Is Fanconi Anemia," National Heart, Lung, and Blood Institute,
National Institutes of Health, November 1, 2011.

What Is Fanconi Anemia?

Fanconi anemia (fan-KO-nee uh-NEE-me-uh), or FA, is a rare, inherited blood disorder that leads to bone marrow failure. The disorder
also is called Fanconi's anemia.

FA prevents your bone marrow from making enough new blood cells
for your body to work normally. FA also can cause your bone marrow to
make many faulty blood cells. This can lead to serious health problems,
such as leukemia (a type of blood cancer).

Although FA is a blood disorder, it also can affect many of your
body's organs, tissues, and systems. Children who inherit FA are at
higher risk of being born with birth defects. FA also increases the risk
of some cancers and other serious health problems.

FA is different from Fanconi syndrome. Fanconi syndrome affects
the kidneys. It's a rare and serious condition that mostly affects
children.

Children who have Fanconi syndrome pass large amounts of key
nutrients and chemicals through their urine. These children may have
serious health and developmental problems.

Bone Marrow and Blood

Bone marrow is the spongy tissue inside the large bones of your
body. Healthy bone marrow contains stem cells that develop into the
three types of blood cells that the body needs:

- Red blood cells, which carry oxygen to all parts of your body. Red
  blood cells also remove carbon dioxide (a waste product) from
  your body's cells and carry it to the lungs to be exhaled.

- White blood cells, which help fight infections.

- Platelets (PLATE-lets), which help your blood clot.

It's normal for blood cells to die. The lifespan of red blood cells is about 120 days. White blood cells live less than one day. Platelets live about six days. As a result, your bone marrow must constantly make new blood cells.

If your bone marrow can't make enough new blood cells to replace the ones that die, serious health problems can occur.

Fanconi Anemia and Your Body

FA is one of many types of anemia. The term "anemia" usually refers to a condition in which the blood has a lower than normal number of red blood cells.

FA is a type of aplastic anemia. In aplastic anemia, the bone marrow stops making or doesn't make enough of all three types of blood cells. Low levels of the three types of blood cells can harm many of the body's organs, tissues, and systems.

With too few red blood cells, your body's tissues won't get enough oxygen to work well. With too few white blood cells, your body may have problems fighting infections. This can make you sick more often and make infections worse. With too few platelets, your blood can't clot normally. As a result, you may have bleeding problems.

Outlook

People who have FA have a greater risk than other people for some cancers. About 10 percent of people who have FA develop leukemia.

People who have FA and survive to adulthood are much more likely than others to develop cancerous solid tumors.

The risk of solid tumors increases with age in people who have FA. These tumors can develop in the mouth, tongue, throat, or esophagus. (The esophagus is the passage leading from the mouth to the stomach.)

Women who have FA are at much greater risk than other women of developing tumors in the reproductive organs.

FA is an unpredictable disease. The average lifespan for people who have FA is between twenty and thirty years. The most common causes of death related to FA are bone marrow failure, leukemia, and solid tumors.

Advances in care and treatment have improved the chances of surviving longer with FA. Blood and marrow stem cell transplant is the major advance in treatment. However, even with this treatment, the risk of some cancers is greater in people who have FA.

What Causes Fanconi Anemia?

Fanconi anemia (FA) is an inherited disease. The term "inherited" means that the disease is passed from parents to children through genes. At least thirteen faulty genes are associated with FA. FA occurs when both parents pass the same faulty FA gene to their child.

People who have only one faulty FA gene are FA "carriers." Carriers don't have FA, but they can pass the faulty gene to their children.

If both of your parents have a faulty FA gene, you have the following:

- A 25 percent chance of having FA

- A 25 percent chance of not having FA

- A 50 percent chance of being an FA carrier and passing the gene to any children you have

If only one of your parents has a faulty FA gene, you won't have the disorder. However, you have a 50 percent chance of being an FA carrier and passing the gene to any children you have.

Who Is at Risk for Fanconi Anemia?

Fanconi anemia (FA) occurs in all racial and ethnic groups and affects men and women equally.

In the United States, about 1 out of every 181 people is an FA carrier. This carrier rate leads to about 1 in 130,000 people being born with FA.

Two ethnic groups, Ashkenazi Jews and Afrikaners, are more likely than other groups to have FA or be FA carriers.

Ashkenazi Jews are people who are descended from the Jewish population of Eastern Europe. Afrikaners are white natives of South Africa who speak a language called Afrikaans. This ethnic group is descended from early Dutch, French, and German settlers.

In the United States, 1 out of 90 Ashkenazi Jews is an FA carrier, and 1 out of 30,000 is born with FA.

Major Risk Factors

FA is an inherited disease—that is, it's passed from parents to children through genes. At least thirteen faulty genes are associated with FA. FA occurs if both parents pass the same faulty FA gene to their child.

Children born into families with histories of FA are at risk of inheriting the disorder. Children whose mothers and fathers both have family histories of FA are at even greater risk. A family history of FA means that it's possible that a parent carries a faulty gene associated with the disorder.

Children whose parents both carry the same faulty gene are at greatest risk of inheriting FA. Even if these children aren't born with FA, they're still at risk of being FA carriers.

Children who have only one parent who carries a faulty FA gene also are at risk of being carriers. However, they're not at risk of having FA.

What Are the Signs and Symptoms of Fanconi Anemia?

Major Signs and Symptoms

Your doctor may suspect you or your child has Fanconi anemia (FA) if you have signs and symptoms of the following:

- Anemia

- Bone marrow failure

- Birth defects

- Developmental or eating problems

FA is an inherited disorder—that is, it's passed from parents to children through genes. If a child has FA, his or her brothers and sisters also should be tested for the disorder.

Anemia: The most common symptom of all types of anemia is fatigue (tiredness). Fatigue occurs because your body doesn't have enough red blood cells to carry oxygen to its various parts. If you have anemia, you may not have the energy to do normal activities.

A low red blood cell count also can cause shortness of breath, dizziness, headaches, coldness in your hands and feet, pale skin, and chest pain.

Bone marrow failure: When your bone marrow fails, it can't make enough red blood cells, white blood cells, and platelets. This can cause many problems that have various signs and symptoms.

With too few red blood cells, you can develop anemia. In FA, the size of your red blood cells also can be much larger than normal. This makes it harder for the cells to work well.

With too few white blood cells, you're at risk for infections. Infections also may last longer and be more serious than normal.

With too few platelets, you may bleed and bruise easily, suffer from internal bleeding, or have petechiae (pe-TEE-kee-ay). Petechiae are tiny red or purple spots on the skin. Bleeding in small blood vessels just below your skin causes these spots.

In some people who have FA, the bone marrow makes a lot of harmful, immature white blood cells called blasts. Blasts don't work like normal blood cells. As they build up, they prevent the bone marrow from making enough normal blood cells.

A large number of blasts in the bone marrow can lead to a type of blood cancer called acute myeloid leukemia (AML).

Birth defects: Many birth defects can be signs of FA. These include the following:

- *Bone or skeletal defects:* FA can cause missing, oddly shaped, or three or more thumbs. Arm bones, hips, legs, hands, and toes may not form fully or normally. People who have FA may have a curved spine, a condition called scoliosis (sco-le-O-sis).

- *Eye and ear defects:* The eyes, eyelids, and ears may not have a normal shape. Children who have FA also might be born deaf.

- *Skin discoloration:* This includes coffee-colored areas or odd-looking patches of lighter skin.

- *Kidney problems:* A child who has FA might be born with a missing kidney or kidneys that aren't shaped normally.

- *Congenital heart defects:* The most common congenital heart defect linked to FA is a ventricular septal defect (VSD). A VSD is a hole or defect in the lower part of the wall that separates the heart's left and right chambers.

Developmental problems: Other signs and symptoms of FA are related to physical and mental development. They include the following:

- Low birth weight
- Poor appetite
- Delayed growth
- Below-average height
- Small head size
- Mental retardation or learning disabilities

Signs and Symptoms of Fanconi Anemia in Adults

Some signs and symptoms of FA may develop as you or your child gets older. Women who have FA may have some or all of the following:

- Sex organs that are less developed than normal

- Menstruating later than women who don't have FA
- Starting menopause earlier than women who don't have FA
- Problems getting pregnant and carrying a pregnancy to full term

Men who have FA may have sex organs that are less developed than normal. They also may be less fertile than men who don't have the disease.

How Is Fanconi Anemia Diagnosed?

People who have Fanconi anemia (FA) are born with the disorder. They may or may not show signs or symptoms of it at birth. For this reason, FA isn't always diagnosed when a person is born. In fact, most people who have the disorder are diagnosed between the ages of two and fifteen years.

The tests used to diagnose FA depend on a person's age and symptoms. In all cases, medical and family histories are an important part of diagnosing FA. However, because FA has many of the same signs and symptoms as other diseases, only genetic testing can confirm its diagnosis.

Specialists Involved

A geneticist is a doctor or scientist who studies how genes work and how diseases and traits are passed from parents to children through genes.

Geneticists do genetic testing for FA. They also can provide counseling about how FA is inherited and the types of prenatal (before birth) testing used to diagnose it.

An obstetrician may detect birth defects linked to FA before your child is born. An obstetrician is a doctor who specializes in providing care for pregnant women.

After your child is born, a pediatrician also can help find out whether your child has FA. A pediatrician is a doctor who specializes in treating children and teens.

A hematologist (blood disease specialist) also may help diagnose FA.

Family and Medical Histories

FA is an inherited disease. Some parents are aware that their family has a medical history of FA, even if they don't have the disease.

Other parents, especially if they're FA carriers, may not be aware of a family history of FA. Many parents may not know that FA can be passed from parents to children.

Knowing your family medical history can help your doctor diagnose whether you or your child has FA or another condition with similar symptoms.

If your doctor thinks that you, your siblings, or your children have FA, he or she may ask you detailed questions about the following:

- Any personal or family history of anemia

- Any surgeries you've had related to the digestive system

- Any personal or family history of immune disorders

- Your appetite, eating habits, and any medicines you take

If you know your family has a history of FA, or if your answers to your doctor's questions suggest a possible diagnosis of FA, your doctor will recommend further testing.

Diagnostic Tests and Procedures

The signs and symptoms of FA aren't unique to the disease. They're also linked to many other diseases and conditions, such as aplastic anemia. For this reason, genetic testing is needed to confirm a diagnosis of FA. Genetic tests for FA include the following.

Chromosome breakage test: This is the most common test for FA. It's available only in special laboratories (labs). It shows whether your chromosomes (long chains of genes) break more easily than normal.

Skin cells sometimes are used for the test. Usually, though, a small amount of blood is taken from a vein in your arm, using a needle. A technician combines some of the blood cells with certain chemicals.

If you have FA, the chromosomes in your blood sample break and rearrange when mixed with the test chemicals. This doesn't happen in the cells of people who don't have FA.

Cytometric flow analysis: Cytometric flow analysis, or CFA, is done in a lab. This test examines how chemicals affect your chromosomes as your cells grow and divide. Skin cells are used for this test.

A technician mixes the skin cells with chemicals that can cause the chromosomes in the cells to act abnormally. If you have FA, your cells are much more sensitive to these chemicals.

The chromosomes in your skin cells will break at a high rate during the test. This doesn't happen in the cells of people who don't have FA.

Mutation screening: A mutation is an abnormal change in a gene or genes. Geneticists and other specialists can examine your genes, usually using a sample of your skin cells. With special equipment and lab processes, they can look for gene mutations that are linked to FA.

Diagnosing Different Age Groups

Before birth (prenatal): If your family has a history of FA and you get pregnant, your doctor may want to test you or your fetus for FA.

Two tests can be used to diagnose FA in a developing fetus: amniocentesis and chorionic villus sampling (CVS). Both tests are done in a doctor's office or hospital.

Amniocentesis is done fifteen to eighteen weeks after a pregnant woman's last period. A doctor uses a needle to remove a small amount of fluid from the sac around the fetus. A technician tests chromosomes (chains of genes) from the fluid sample to see whether they have faulty genes associated with FA.

CVS is done ten to twelve weeks after a pregnant woman's last period. A doctor inserts a thin tube through the vagina and cervix to the placenta (the temporary organ that connects the fetus to the mother).

The doctor removes a tissue sample from the placenta using gentle suction. The tissue sample is sent to a lab to be tested for genetic defects associated with FA.

At birth: Three out of four people who inherit FA are born with birth defects. If your baby is born with certain birth defects, your doctor may recommend genetic testing to confirm a diagnosis of FA.

Childhood and later: Some people who have FA are not born with birth defects. Doctors may not diagnose them with the disorder until signs of bone marrow failure or cancer occur. This usually happens within the first ten years of life.

Signs of bone marrow failure most often begin between the ages of three and twelve years, with seven to eight years as the most common ages. However, 10 percent of children who have FA aren't diagnosed until after sixteen years of age.

If your bone marrow is failing, you may have signs of aplastic anemia. FA is one type of aplastic anemia.

In aplastic anemia, your bone marrow stops making or doesn't make enough of all three types of blood cells: red blood cells, white blood cells, and platelets.

Aplastic anemia can be inherited or acquired after birth through exposure to chemicals, radiation, or medicines.

Doctors diagnose aplastic anemia using the following methods:

- Family and medical histories and a physical exam.

- A complete blood count (CBC) to check the number, size, and condition of your red blood cells. The CBC also checks numbers of white blood cells and platelets.

- A reticulocyte (re-TIK-u-lo-site) count. This test counts the number of new red blood cells in your blood to see whether your bone marrow is making red blood cells at the proper rate.

- Bone marrow tests. For a bone marrow aspiration, a small amount of liquid bone marrow is removed and tested to see whether it's making enough blood cells. For a bone marrow biopsy, a small amount of bone marrow tissue is removed and tested to see whether it's making enough blood cells.

If you or your child is diagnosed with aplastic anemia, your doctor will want to find the cause. If your doctor suspects you have FA, he or she may recommend genetic testing.

How Is Fanconi Anemia Treated?

Doctors decide how to treat Fanconi anemia (FA) based on a person's age and how well the person's bone marrow is making new blood cells.

Goals of Treatment

Long-term treatments for FA can do the following things:

- **Cure the anemia:** Damaged bone marrow cells are replaced with healthy ones that can make enough of all three types of blood cells on their own; or

- **Treat the symptoms without curing the cause:** This is done using medicines and other substances that can help your body make more blood cells for a limited time.

Screening and Short-Term Treatment

Even if you or your child has FA, your bone marrow might still be able to make enough new blood cells. If so, your doctor might suggest frequent blood count checks so he or she can watch your condition.

Your doctor will probably want you to have bone marrow tests once a year. He or she also will screen you for any signs of cancer or tumors.

If your blood counts begin to drop sharply and stay low, your bone marrow might be failing. Your doctor may prescribe antibiotics to help your body fight infections. In the short term, he or she also may want to give you blood transfusions to increase your blood cell counts to normal levels.

However, long-term use of blood transfusions can reduce the chance that other treatments will work.

Long-Term Treatment

The four main types of long-term treatment for FA are as follows:

- Blood and marrow stem cell transplant
- Androgen therapy
- Synthetic growth factors
- Gene therapy

Blood and marrow stem cell transplant: A blood and marrow stem cell transplant is the current standard treatment for patients who have FA that's causing major bone marrow failure. Healthy stem cells from another person, called a donor, are used to replace the faulty cells in your bone marrow.

If you're going to receive stem cells from another person, your doctor will want to find a donor whose stem cells match yours as closely as possible.

Stem cell transplants are most successful in younger people who:

- have few or no serious health problems;
- receive stem cells from a brother or sister who is a good donor match;
- have had few or no previous blood transfusions.

During the transplant, you'll get donated stem cells in a procedure that's like a blood transfusion. Once the new stem cells are in your body, they travel to your bone marrow and begin making new blood cells.

A successful stem cell transplant will allow your body to make enough of all three types of blood cells.

Even if you've had a stem cell transplant to treat FA, you're still at risk for some types of blood cancer and cancerous solid tumors. Your doctor will check your health regularly after the procedure.

Androgen therapy: Before improvements made stem cell transplants more effective, androgen therapy was the standard treatment for people who had FA. Androgens are man-made male hormones that can help your body make more blood cells for long periods.

Androgens increase your red blood cell and platelet counts. They don't work as well at raising your white blood cell count.

Unlike a stem cell transplant, androgens don't allow your bone marrow to make enough of all three types of blood cells on its own. You may need ongoing treatment with androgens to control the effects of FA.

Also, over time, androgens lose their ability to help your body make more blood cells, which means you'll need other treatments.

Androgen therapy can have serious side effects, such as liver disease. This treatment also can't prevent you from developing leukemia (a type of blood cancer).

Synthetic growth factors: Your doctor may choose to treat your FA with growth factors. These are substances found in your body, but they also can be man-made.

Growth factors help your body make more red and white blood cells. Growth factors that help your body make more platelets still are being studied.

More research is needed on growth factor treatment for FA. Early results suggest that growth factors may have fewer and less serious side effects than androgens.

Gene therapy: Researchers are looking for ways to replace faulty FA genes with normal, healthy genes. They hope these genes will make proteins that can repair and protect your bone marrow cells. Early results of this therapy hold promise, but more research is needed.

Surgery: FA can cause birth defects that affect the arms, thumbs, hips, legs, and other parts of the body. Doctors may recommend surgery to repair some defects.

For example, your child might be born with a ventricular septal defect—a hole or defect in the wall that separates the lower chambers of the heart. His or her doctor may recommend surgery to close the hole so the heart can work properly.

Children who have FA also may need surgery to correct digestive system problems that can harm their nutrition, growth, and survival.

One of the most common problems is an FA-related birth defect in which the trachea (windpipe), which carries air to the lungs, is connected to the esophagus, which carries food to the stomach.

This can cause serious breathing, swallowing, and eating problems and can lead to lung infections. Surgery is needed to separate the two organs and allow normal eating and breathing.

How Can Fanconi Anemia Be Prevented?

You can't prevent Fanconi anemia (FA) because it's an inherited disease. If a child gets two copies of the same faulty FA gene, he or she will have the disease.

If you're at high risk for FA and are planning to have children, you may want to consider genetic counseling. A counselor can help you understand your risk of having a child who has FA. He or she also can explain the choices that are available to you.

If you're already pregnant, genetic testing can show whether your child has FA.

In the United States, Ashkenazi Jews (Jews of Eastern European descent) are at higher risk for FA than other ethnic groups. For Ashkenazi Jews, it's recommended that prospective parents get tested for FA-related gene mutations before getting pregnant.

Preventing Complications

If you or your child has FA, you can prevent some health problems related to the disorder. Pneumonia, hepatitis, and chicken pox can occur more often and more severely in people who have FA compared with those who don't. Ask your doctor about vaccines for these conditions.

People who have FA also are at higher risk than other people for some cancers. These cancers include leukemia (a type of blood cancer), myelodysplastic syndrome (abnormal levels of all three types of blood cells), and liver cancer. Screening and early detection can help manage these life-threatening diseases.

Living with Fanconi Anemia

Improvements in blood and marrow stem cell transplants have increased the chances of living longer with FA. Also, researchers are studying new and promising treatments for FA. However, the disorder still presents serious challenges to patients and their families.

What to Expect

FA is a life-threatening illness. If you or your child is diagnosed with FA, you and your family members may feel shock, anger, grief, and depression. If you're the parent or grandparent of a child who has FA, you may blame yourself for causing the disease.

Your doctor will want to test all of your children for FA if one of your children is born with the disorder. If you're diagnosed with FA as an adult, your doctor may suggest testing your brothers and sisters for the disorder.

All of these things can create stress and anxiety for your entire family. Family counseling for FA may give you and other relatives important support, comfort, and advice.

One of the hardest issues to deal with is telling children that they have FA and what effect it will have on their lives.

Most FA support groups believe that parents need to give children information about the disorder in terms they can understand. These groups recommend answering questions honestly and directly, stressing the positive developments in treatment and survival.

If your child becomes upset or begins to act out after learning that he or she has FA, you may want to seek counseling.

Special Concerns and Needs

Many people who have FA survive to adulthood. If you have FA, you'll need ongoing medical care. Your blood counts will need to be checked regularly.

Even if you have a blood and marrow stem cell transplant, you remain at risk for many cancers. You'll need to be screened for cancer more often than people who don't have FA.

If FA has left you with a very low platelet count, your doctor may advise you to avoid contact sports and other activities that can lead to injuries.

If your child has FA, he or she may have problems eating or keeping food down. Your doctor may recommend additional, special feedings to support growth and good health.

Support Groups

You or your family members may find it helpful to know about resources that can give you emotional support and helpful information about FA and its treatments.

Your doctor or hospital social worker may have information about counseling and support services. They also may be able to refer you to support groups that offer help with financial planning (treatment for FA can be costly).

Clinical Trials

The National Heart, Lung, and Blood Institute (NHLBI) is strongly committed to supporting research aimed at preventing and treating heart, lung, and blood diseases and conditions and sleep disorders.

Researchers have learned a lot about anemia and other blood diseases and conditions over the years. That knowledge has led to advances in medical knowledge and care.

Many questions remain about blood diseases and conditions, including Fanconi anemia. The NHLBI continues to support research aimed at learning more about these illnesses.

For example, the NHLBI currently is taking part in a research study to examine gene therapy as a treatment for Fanconi anemia.

Much of the NHLBI's research depends on the willingness of volunteers to take part in clinical trials. Clinical trials test new ways to prevent, diagnose, or treat various diseases and conditions.

For example, new treatments for a disease or condition (such as medicines, medical devices, surgeries, or procedures) are tested in volunteers who have the illness. Testing shows whether a treatment is safe and effective in humans before it is made available for widespread use.

By taking part in a clinical trial, you can gain access to new treatments before they're widely available. You also will have the support of a team of health care providers, who will likely monitor your health closely. Even if you don't directly benefit from the results of a clinical trial, the information gathered can help others and add to scientific knowledge.

If you volunteer for a clinical trial, the research will be explained to you in detail. You'll learn about treatments and tests you may receive, and the benefits and risks they may pose. You'll also be given a chance to ask questions about the research. This process is called informed consent.

If you agree to take part in the trial, you'll be asked to sign an informed consent form. This form is not a contract. You have the right to withdraw from a study at any time, for any reason. Also, you have the right to learn about new risks or findings that emerge during the trial.

Section 11.2

Hemochromatosis

Reprinted from "Hemochromatosis," National Institute
of Diabetes and Digestive and Kidney Diseases, National
Institutes of Health, May 10, 2012.

What is hemochromatosis?

Hemochromatosis is the most common form of iron overload disease. Primary hemochromatosis, also called hereditary hemochromatosis, is an inherited disease. Secondary hemochromatosis is caused by anemia, alcoholism, and other disorders.

Juvenile hemochromatosis and neonatal hemochromatosis are two additional forms of the disease. Juvenile hemochromatosis leads to severe iron overload and liver and heart disease in adolescents and young adults between the ages of fifteen and thirty. The neonatal form causes rapid iron buildup in a baby's liver that can lead to death.

Hemochromatosis causes the body to absorb and store too much iron. The extra iron builds up in the body's organs and damages them. Without treatment, the disease can cause the liver, heart, and pancreas to fail.

Iron is an essential nutrient found in many foods. The greatest amount is found in red meat and iron-fortified breads and cereals. In the body, iron becomes part of hemoglobin, a molecule in the blood that transports oxygen from the lungs to all body tissues.

Healthy people usually absorb about 10 percent of the iron contained in the food they eat, which meets normal dietary requirements. People with hemochromatosis absorb up to 30 percent of iron. Over time, they absorb and retain between five and twenty times more iron than the body needs.

Because the body has no natural way to rid itself of the excess iron, it is stored in body tissues, specifically the liver, heart, and pancreas.

What causes hemochromatosis?

Hereditary hemochromatosis is mainly caused by a defect in a gene called HFE, which helps regulate the amount of iron absorbed from food. The two known mutations of HFE are C282Y and H63D. C282Y is the most important. In people who inherit C282Y from both parents, the body absorbs too much iron and hemochromatosis can result. Those who inherit the defective gene from only one parent are carriers for the disease but usually do not develop it; however, they still may have higher than average iron absorption. Neither juvenile hemochromatosis nor neonatal hemochromatosis are caused by an HFE defect. Juvenile and neonatal hemochromatosis are caused by a mutation in a gene called hemojuvelin.

What are the risk factors of hemochromatosis?

Hereditary hemochromatosis is one of the most common genetic disorders in the United States. It most often affects Caucasians of Northern European descent, although other ethnic groups are also affected. About five people out of one thousand—0.5 percent—of the U.S. Caucasian population carry two copies of the hemochromatosis gene and are susceptible to developing the disease. One out of every eight to twelve people is a carrier of one abnormal gene. Hemochromatosis is less common in African Americans, Asian Americans, Hispanics/Latinos, and American Indians.

Although both men and women can inherit the gene defect, men are more likely than women to be diagnosed with hereditary hemochromatosis at a younger age. On average, men develop symptoms and are diagnosed between thirty and fifty years of age. For women, the average age of diagnosis is about fifty.

What are the symptoms of hemochromatosis?

Joint pain is the most common complaint of people with hemochromatosis. Other common symptoms include fatigue, lack of energy, abdominal pain, loss of sex drive, and heart problems. However, many people have no symptoms when they are diagnosed.

If the disease is not detected and treated early, iron may accumulate in body tissues and eventually lead to serious problems such as the following:

- Arthritis

- Liver disease, including an enlarged liver, cirrhosis, cancer, and liver failure

- Damage to the pancreas, possibly causing diabetes

- Heart abnormalities, such as irregular heart rhythms or congestive heart failure

- Impotence
- Early menopause
- Abnormal pigmentation of the skin, making it look gray or bronze
- Thyroid deficiency
- Damage to the adrenal glands

How is hemochromatosis diagnosed?

A thorough medical history, physical examination, and routine blood tests help rule out other conditions that could be causing the symptoms. This information often provides helpful clues, such as a family history of arthritis or unexplained liver disease.

Blood tests can determine whether the amount of iron stored in the body is too high. The transferrin saturation test reveals how much iron is bound to the protein that carries iron in the blood. Transferrin saturation values higher than 45 percent are considered too high.

The total iron binding capacity test measures how well your blood can transport iron, and the serum ferritin test shows the level of iron in the liver. If either of these tests shows higher than normal levels of iron in the body, doctors can order a special blood test to detect the HFE mutation, which will confirm the diagnosis. If the mutation is not present, hereditary hemochromatosis is not the reason for the iron buildup and the doctor will look for other causes.

A liver biopsy may be needed, in which case a tiny piece of liver tissue is removed and examined with a microscope. The biopsy will show how much iron has accumulated in the liver and whether the liver is damaged.

Hemochromatosis is considered rare and doctors may not think to test for it. Thus, the disease is often not diagnosed or treated. The initial symptoms can be diverse, vague, and mimic the symptoms of many other diseases. The doctors also may focus on the conditions caused by hemochromatosis—arthritis, liver disease, heart disease, or diabetes—rather than on the underlying iron overload. However, if the iron overload caused by hemochromatosis is diagnosed and treated before organ damage has occurred, a person can live a normal, healthy life.

Hemochromatosis is usually treated by a specialist in liver disorders called a hepatologist, a specialist in digestive disorders called a gastroenterologist, or a specialist in blood disorders called a hematologist. Because of the other problems associated with hemochromatosis, other specialists may be involved in treatment, such as an endocrinologist, cardiologist, or rheumatologist. Internists or family practitioners can also treat the disease.

How is hemochromatosis treated?

Treatment is simple, inexpensive, and safe. The first step is to rid the body of excess iron. This process is called phlebotomy, which means removing blood the same way it is drawn from donors at blood banks. Based on the severity of the iron overload, a pint of blood will be taken once or twice a week for several months to a year, and occasionally longer. Blood ferritin levels will be tested periodically to monitor iron levels. The goal is to bring blood ferritin levels to the low end of normal and keep them there. Depending on the lab, that means twenty-five to fifty micrograms of ferritin per liter of serum.

Once iron levels return to normal, maintenance therapy begins, which involves giving a pint of blood every two to four months for life. Some people may need phlebotomies more often. An annual blood ferritin test will help determine how often blood should be removed. Regular follow-up with a specialist is also necessary.

If treatment begins before organs are damaged, associated conditions—such as liver disease, heart disease, arthritis, and diabetes—can be prevented. The outlook for people who already have these conditions at diagnosis depends on the degree of organ damage. For example, treating hemochromatosis can stop the progression of liver disease in its early stages, which leads to a normal life expectancy. However, if cirrhosis, or scarring of the liver, has developed, the person's risk of developing liver cancer increases, even if iron stores are reduced to normal levels.

People with complications of hemochromatosis may want to receive treatment from a specialized hemochromatosis center. These centers are located throughout the country.

People with hemochromatosis should not take iron or vitamin C supplements, and those who have liver damage should not consume alcoholic beverages or raw seafood because they may further damage the liver.

Treatment cannot cure the conditions associated with established hemochromatosis, but it will help most of them improve. The main exception is arthritis, which does not improve even after excess iron is removed.

How is hemochromatosis tested?

Screening for hemochromatosis—testing people who have no symptoms—is not a routine part of medical care or checkups. However, researchers and public health officials do have some suggestions.

Siblings of people who have hemochromatosis should have their blood tested to see if they have the disease or are carriers.

Parents, children, and other close relatives of people who have the disease should consider being tested.

Doctors should consider testing people who have joint disease, severe and continuing fatigue, heart disease, elevated liver enzymes, impotence, and diabetes because these conditions may result from hemochromatosis.

Since the genetic defect is common and early detection and treatment are so effective, some researchers and education and advocacy groups have suggested that widespread screening for hemochromatosis would be cost-effective and should be conducted. However, a simple, inexpensive, and accurate test for routine screening does not yet exist and the available options have limitations. For example, the genetic test provides a definitive diagnosis, but it is expensive. The blood test for transferrin saturation is widely available and relatively inexpensive, but it may have to be done twice with careful handling to confirm a diagnosis and show that the result is the consequence of iron overload.

Hope through Research

Scientists hope further study of the HFE gene will reveal how the body normally metabolizes iron. They also want to learn how iron injures cells and contributes to organ damage in other diseases, such as alcoholic liver disease, hepatitis C, porphyria cutanea tarda, heart disease, reproductive disorders, cancer, autoimmune hepatitis, diabetes, and joint disease.

Scientists are working to find out why only some patients with HFE mutations develop the disease. In addition, hemochromatosis research includes the following areas:

- **Genetics:** Researchers are examining how the HFE gene normally regulates iron levels and why not everyone with an abnormal pair of genes develops the disease.

- **Pathogenesis:** Scientists are studying how iron injures body cells. Iron is an essential nutrient, but above a certain level it can damage or even kill cells.

- **Epidemiology:** Research is underway to explain why the amounts of iron people normally store in their bodies differ. Research is also being conducted to determine how many people with the defective HFE gene go on to develop symptoms and why some people develop symptoms and others do not.

- **Screening and testing:** Scientists are working to determine at what age testing is most effective, which groups should be tested, and which are the best tests for widespread screening.

Section 11.3

Sickle Cell Disease

Sickle cell disease is an inherited disorder in which red blood cells (RBCs) are abnormally shaped. This abnormality can result in painful episodes, serious infections, chronic anemia, and damage to body organs.

These complications can, however, vary from person to person depending on the type of sickle cell disease each has. Some people are relatively healthy and others are hospitalized frequently.

But thanks to advancements in early diagnosis and treatment, most kids born with this disorder grow up to live relatively healthy and productive lives.

A Closer Look at Sickle Cell Disease

The different forms of sickle cell disease are determined by the genes inherited from the person's parents.

Someone who inherits a sickle cell gene from each parent has hemoglobin SS disease, also called sickle cell anemia.

A person can also inherit a sickle cell gene from one parent and a different kind of abnormal gene from the other and end up with a different form of sickle cell disease, such as hemoglobin SC disease or hemoglobin S beta thalassemia.

Someone who inherits only one sickle cell gene and a normal gene from the other parent will have the sickle cell trait, but not the disease.

A blood test can determine whether someone has a form of sickle cell disease or carries the sickle cell trait.

People with sickle cell trait don't have sickle cell disease and usually don't exhibit signs of the disorder, but they can pass the gene for the disease to their children. Many people don't know they have sickle cell trait, but most babies in the United States are now tested as part of their newborn screening. When both parents have the sickle cell trait, there's a 25 percent chance that a child will have sickle cell disease. But when one parent is carrying the trait and the other actually has the disease, the odds increase to 50 percent that their child will inherit the disease.

Who Is Affected?

In the United States, hemoglobin SS disease (sickle cell anemia) affects mostly African Americans. However, forms of sickle cell disease may occur in people with different ethnic backgrounds, such as those whose ancestors came from Mediterranean countries (including Turkey, Greece, and Italy), East India, or Middle Eastern countries.

Causes of Sickle Cell Disease

Hemoglobin allows red blood cells to carry oxygen. It is made up of alpha chains and beta chains. A child with sickle cell disease has inherited two defective genes for the beta chain of hemoglobin.

The hemoglobin can take on an abnormal shape, distorting the shape of RBCs. The cells change from a normal round, doughnut shape to the elongated shape of a sickle, or the shape of the letter "C."

Unlike normal RBCs, which move easily through small blood vessels, sickle cells are stiff and pointed. They have a tendency to get stuck in narrow blood vessels and block the flow of blood. This can cause episodes of pain and can also lead to organ damage because the tissues aren't getting enough oxygen.

Sickle cells have a shorter-than-normal life span, which leads to anemia (low RBC count). A normal red blood cell lives for about 120 days in circulation, whereas a sickle cell lives for only 10 to 20 days.

Diagnosis

Sickle cell disease usually is diagnosed at birth with a blood test during routine newborn screening tests. If a child tests positive on the screening test, a second blood test (called a hemoglobin electrophoresis) should be performed to confirm the diagnosis.

Because kids with sickle cell disease are at an increased risk of infection and other health complications, early diagnosis and treatment to prevent problems is important. Currently, more than forty states require newborn screening programs for sickle cell disease.

Signs and Symptoms

Symptoms of sickle cell disease vary, ranging from mild to severe, and may be less severe or different in kids who have inherited a sickle cell gene from one parent and a different abnormal hemoglobin gene from the other.

Most kids with sickle cell disease have some degree of anemia and might develop one or more of the following conditions and symptoms as part of the disorder:

- **Acute chest syndrome:** Inflammation, infection, and occlusion of small vessels may cause this syndrome. Signs include chest pain, coughing, difficulty breathing, and fever.

- **Aplastic crisis:** This is when the bone marrow temporarily slows its production of RBCs due to infection or another cause, resulting in a serious drop in RBCs and severe anemia. Signs include paleness, fatigue, and rapid pulse.

- **Hand-foot syndrome (also called dactylitis):** This painful swelling of the hands and feet may be the first sign of sickle cell anemia in some infants.

- **Infection:** Kids with sickle cell disease are at increased risk for certain bacterial infections. It's important to watch for fevers of 101° F (38° C) or higher, which could signal an infection. Children with sickle cell disease and fever should be seen by a doctor immediately.

- **Painful crises:** These may occur in any part of the body and may be brought on by cold or dehydration. The pain may last a few hours, a few days, or sometimes much longer. Pain may be so severe that a child needs to be hospitalized.

- **Splenic sequestration crises:** The spleen becomes enlarged by trapping (or "sequestering") the abnormal RBCs. This can lead to a serious and rapid drop in the red cell count (severe anemia). Early signs include paleness, weakness or fatigue, an enlarged spleen, and pain in the abdomen.

- **Stroke:** Impaired blood flow in the brain can occur when the sickle-shaped cells block small blood vessels, which may lead to a stroke. Signs can include headache, seizures, weakness of the arms and legs, speech problems, a facial droop, or loss of consciousness.

Other possible complications include leg ulcers, bone or joint damage, gallstones, kidney damage, painful prolonged erections in males (priapism), eye damage, and delayed growth.

Treatment

Bone marrow transplant is the only known cure for sickle cell disease. Transplants are complex and risky procedures and currently are an option only for a carefully selected subset of patients with severe complications.

To be eligible, a child would need bone marrow or stem cells from a "matched" donor with a low risk of rejection. Even then, the procedure has significant risks and there's always the chance of rejection of the transplanted marrow.

But even without a cure, kids with sickle cell disease can lead relatively normal lives. Medicines are available to help manage the pain, and immunizations and daily doses of penicillin (an antibiotic) can help prevent infection.

Infection used to cause many deaths in infants and young children with sickle cell disease, but thanks to penicillin (or a similar antibiotic, amoxicillin) and appropriate immunizations, kids are much more likely to live longer, healthier lives. Although penicillin isn't a cure, it can help prevent life-threatening infections due to bacteria that cause serious infections in the blood, meningitis, and pneumonia.

Most kids will require two daily doses of penicillin, as prescribed by their doctors, until they're at least five years old (and often older). They also should be fully immunized with the regular childhood vaccinations, as well as the pneumococcal vaccine and influenza and meningococcal vaccines. Folic acid supplements can help them continue to produce new RBCs.

Sometimes, kids who develop serious complications (such as recurrent acute chest syndrome, especially severe anemia, or stroke) may receive regular transfusions of red blood cells to prevent or treat these complications.

In 1998 the U.S. Food and Drug Administration (FDA) approved the drug hydroxyurea for use in adults with sickle cell disease; while it still has not been officially approved for use in children, it is now commonly used by pediatric specialists in certain circumstances.

Hydroxyurea increases the amount of fetal hemoglobin in blood cells, which interferes with the sickling process and makes RBCs less sticky. This helps decrease the frequency and intensity of painful episodes and other complications such as acute chest syndrome. Hydroxyurea has been proved to decrease pain and other complications in kids and adults.

When to Call the Doctor

Seek emergency medical attention immediately if your child develops any of the following:

- Fever of 101 °F (38 °C) or higher
- Pain that isn't relieved by oral medication
- Chest pain
- Shortness of breath or trouble breathing
- Extreme fatigue
- Severe headaches or dizziness
- Severe stomach pain or swelling
- Jaundice or extreme paleness
- Painful erection in males
- Sudden change in vision
- Seizures
- Weakness or inability to move any part of the body
- Slurring of speech
- Loss of consciousness
- Numbness or tingling

Caring for Your Child

Your child should receive regular care from your primary care doctor as well as a hematologist (a blood specialist) or a sickle cell specialty clinic. It's important to share your concerns and discuss any new symptoms or complications with your child's health care team.

Your child also should drink lots of fluids, get plenty of rest, and avoid extreme temperatures.

Most people with sickle cell disease now live into middle age and often well beyond. A critical time is the first few years of life, which is why early diagnosis and treatment are so important.

Section 11.4

Thalassemia

Thalassemia is a blood disorder passed down through families (inherited) in which the body makes an abnormal form of hemoglobin, the protein in red blood cells that carries oxygen. The disorder results in excessive destruction of red blood cells, which leads to anemia.

Causes

Hemoglobin is made of two proteins: Alpha globin and beta globin. Thalassemia occurs when there is a defect in a gene that helps control production of one of these proteins.

There are two main types of thalassemia:

- Alpha thalassemia occurs when a gene or genes related to the alpha globin protein are missing or changed (mutated).

- Beta thalassemia occurs when similar gene defects affect production of the beta globin protein.

Alpha thalassemias occur most commonly in persons from southeast Asia, the Middle East, China, and in those of African descent.

Beta thalassemias occur in persons of Mediterranean origin, and to a lesser extent, Chinese, other Asians, and African Americans.

There are many forms of thalassemia. Each type has many different subtypes. Both alpha and beta thalassemia include the following two forms:

- Thalassemia major

- Thalassemia minor

You must inherit the defective gene from both parents to develop thalassemia major.

Thalassemia minor occurs if you receive the defective gene from only one parent. Persons with this form of the disorder are carriers of the disease and usually do not have symptoms.

Beta thalassemia major is also called Cooley anemia.

Risk factors for thalassemia include:

- Asian, Chinese, Mediterranean, or African American ethnicity;
- family history of the disorder.

Symptoms

The most severe form of alpha thalassemia major causes stillbirth (death of the unborn baby during birth or the late stages of pregnancy).

Children born with thalassemia major (Cooley anemia) are normal at birth, but develop severe anemia during the first year of life.

Other symptoms can include:

- bone deformities in the face;
- fatigue;
- growth failure;
- shortness of breath;
- yellow skin (jaundice).

Persons with the minor form of alpha and beta thalassemia have small red blood cells (which are identified by looking at their red blood cells under a microscope), but no symptoms.

Exams and Tests

A physical exam may reveal a swollen (enlarged) spleen.

A blood sample will be taken and sent to a laboratory for examination:

- Red blood cells will appear small and abnormally shaped when looked at under a microscope.
- A complete blood count (CBC) reveals anemia.
- A test called hemoglobin electrophoresis shows the presence of an abnormal form of hemoglobin.

A test called mutational analysis can help detect alpha thalassemia that cannot be seen with hemoglobin electrophoresis.

Treatment

Treatment for thalassemia major often involves regular blood transfusions and folate supplements.

If you receive blood transfusions, you should not take iron supplements. Doing so can cause a high amount of iron to build up in the body, which can be harmful.

Persons who receive significant numbers of blood transfusions need a treatment called chelation therapy to remove excess iron from the body.

A bone marrow transplant may help treat the disease in some patients, especially children.

Outlook (Prognosis)

Severe thalassemia can cause early death due to heart failure, usually between ages twenty and thirty. Getting regular blood transfusions and therapy to remove iron from the body helps improve the outcome.

Less severe forms of thalassemia usually do not shorten lifespan.

Genetic counseling and prenatal screening may help people with a family history of this condition who are planning to have children.

Possible Complications

Untreated, thalassemia major leads to heart failure and liver problems, and makes a person more likely to develop infections.

Blood transfusions can help control some symptoms. However, they may result in too much iron, which can damage the heart, liver, and endocrine system.

When to Contact a Medical Professional

Call for an appointment with your health care provider if:

- you or your child has symptoms of thalassemia;

- you are being treated for the disorder and new symptoms develop.

Alternative Names

Mediterranean anemia; Cooley anemia; Beta thalassemia; Alpha thalassemia

References

Giardina PJ, Forget BG. Thalassemia syndromes. In: Hoffman R, Benz EJ, Shattil SS, et al., eds. *Hematology: Basic Principles and Practice. 5th ed*. Philadelphia, Pa: Elsevier Churchill Livingstone; 2008:chap 41.

DeBaun MR, Frei-Jones M, Vichinsky E. Hemoglobinopathies. In: Kliegman RM, Behrman RE, Jenson HB, Stanton BF, eds. *Nelson Textbook of Pediatrics. 19th ed*. Philadelphia, Pa: Saunders Elsevier; 2011:chap 456.

Chapter 12

CHARGE Syndrome

What is CHARGE syndrome?

CHARGE syndrome is a disorder that affects many areas of the body. CHARGE stands for coloboma, heart defect, atresia choanae (also known as choanal atresia), retarded growth and development, genital abnormality, and ear abnormality. The pattern of malformations varies among individuals with this disorder, and infants often have multiple life-threatening medical conditions. The diagnosis of CHARGE syndrome is based on a combination of major and minor characteristics.

The major characteristics of CHARGE syndrome are more specific to this disorder than are the minor characteristics. Many individuals with CHARGE syndrome have a hole in one of the structures of the eye (coloboma), which forms during early development. A coloboma may be present in one or both eyes and can affect a person's vision, depending on its size and location. Some people also have small eyes (microphthalmia). One or both nasal passages may be narrowed (choanal stenosis) or completely blocked (choanal atresia). Individuals with CHARGE syndrome frequently have cranial nerve abnormalities. The cranial nerves emerge directly from the brain and extend to various areas of the head and neck, controlling muscle movement and transmitting sensory information. Abnormal function of certain cranial nerves can cause swallowing problems, facial paralysis, a sense of smell that is

Excerpted from "CHARGE Syndrome," Genetics Home Reference (http://ghr .nlm.nih.gov), May 2008. Reviewed by David A. Cooke, M.D., FACP, April 2013.

diminished (hyposmia) or completely absent (anosmia), and mild to profound hearing loss. People with CHARGE syndrome also typically have middle and inner ear abnormalities and unusually shaped ears.

The minor characteristics of CHARGE syndrome are not specific to this disorder; they are frequently present in people without CHARGE syndrome. The minor characteristics include heart defects, slow growth starting in late infancy, developmental delay, and an opening in the lip (cleft lip) with or without an opening in the roof of the mouth (cleft palate). Individuals frequently have hypogonadotropic hypogonadism, which affects the production of hormones that direct sexual development. Males are often born with an unusually small penis (micropenis) and undescended testes (cryptorchidism). External genitalia abnormalities are seen less often in females with CHARGE syndrome. Puberty can be incomplete or delayed. Individuals may have a tracheoesophageal fistula, which is an abnormal connection (fistula) between the esophagus and the trachea. People with CHARGE syndrome also have distinctive facial features, including a square-shaped face and difference in the appearance between the right and left sides of the face (facial asymmetry). Individuals have a wide range of cognitive function, from normal intelligence to major learning disabilities with absent speech and poor communication.

How common is CHARGE syndrome?

CHARGE syndrome occurs in approximately 1 in 8,500 to 10,000 individuals.

What genes are related to CHARGE syndrome?

Mutations in the CHD7 gene cause more than half of all cases of CHARGE syndrome. The CHD7 gene provides instructions for making a protein that most likely regulates gene activity (expression) by a process known as chromatin remodeling. Chromatin is the complex of deoxyribonucleic acid (DNA) and protein that packages DNA into chromosomes. The structure of chromatin can be changed (remodeled) to alter how tightly DNA is packaged. Chromatin remodeling is one way gene expression is regulated during development. When DNA is tightly packed, gene expression is lower than when DNA is loosely packed.

Most mutations in the CHD7 gene lead to the production of an abnormally short, nonfunctional CHD7 protein, which presumably disrupts chromatin remodeling and the regulation of gene expression. Changes in gene expression during embryonic development likely cause the signs and symptoms of CHARGE syndrome.

About one-third of individuals with CHARGE syndrome do not have an identified mutation in the CHD7 gene. Researchers suspect that other genetic and environmental factors may be involved in these individuals.

How do people inherit CHARGE syndrome?

CHARGE syndrome is inherited in an autosomal dominant pattern, which means one copy of the altered gene in each cell is sufficient to cause the disorder. Most cases result from new mutations in the CHD7 gene and occur in people with no history of the disorder in their family. In rare cases, an affected person inherits the mutation from an affected parent.

Chapter 13

Connective Tissue Disorders

Chapter Contents

Section 13.1

What Are Heritable Disorders of Connective Tissue?

Excerpted from "Questions and Answers about Heritable Disorders of Connective Tissue," National Institute of Arthritis and Musculoskeletal and Skin Diseases, National Institutes of Health, NIH Publication No. 12-7843, October 2011.

Heritable (genetic) disorders of connective tissue (HDCTs) are a family of more than two hundred disorders that affect connective tissues. These disorders result from alterations (mutations) in genes, and thus are called "heritable." All of these diseases are directly related to mutations in genes that are responsible for building tissues. Alterations in these genes may change the structure and development of skin, bones, joints, the heart, blood vessels, lungs, eyes, and ears. Some mutations also change how these tissues work.

Some other connective tissue problems are not directly linked to mutations in tissue-building genes, although some people may be genetically predisposed to becoming affected. Many, but not all, of the disorders discussed in this section are rare.

What is connective tissue and what does heritable disorders mean?

Connective tissue is the material between the cells of the body that gives tissues form and strength. This "cellular glue" is also involved in delivering nutrients to the tissue, and in the special functioning of certain tissues. Connective tissue is made up of dozens of proteins, including collagens, proteoglycans, and glycoproteins. The combination of these proteins can vary between tissues.

The genes that encode these proteins can harbor defects or mutations, which can affect the functioning of certain properties of connective tissue in selected tissues. When this occurs, the result can be a heritable disorder—one that can be inherited, or passed from parent to child—of connective tissue.

How do people get gene alterations?

People with heritable disorders of connective tissue inherit an altered gene either from one or from both parents. We have two copies of most genes: one inherited from each parent. Males have one copy of each gene on the X chromosome, because they have only one X chromosome, and one copy of each gene on the Y chromosome. In contrast, females have two copies of X chromosome genes because they have two X chromosomes.

Some genetic disorders require that only a single copy of a gene be altered. These disorders can be seen in many generations of a family because the altered copy of the gene is passed from parent to child (dominant inheritance). The same disorder can occur in a person without a family history of the condition if there is a new mutation in the right gene at conception. Some disorders are seen only when the person has received an altered copy of the gene from each parent (recessive inheritance); in these families, the person with only a single copy is called a "carrier" and is not actually affected.

If a mutation occurs on an X chromosome, it generally produces a condition in which the pattern of affected individuals in a family is unusual. Often, women are carriers (that is, they have only a single altered copy of the gene), but males show the condition because they do not have a second protective copy of the gene. Such a condition is referred to as "X-linked."

Who gets HDCTs?

By one estimate, more than a half million people in the United States are affected by the more than two hundred HDCTs. Generally, these conditions affect people of all ethnic groups. All ages and both sexes are affected. Many of these disorders are rare. Some may not be evident at birth, but only appear after a certain age or after exposure to a particular environmental stress.

Does anything increase the chances of having a genetic disease?

Several factors increase the likelihood that a person will inherit an alteration in a gene. If you are concerned about your risk—or the risk to your children or future children—you should talk to your health care provider or a genetic counselor.

The following factors may increase the chance of getting or passing on a genetic disease:

133

- Parents who have a genetic disease
- A family history of a genetic disease
- Parents who are closely related or part of a distinct ethnic or geographic community
- Parents who do not show disease symptoms, but "carry" a disease gene in their genetic makeup (this can be discovered through genetic testing).

How does genetic counseling help?

People seek genetic counseling to make better decisions about their lives and families. Because genetic counselors understand how genetic disorders are passed on through families, they can help couples estimate the risks of having children with genetic diseases. They can also tell parents about tests to determine if they are carrying certain altered genes, tests for newborns who may have inherited certain altered genes, and tests that can be done in early pregnancy to determine if a fetus either carries an altered copy of a gene or is affected with a disorder. The information derived from all these studies can facilitate family planning.

Your health care team can help you find genetic counseling if you wish to better understand your or your child's disease or risk of disease.

What are the symptoms of a HDCT?

The symptoms are different for different disorders. Some of them cause bone growth problems. People with bone growth disorders may have brittle bones or bones that are too long or too short. Some cause people to be unusually tall (Marfan syndrome) or short (chondrodysplasias, osteogenesis imperfecta), or to have head and facial structure malformations (Apert syndrome, Pfeiffer syndrome). In others, joints may be stiff or immobile (fibrodysplasia ossificans progressiva, or FOP).

Some disorders affect the skin. For example, Ehlers-Danlos syndrome results in stretchy or loose skin, while in another connective tissue disorder, cutis laxa, deficient elastic fibers cause the skin to hang in folds. Epidermolysis bullosa results in blistered skin.

Other tissues can be affected as well. Pseudoxanthoma elasticum causes skin, eye, and heart problems, and closed-off or blocked blood vessels. Marfan syndrome and some forms of Ehlers-Danlos syndrome lead to weak blood vessels.

It is critical for people with these disorders and their family members to work closely with their health care teams to get a proper diagnosis and the best treatment. Symptoms of HDCTs are extremely variable, and some disorders can pose severe health risks even when affected individuals have no symptoms.

How do doctors diagnose HDCTs?

Diagnosis always rests first on a combination of family history, medical history, and physical examination. Because many of these conditions are uncommon, the family physician may suspect a diagnosis but be uncertain about how to confirm it. At this point, referral to experienced clinicians, often medical geneticists, can be extremely valuable to either confirm or exclude the suspected diagnosis. Laboratory tests are available to confirm the diagnosis for many HDCTs, but not for all. Once a diagnosis is made, laboratory studies may be available to provide some or all of the following:

- Prenatal testing to identify an affected fetus and assist in family planning.

- Newborn screening to spot a condition that may become evident later in life.

- Carrier testing to identify adults who, without symptoms, carry a genetic mutation for a disease.

- Predictive testing to spot people at risk for developing a genetic connective tissue disease later in life. These tests are helpful for diseases that run in the family.

What treatments are available?

The term "heritable disorders of connective tissue" refers to a wide range of disorders, each requiring a specific program for management and treatment. In most instances, regular monitoring is important to assess, for example, the diameter of the aorta in people with Marfan syndrome, the extent of scoliosis (spine curvature) in people with osteogenesis imperfecta (OI) and those with some forms of Ehlers-Danlos syndrome (EDS), and whether there is protrusion of the spine into the base of the skull in people with OI. For some conditions, specific metabolic treatment is useful, for example, vitamin B6 in people with homocystinuria, a metabolic disorder resulting from a liver enzyme deficiency. In others, drugs like beta blockers are useful for slowing the dilation of the aorta, and bone-building drugs called bisphosphonates may help strengthen fragile bones. Maintaining general health though a nutritious diet, exercise, and healthy lifestyle habits is also important for people with all HDCTs.

What research is being done on HDCTs?

Scientists are working to better understand these disorders at several levels: (1) to identify the genes in which the mutations reside, (2) to identify the mutations that result in the clinical condition, (3) to understand how these mutations result in the condition, and (4) to use all available information about the condition to plan new therapies and test their use and value, both in animal models and in affected individuals. Because most of these conditions are uncommon, and individuals with them are widely scattered, it is often difficult to gather information about the clinical course of the disorder and assemble enough people to plan effective clinical trials.

The National Institute of Arthritis and Musculoskeletal and Skin Diseases (NIAMS), a part of the Department of Health and Human Services' National Institutes of Health (NIH), is the lead federal agency for connective tissue research. Several other NIH institutes are also studying HDCTs. NIAMS supports research through grants to scientists around the country, in national and international clinical trials, and at the NIH campus. This is some of the research underway:

- NIAMS is conducting an in-depth natural history study of people who have Marfan syndrome (which leads to abnormally long bones), nail-patella syndrome (a congenital skeletal disorder), Stickler syndrome (which causes eye and joint problems), and Ehlers-Danlos syndrome (which causes skin and blood vessel problems). All of these disorders have multiple, interrelated symptoms. NIAMS scientists are closely observing the people in this study over a long period to get a more complete picture of the diseases. They hope to improve their understanding of the genetic origins of the symptoms, of disease progression, and of mutations in patients and their relatives. Scientists expect their findings to apply to other HDCTs as well. Specific areas of research and findings arising from this long-term study include the following:

  - Examining the efficacy of screening for dural ectasia (an enlargement of the membrane that surrounds the spinal cord) in the diagnosis of Marfan syndrome

  - Analyzing the prevalence of spinal and hip abnormalities in Stickler syndrome and their relationship to chronic pain

  - Documenting an increased risk of failure of the femoral head (the ball portion at the top of the thigh bone) in children with Stickler syndrome

- Developing proposed diagnostic criteria for Stickler syndrome based on clinical and molecular studies in this population

- Identifying a connective tissue disorder with features resembling Marfan syndrome, Stickler syndrome, and Ehlers-Danlos syndrome

- Studying the mechanism of chronic musculoskeletal pain in people with HDCTs and exploring ways, including mindfulness-based stress reduction, to ameliorate it

- Looking at some specific musculoskeletal complications of aging in patients with HDCTs, such as the prevalence and severity of osteoporosis and osteoarthritis

- Using molecular genetic studies to identify both new genes contributing to Stickler syndrome and Ehlers-Danlos syndrome, and mutations in previously recognized genes

- NIAMS-supported researchers have succeeded in healing wounds in a mouse model of a particularly severe form of epidermolysis bullosa called recessive dystrophic epidermolysis bullosa (RDEB) by injecting the mice with RDEB patient cells in which the gene defect has been corrected. This approach may be useful in developing therapies for the disease. Other NIAMS-supported research shows it may be possible to grow healthy new skin in the lab for people with RDEB by using skin cells from patients that were modified to express a normal gene for type VII collagen. Having successfully transplanted the modified skin on mice, scientists can now try to grow larger sheets of skin and graft them back onto people affected by RDEB.

- NIAMS is examining gene defects that lead to abnormal elastin, the connective tissue protein that allows arteries, muscles, and other organs to respond in certain ways to movement. So far, the investigators have shown how elastin gene mutations cause two specific diseases: a skin disease (cutis laxa) and a blood vessel disease (supravalvular aortic stenosis). Scientists hope to learn more about how mutations affect elastin fiber and tissue growth. They also hope to find out how gene defects lead to the development of elastin disease.

- NIAMS is supporting research looking for ways to treat diseases such as osteogenesis imperfecta by using gene therapy. Stem cells, which have the potential to develop into more specialized cells, would replace bone cells that have gene defects. This research is being conducted on specially bred mice. Other research on osteogenesis imperfecta treatment focuses on the use of growth hormone therapy to promote height increases and bone density. In some cases, growth hormone therapy is being used in combination with medications known as bisphosphonates.

- NIAMS is encouraging the establishment of new research registries for connective tissue disorders and other conditions. Through these registries, demographic and medical data from patients and families could be collected and used in research on disorders. Epidermolysis bullosa is one of the disorders for which the Institute has already established a research registry.

- Other NIAMS-supported research is focused on the following:

  - The chemistry and biology of elastin genes

  - Collagen gene defects (several types) that cause bone diseases

  - Collagen IV gene defects in mice and humans (Alport syndrome)

  - Proteoglycans, a group of proteins that maintain tissue stiffness

  - Fibroblasts, cells that form the fibrous tissues in the body

  - Cartilage, joints, and skin layers

- Ongoing studies of aneurysms (weak spots in blood vessel walls that threaten to burst) are taking place at several NIH institutes. Aneurysms can prove deadly to people with Marfan syndrome and other HDCTs. NIAMS has supported these studies by pioneering development of a breed of mice prone to aneurysms. Scientists hope the mutant mice will improve understanding of aneurysms and ways to prevent them.

- The National Institutes of Health supports the annual Gordon Research Conference on Elastin and Elastic Fibers, which brings together basic scientists and clinicians to exchange data on the makeup of and problems associated with these critical components of connective tissue.

- Studies have shown that the blood pressure medication losartan prevents aortic aneurysms in a mouse model of Marfan syndrome, and one small study of eighteen patients with Marfan syndrome showed that losartan slowed the enlargement of the aorta. A large multicenter trial receiving funding from the National Heart, Lung, and Blood Institute is now under way to further evaluate the use of losartan in people with Marfan syndrome.

- At the Eunice Kennedy Shriver National Institute of Child Health and Human Development, scientists are working with young patients who have osteogenesis imperfecta. They hope to learn more about the genetics of the disease and the natural history of the many secondary features involved, as well as rehabilitation techniques.

- Clinical trials organized by the National Eye Institute are comparing different antiangiogenic compounds (drugs that inhibit blood vessel formation) for pseudoxanthoma elasticum (PXE). New antiangiogenic agents are also in development.

- Scientists at the National Institute of Dental and Craniofacial Research are carrying out clinical studies on fibrous dysplasia of bone.

Section 13.2

Beals Syndrome (Congenital Contractural Arachnodactyly)

Beals syndrome is similar to Marfan syndrome in many ways, but has distinct differences that should be noted. It is also caused by a mutation on the FBN2 gene rather than FBN1.

What is Beals syndrome?

Beals syndrome, or congenital contractural arachnodactyly (CCA), is a genetic condition caused by an alteration (mutation) in a gene (FBN2) that is closely related to the gene (FBN1) that causes Marfan syndrome. It is similar but distinct from Marfan syndrome.

Beals syndrome can cause contractures of the joints (an inability to fully extend a joint) and abnormally shaped ears. People with Beals syndrome have many of the skeletal problems and aortic enlargement that affect people with Marfan syndrome, and the treatment of these problems is the same. The eyes are not affected.

What are the symptoms of Beals syndrome?

Following are features commonly associated with Beals syndrome:

- Inability to fully extend multiple joints such as fingers, elbows, knees, toes, and hips (contractures)

- Delay in motor development often occurs (due to congenital contractures)

- Crumpled appearance to the top of the ear

- Long, slender fingers and toes (arachnodactyly)

- Curvature of the spine (scoliosis)

- Backward and lateral curvature of the spine at birth or early childhood (kyphoscoliosis)

- Reduced bone mass (osteopenia)

- Long, narrow body type (dolichostenomelia)

- Chest abnormalities—concave chest (pectus excavatum) or pigeon chest (pectus carinatum)

- Underdevelopment of muscles—particularly calves (muscular hypoplasia)

- Facial abnormalities, such as unusually small jaws (micrognathia) and highly arched palate

- Occasionally aortic enlargement and/or mitral valve regurgitation

What is the treatment for Beals syndrome?

People with Beals Syndrome benefit from physical therapy that can improve mobility of joints. Sometimes braces are used to provide stability.

People with Beals syndrome should have their heart monitored on a yearly basis to check for cardiovascular complications that may arise.

Section 13.3

Ehlers-Danlos Syndrome

© 2013 A.D.A.M., Inc. Reprinted with permission.

Ehlers-Danlos syndrome (EDS) is a group of inherited disorders marked by extremely loose joints, hyperelastic skin that bruises easily, and easily damaged blood vessels.

Causes

There are six major types and at least five minor types of Ehlers-Danlos syndrome.

A variety of gene mutations (changes) cause problems with collagen. This is the material that provides strength and structure to skin, bone, blood vessels, and internal organs.

The abnormal collagen leads to the symptoms associated with EDS. In some forms of the condition this can include rupture of internal organs or abnormal heart valves.

Family history is a risk factor in some cases.

Symptoms

Symptoms of EDS include:

- back pain;
- double-jointedness;
- easily damaged, bruised, and stretchy skin;
- easy scarring and poor wound healing;
- flat feet;
- increased joint mobility, joints popping, early arthritis;
- joint dislocation;
- joint pain;
- premature rupture of membranes during pregnancy;

- very soft and velvety skin;
- vision problems.

Exams and Tests

Examination by the health care provider may show:

- deformed surface of the eye (cornea);
- excess joint laxity and joint hypermobility;
- mitral valve prolapse;
- periodontitis;
- rupture of intestines, uterus, or eyeball (seen only in vascular EDS, which is rare);
- soft, thin, or very stretchy (hyperextensible) skin.

Tests performed to diagnose EDS include:

- collagen typing (performed on a skin biopsy sample);
- collagen gene mutation testing;
- echocardiogram (heart ultrasound);
- lysyl hydroxylase or oxidase activity.

Treatment

There is no specific cure for Ehlers-Danlos syndrome. Individual problems and symptoms are evaluated and cared for appropriately. Physical therapy or evaluation by a doctor specializing in rehabilitation medicine is often needed.

Outlook (Prognosis)

People with EDS generally have a normal life span. Intelligence is normal.

Those with the rare vascular type of EDS are at greater risk of rupture of a major organ or blood vessel. These individuals, therefore, have a high risk of sudden death.

Possible Complications

Possible complications of Ehlers-Danlos syndrome include:

- chronic joint pain;

- early-onset arthritis;

- failure of surgical wounds to close (or stitches tear out);

- premature rupture of membranes during pregnancy;

- rupture of major vessels, including a ruptured aortic aneurysm (only in vascular EDS);

- rupture of a hollow organ such as the uterus or bowel (only in vascular EDS);

- rupture of the eyeball.

When to Contact a Medical Professional

Call for an appointment with your health care provider if you have a family history of Ehlers-Danlos syndrome and you are concerned about your risk or are planning to start a family.

Call for an appointment with your health care provider if you or your child have symptoms of EDS.

Prevention

Genetic counseling is recommended for prospective parents with a family history of Ehlers-Danlos syndrome. Those planning to start a family should be aware of the type of EDS they have and its mode of inheritance (how it is passed down to children). This can be determined through testing and evaluation suggested by your health care provider or genetic counselor.

Identifying any significant health risks may help prevent severe complications by vigilant screening and lifestyle alterations.

References

Krakow D. Heritable diseases of connective tissue. In: Firestein GS, Budd RC, Gabriel SE, et al, eds. *Kelley's Textbook of Rheumatology. 9th ed*. Philadelphia, PA: Elsevier Saunders; 2012:chap 105.

Pyeritz RE. Inherited diseases of connective tissue. In: Goldman L, Schafer AI, eds. *Goldman's Cecil Medicine. 24th ed*. Philadelphia, PA: Elsevier Saunders; 2011:chap 268.

Section 13.4

Marfan Syndrome

"Learning about Marfan Syndrome," National Human Genome Research Institute (www.genome.gov), National Institutes of Health, May 14, 2012.

What is Marfan syndrome?

Marfan syndrome is one of the most common inherited disorders of connective tissue. It is an autosomal dominant condition occurring once in every ten thousand to twenty thousand individuals. There is a wide variability in clinical symptoms in Marfan syndrome, with the most notable occurring in eye, skeleton, connective tissue, and cardio-vascular systems.

Marfan syndrome is caused by mutations in the FBN1 gene. FBN1 mutations are associated with a broad continuum of physical features ranging from isolated features of Marfan syndrome to a severe and rapidly progressive form in newborns.

What are the symptoms of Marfan syndrome?

The most common symptom of Marfan syndrome is myopia (near-sightedness from the increased curve of the retina due to connective tissue changes in the globe of the eye). About 60 percent of individuals who have Marfan syndrome have lens displacement from the center of the pupil (ectopia lentis). Individuals who have Marfan syndrome also have an increased risk for retinal detachment, glaucoma, and early cataract formation.

Other common symptoms of Marfan syndrome involve the skeleton and connective tissue systems. These include bone overgrowth and loose joints (joint laxity). Individuals who have Marfan syndrome have long thin arms and legs (dolichostenomelia). Overgrowth of the ribs can cause the chest bone (sternum) to bend inward (pectus excavatum or funnel chest) or push outward (pectus carinatum or pigeon breast). Curvature of the spine (scoliosis) is another common skeletal symptom that can be mild or severe and progressively worsen with age. Scoliosis shortens the trunk and also contributes to the arms and legs appearing too long.

Cardiovascular malformations are the most life-threatening symptom of Marfan syndrome. They include dilated aorta just as it leaves the heart (at the level of the sinuses of Valsalva), mitral valve prolapse, tricuspid valve prolapse, enlargement of the proximal pulmonary artery, and a high risk for aortic tear and rupture(aortic dissection).

How is Marfan syndrome diagnosed?

The diagnosis of Marfan syndrome is a clinical diagnosis that is based on family history and the presence of characteristic clinical findings in the ocular, skeletal, and cardiovascular systems. There are four major clinical diagnostic features:

1. Dilatation or dissection of the aorta at the level of the sinuses of Valsalva

2. Ectopia lentis (dislocated lens of the eye)

3. Lumbosacral dural ectasia determined by computed tomography (CT) scan or magnetic resonance imaging (MRI)

4. Four of the eight typical skeletal features

Major criteria for establishing the diagnosis in a family member also include having a parent, child, or sibling who meets major criteria independently, the presence of an FBN-1 mutation known to cause the syndrome, or a haplotype around FBN-1 inherited by descent and identified in a familial Marfan patient (also known as genetic linkage to the gene).

The FBN1 gene is the gene associated with the true Marfan syndrome. Genetic testing of the FBN1 gene identifies 70 to 93 percent of the mutations and is available in clinical laboratories. However patients negative for the test for gene mutation should be considered for evaluation for other conditions that have similar features of Marfan syndrome, such as Dietz syndrome, Ehlers-Danlos syndrome, and homocystinuria. To unequivocally establish the diagnosis in the absence of a family history requires a major manifestation from two systems and involvement of a third system. If a mutation known to cause Marfan syndrome is identified, the diagnosis requires one major criterion and involvement of a second organ system.

To establish the diagnosis in a relative of a patient known to have Marfan syndrome (index case) requires the presence of a major criterion in the family history and one major criterion in an organ system with involvement of a second organ system.

What is the treatment for Marfan syndrome?

Individuals who have Marfan syndrome are treated by a multidisciplinary medical team that includes a geneticist, cardiologist, ophthalmologist, orthopedist, and cardiothoracic surgeon.

Eye problems are generally treated with eyeglasses. When lens dislocation interferes with vision or causes glaucoma, surgery can be performed and an artificial lens implanted.

Skeletal problems such as scoliosis and pectus excavatum may require surgery. For those individuals who have pes planus (flat feet), arch supports and orthotics can be used to decrease leg fatigue and muscle cramps.

Medication, such as beta blockers, is used to decrease the stress on the aorta at the time of diagnosis or when there is progressive aortic dilatation. Surgery to repair the aorta is done when the aortic diameter is greater than 5 mm in adults and older children, when the aortic diameter increases by 1.0 mm per year, or when there is progressive aortic regurgitation.

Cardiovascular surveillance includes yearly echocardiograms to monitor the status of the aorta. Currently the use of beta blocker medications has delayed but not prevented the need to eventually perform aortic surgery.

Recent work on angiotensin II receptor blockers, another blood pressure medication like beta blockers, has shown additional promise to protect the aorta from dilatation. Clinical trials will be starting soon to see if this drug can prevent the need for surgery better than beta blockers have.

Individuals who have Marfan syndrome are advised to avoid contact and competitive sports and isometric exercise like weight lifting and other static forms of exercise. They can participate in aerobic exercises like swimming. They are also advised to avoid medications such as decongestants and foods that contain caffeine, which can lead to chronic increases in blood pressure and stretch the connective tissue in the cardiovascular system.

Is Marfan syndrome inherited?

Marfan syndrome is inherited in families in an autosomal dominant manner. Approximately 75 percent of individuals who have Marfan syndrome have a parent who also has the condition (inherited). Approximately 25 percent of individuals who have Marfan syndrome, have the condition as a result of a new (de novo) mutation. When a parent has Marfan syndrome, each of his or her children has a 50 percent chance (one chance in two) to inherit the FBN1 gene. While Marfan syndrome is not always inherited, it is always heritable.

When a child with Marfan syndrome is born to parents who do not show features of the Marfan syndrome, it is likely the child has a new mutation. In this family situation, the chance for future siblings (brothers and sisters of the child with Marfan syndrome) to be born with Marfan syndrome is less than 50 percent. But the risk is still greater than the general population risk of one in ten thousand. The risk is higher for siblings because there are rare families where a Marfan gene mutation is in some percentage of the germline cells of one of the parents (testes or ovaries).

Prenatal testing for Marfan syndrome is available when the gene mutation is known, and also using a technique called linkage analysis (tracking the gene for Marfan syndrome in a family using genetic markers).

Section 13.5

Osteogenesis Imperfecta

Excerpted from "What Is Osteogenesis Imperfecta?" National Institute of Arthritis and Musculoskeletal and Skin Diseases, National Institutes of Health, May 2009.

Osteogenesis imperfecta (OI) is a disease that causes weak bones that break easily. It is known as brittle bone disease. Sometimes the bones break for no known reason. OI can also cause many other problems such as weak muscles, brittle teeth, and hearing loss. About twenty thousand to fifty thousand people in the United States have OI.

What causes osteogenesis imperfecta?

Osteogenesis imperfecta is caused by one of several genes that aren't working properly. Genes carry our hereditary (family) information. We each have two copies of most genes: one set from each parent. Genes are what make you look like your biological family.

Each of the genes that cause OI plays a role in how the body makes collagen. Collagen is a material in bones that helps make them strong. When these genes aren't working properly, there isn't enough collagen, or the collagen doesn't work properly. This leads to weak bones that break easily.

Most children inherit the gene that doesn't work properly from one parent. Some inherit it from both parents. In some cases, neither parent passes on this gene. Instead, the gene stops working properly soon after the child is conceived.

What are the symptoms of osteogenesis imperfecta?

All people with osteogenesis imperfecta have brittle bones. OI can range from mild to severe, and symptoms vary from person to person. Some of the symptoms that people with OI may have are as follows:

- Malformed bones
- Short, small body
- Loose joints
- Muscle weakness
- Sclera (whites of the eyes) that look blue, purple, or gray
- Triangular face
- Barrel-shaped rib cage
- Curved spine
- Brittle teeth
- Hearing loss (often starting in twenties or thirties)
- Breathing problems
- Type 1 collagen that does not work well
- Not enough collagen

What are some types of osteogenesis imperfecta?

There are eight main types of osteogenesis imperfecta. People with types 2, 3, 7, and 8 tend to have severe symptoms. People with types 4, 5, and 6 tend to have more moderate symptoms. People with type 1 tend to have mild symptoms. There used to be only four types of OI, but then scientists found that even when symptoms look similar in a group of patients, they can be caused by problems in different genes. This is why there are now eight main types of OI instead of four.

How is osteogenesis imperfecta diagnosed?

No single test can identify osteogenesis imperfecta. To diagnose OI, doctors look at the following:

- Family history
- Medical history
- Results from a physical exam
- X-rays

Your doctor may also test your collagen (from skin) or genes (from blood). It may take a few weeks to learn the results of the tests. These tests spot OI in nine out of ten people who have it.

How is osteogenesis imperfecta treated?

Although there is no cure for OI, symptoms can be managed. Treatments for OI may include the following:

- Care for broken bones
- Care for brittle teeth
- Pain medication
- Physical therapy
- Use of wheelchairs, braces, and other aids
- Surgery

One type of surgery is called "rodding." Metal rods are put inside the long bones to do the following things:

- Strengthen them
- Fix bone malformations
- Prevent bone malformations

A healthy lifestyle also helps people with OI.

Section 13.6

Stickler Syndrome

What is Stickler syndrome?

Stickler syndrome is a progressive genetic disorder of connective
tissue throughout out the body. The condition was first described by
Dr. Gunnar B. Stickler in 1965 and was originally called "hereditary
progressive arthroophthalmopathy" because of its tendency to affect
the joints and the eyes.

What are the features of Stickler syndrome?

Stickler syndrome is associated with problems of vision (severe
nearsightedness and retinal detachments), hearing (hearing loss and
frequent ear infections), craniofacial abnormalities (small noses and
chins, cleft palates) musculoskeletal abnormalities (arthritis and loose
joints) as well as other problems caused by abnormal collagen.

What causes Stickler syndrome?

Stickler syndrome is usually caused by a mutation in the Type II
pro-collagen (COL2A1) gene, although several other mutations have
also been identified. These mutations cause abnormalities in the formation of connective tissues throughout the body and give rise to the
features of Stickler syndrome.

How is Stickler syndrome inherited?

Stickler syndrome is usually inherited in an autosomal dominant
pattern (50 percent chance of passing that mutation on to each child).
Less commonly, Stickler syndrome can occur sporadically, which means
that there is no family history of the disease, and that the individual
is the first one in the family to have the mutation. Genetic counseling

is recommended, and children of affected parents should be evaluated by an eye doctor (ophthalmologist) in early childhood.

How does Stickler syndrome affect vision?

Extreme myopia (nearsightedness) is one of the earliest and most characteristic signs of Stickler syndrome. The associated thin peripheral retina can lead to retinal breaks, holes, detachment, and scarring which can permanently reduce vision. Cataracts (clouding of the lens in the eye) can reduce vision, and typically occur at a younger age in individuals with Stickler syndrome.

How is Stickler syndrome diagnosed?

A point system is used to diagnose Stickler syndrome based on the number of oral-facial, ocular, auditory, and skeletal abnormalities detected. In addition, points are given for family history or the presence of a mutation in one of the genes known to be associated with Stickler syndrome. There are twelve points possible on nine criteria. Diagnosis requires five points minimum and presence of cleft palate, ocular abnormalities, or high-frequency hearing loss.

How is Stickler syndrome treated?

Early, regular, long-term evaluation is essential. Glasses and/or contact lenses are utilized for myopia. Laser may be applied to areas of thin retina to reduce the risk of detachment. Additional retina surgery may be necessary to repair detachment. Significant cataract may require lens removal.

Chapter 14

Cornelia de Lange Syndrome

What is Cornelia de Lange syndrome?

Cornelia de Lange syndrome is a developmental disorder that affects many parts of the body. The features of this disorder vary widely among affected individuals and range from relatively mild to severe.

Cornelia de Lange syndrome is characterized by slow growth before and after birth, intellectual disability that is usually severe to profound, skeletal abnormalities involving the arms and hands, and distinctive facial features. The facial differences include arched eyebrows that often grow together in the middle (synophrys); long eyelashes; low-set ears; small, widely spaced teeth; and a small, upturned nose. Many affected individuals also have behavior problems similar to autism, a developmental condition that affects communication and social interaction.

Additional signs and symptoms of Cornelia de Lange syndrome can include excessive body hair (hirsutism), an unusually small head (microcephaly), hearing loss, short stature, and problems with the digestive tract. Some people with this condition are born with an opening in the roof of the mouth called a cleft palate. Seizures, heart defects, eye problems, and skeletal abnormalities also have been reported in people with this condition.

How common is Cornelia de Lange syndrome?

Although the exact incidence is unknown, Cornelia de Lange syndrome likely affects one in ten thousand to thirty thousand newborns.

Excerpted from "Cornelia de Lange Syndrome," Genetics Home Reference (http://ghr.nlm.nih.gov), July 2012.

153

What genes are related to Cornelia de Lange syndrome?

Mutations in the NIPBL, SMC1A, and SMC3 genes can cause Cornelia de Lange syndrome. NIPBL gene mutations have been identified in more than half of all people with this condition; mutations in the other two genes are much less common. The proteins produced from all three genes play important roles in directing development before birth. Within cells, these proteins help regulate the structure and organization of chromosomes and are involved in the repair of damaged deoxyribonucleic acid (DNA). They also regulate the activity of certain genes in the developing limbs, face, and other parts of the body.

Mutations in the NIPBL, SMC1A, and SMC3 genes can cause Cornelia de Lange syndrome by disrupting gene regulation during critical stages of early development. Studies suggest that SMC1A and SMC3 gene mutations tend to cause somewhat milder signs and symptoms than those seen with mutations in the NIPBL gene.

In about 35 percent of cases, the cause of Cornelia de Lange syndrome is unknown. Researchers are looking for additional changes in the NIPBL, SMC1A, and SMC3 genes, as well as mutations in other genes, that may be responsible for this condition.

How do people inherit Cornelia de Lange syndrome?

When Cornelia de Lange syndrome is caused by mutations in the NIPBL or SMC3 gene, this condition is considered to have an autosomal dominant pattern of inheritance. Autosomal dominant inheritance means one copy of the altered gene in each cell is sufficient to cause the disorder. Almost all cases result from new gene mutations and occur in people with no history of the condition in their family.

Cases of Cornelia de Lange syndrome caused by SMC1A gene mutations have an X-linked pattern of inheritance. A condition is considered X-linked if the mutated gene that causes the disorder is located on the X chromosome, one of the two sex chromosomes. Studies of X-linked Cornelia de Lange syndrome indicate that one copy of the altered gene in each cell may be sufficient to cause the condition. Unlike most X-linked conditions, in which males are more frequently affected or experience more severe symptoms than females, X-linked Cornelia de Lange syndrome appears to affect males and females similarly. Most cases result from new mutations in the SMC1A gene and occur in people with no history of the condition in their family.

Chapter 15

Cystic Fibrosis

Cystic fibrosis, or CF, is an inherited disease of the secretory glands. Secretory glands include glands that make mucus and sweat.

"Inherited" means the disease is passed from parents to children through genes. People who have CF inherit two faulty genes for the disease—one from each parent. The parents likely don't have the disease themselves.

CF mainly affects the lungs, pancreas, liver, intestines, sinuses, and sex organs.

What causes cystic fibrosis?

A defect in the CFTR gene causes cystic fibrosis (CF). This gene makes a protein that controls the movement of salt and water in and out of your body's cells. In people who have CF, the gene makes a protein that doesn't work well. This causes thick, sticky mucus and very salty sweat.

Research suggests that the CFTR protein also affects the body in other ways. This may help explain other symptoms and complications of CF.

More than a thousand known defects can affect the CFTR gene. The type of defect you or your child has may affect the severity of CF. Other genes also may play a role in the severity of the disease.

Excerpted from "Cystic Fibrosis," National Heart, Lung, and Blood Institute, National Institutes of Health, June 2011.

How is cystic fibrosis inherited?

Every person inherits two CFTR genes—one from each parent. Children who inherit a faulty CFTR gene from each parent will have CF.

Children who inherit one faulty CFTR gene and one normal CFTR gene are "CF carriers." CF carriers usually have no symptoms of CF and live normal lives. However, they can pass the faulty CFTR gene to their children.

Who is at risk for cystic fibrosis?

Cystic fibrosis (CF) affects both males and females and people from all racial and ethnic groups. However, the disease is most common among Caucasians of Northern European descent.

CF also is common among Latinos and American Indians, especially the Pueblo and Zuni. The disease is less common among African Americans and Asian Americans.

More than ten million Americans are carriers of a faulty CF gene. Many of them don't know that they're CF carriers.

What are the signs and symptoms of cystic fibrosis?

The signs and symptoms of cystic fibrosis (CF) vary from person to person and over time. Sometimes you'll have few symptoms. Other times, your symptoms may become more severe.

One of the first signs of CF that parents may notice is that their baby's skin tastes salty when kissed, or the baby doesn't pass stool when first born.

Most of the other signs and symptoms of CF happen later. They're related to how CF affects the respiratory, digestive, or reproductive systems of the body.

Respiratory system signs and symptoms: People who have CF have thick, sticky mucus that builds up in their airways. This buildup of mucus makes it easier for bacteria to grow and cause infections. Infections can block the airways and cause frequent coughing that brings up thick sputum (spit) or mucus that's sometimes bloody.

People who have CF tend to have lung infections caused by unusual germs that don't respond to standard antibiotics. For example, lung infections caused by bacteria called mucoid *Pseudomonas* are much more common in people who have CF than in those who don't. An infection caused by these bacteria may be a sign of CF.

People who have CF have frequent bouts of sinusitis, an infection of the sinuses. The sinuses are hollow air spaces around the eyes, nose, and forehead. Frequent bouts of bronchitis and pneumonia also can occur. These infections can cause long-term lung damage.

As CF gets worse, you may have more serious problems, such as pneumothorax or bronchiectasis.

Some people who have CF also develop nasal polyps (growths in the nose) that may require surgery.

Digestive system signs and symptoms: In CF, mucus can block tubes, or ducts, in your pancreas (an organ in your abdomen). These blockages prevent enzymes from reaching your intestines.

As a result, your intestines can't fully absorb fats and proteins. This can cause ongoing diarrhea or bulky, foul-smelling, greasy stools. Intestinal blockages also may occur, especially in newborns. Too much gas or severe constipation in the intestines may cause stomach pain and discomfort.

A hallmark of CF in children is poor weight gain and growth. These children are unable to get enough nutrients from their food because of the lack of enzymes to help absorb fats and proteins.

As CF gets worse, other problems may occur, such as the following:

- Pancreatitis. This is a condition in which the pancreas become inflamed, which causes pain.
- Rectal prolapse. Frequent coughing or problems passing stools may cause rectal tissue from inside you to move out of your rectum.
- Liver disease due to inflamed or blocked bile ducts.
- Diabetes.
- Gallstones.

Reproductive system signs and symptoms: Men who have CF are infertile because they're born without a vas deferens. The vas deferens is a tube that delivers sperm from the testes to the penis.

Women who have CF may have a hard time getting pregnant because of mucus blocking the cervix or other CF complications.

Other signs, symptoms, and complications: Other signs and symptoms of CF are related to an upset of the balance of minerals in your blood.

CF causes your sweat to become very salty. As a result, your body loses large amounts of salt when you sweat. This can cause dehydration (a lack of fluid in your body), increased heart rate, fatigue (tiredness), weakness, decreased blood pressure, heat stroke, and, rarely, death.

CF also can cause clubbing and low bone density. Clubbing is the widening and rounding of the tips of your fingers and toes. This sign develops late in CF because your lungs aren't moving enough oxygen into your bloodstream.

Low bone density also tends to occur late in CF. It can lead to a bone-thinning disorder called osteoporosis.

How is cystic fibrosis diagnosed?

Doctors diagnose cystic fibrosis (CF) based on the results from various tests.

Newborn screening: All states screen newborns for CF using a genetic test or a blood test. The genetic test shows whether a newborn has faulty CFTR genes. The blood test shows whether a newborn's pancreas is working properly.

Sweat test: If a genetic test or blood test suggests CF, a doctor will confirm the diagnosis using a sweat test. This test is the most useful test for diagnosing CF. A sweat test measures the amount of salt in sweat.

For this test, the doctor triggers sweating on a small patch of skin on an arm or leg. He or she rubs the skin with a sweat-producing chemical and then uses an electrode to provide a mild electrical current. This may cause a tingling or warm feeling.

Sweat is collected on a pad or paper and then analyzed. The sweat test usually is done twice. High salt levels confirm a diagnosis of CF.

Other tests: If you or your child has CF, your doctor may recommend other tests, such as the following:

- *Genetic tests:* These tests are used to find out what type of CFTR defect is causing your CF.

- *A chest x-ray:* This test creates pictures of the structures in your chest, such as your heart, lungs, and blood vessels. A chest x-ray can show whether your lungs are inflamed or scarred, or whether they trap air.

- *A sinus x-ray:* This test may show signs of sinusitis, a complication of CF.

- *Lung function tests:* These tests measure how much air you can breathe in and out, how fast you can breathe air out, and how well your lungs deliver oxygen to your blood.

- *A sputum culture:* For this test, your doctor will take a sample of your sputum (spit) to see whether bacteria are growing in it. If you have bacteria called mucoid *Pseudomonas*, you may have more advanced CF that needs aggressive treatment.

Prenatal screening: If you're pregnant, prenatal genetic tests can show whether your fetus has CF. These tests include amniocentesis and chorionic villus sampling (CVS).

In amniocentesis, your doctor inserts a hollow needle through your abdominal wall into your uterus. He or she removes a small amount of fluid from the sac around the baby. The fluid is tested to see whether both of the baby's CFTR genes are normal.

In CVS, your doctor threads a thin tube through the vagina and cervix to the placenta. The doctor removes a tissue sample from the placenta using gentle suction. The sample is tested to see whether the baby has CF.

Cystic fibrosis carrier testing: People who have one normal CFTR gene and one faulty CFTR gene are CF carriers. CF carriers usually have no symptoms of CF and live normal lives. However, carriers can pass faulty CFTR genes on to their children.

If you have a family history of CF or a partner who has CF (or a family history of it) and you're planning a pregnancy, you may want to find out whether you're a CF carrier.

A genetics counselor can test a blood or saliva sample to find out whether you have a faulty CF gene. This type of testing can detect faulty CF genes in nine out of ten cases.

How is cystic fibrosis treated?

Cystic fibrosis (CF) has no cure. However, treatments have greatly improved in recent years. The goals of CF treatment include the following:

- Preventing and controlling lung infections
- Loosening and removing thick, sticky mucus from the lungs
- Preventing or treating blockages in the intestines
- Providing enough nutrition
- Preventing dehydration (a lack of fluid in the body)

Depending on the severity of CF, you or your child may be treated in a hospital.

What is the treatment for lung problems?

The main treatments for lung problems in people who have CF are chest physical therapy (CPT), exercise, and medicines. Your doctor also may recommend a pulmonary rehabilitation (PR) program.

Chest physical therapy: CPT also is called chest clapping or percussion. It involves pounding your chest and back over and over with your hands or a device to loosen the mucus from your lungs so that you can cough it up.

You might sit down or lie on your stomach with your head down while you do CPT. Gravity and force help drain the mucus from your lungs.

Some people find CPT hard or uncomfortable to do. Several devices have been developed that may help with CPT, such as the following:

- An electric chest clapper, known as a mechanical percussor.

- An inflatable therapy vest that uses high-frequency airwaves to force the mucus that's deep in your lungs toward your upper airways so you can cough it up.

- A small, handheld device that you exhale through. The device causes vibrations that dislodge the mucus.

- A mask that creates vibrations that help break the mucus loose from your airway walls.

Breathing techniques also may help dislodge mucus so you can cough it up. These techniques include forcing out a couple of short breaths or deeper breaths and then doing relaxed breathing. This may help loosen the mucus in your lungs and open your airways.

Exercise: Aerobic exercise that makes you breathe harder can help loosen the mucus in your airways so you can cough it up. Exercise also helps improve your overall physical condition.

However, CF causes your sweat to become very salty. As a result, your body loses large amounts of salt when you sweat. Thus, your doctor may recommend a high-salt diet or salt supplements to maintain the balance of minerals in your blood.

If you exercise regularly, you may be able to cut back on your CPT. However, you should check with your doctor first.

Medicines: If you have CF, your doctor may prescribe antibiotics, anti-inflammatory medicines, bronchodilators, or mucus-thinning medicines. These medicines help treat or prevent lung infections, reduce swelling, open up the airways, and thin mucus.

What are the treatments for advanced lung disease?

If you have advanced lung disease, you may need oxygen therapy. Oxygen usually is given through nasal prongs or a mask.

If other treatments haven't worked, a lung transplant may be an option if you have severe lung disease. A lung transplant is surgery to remove a person's diseased lung and replace it with a healthy lung from a deceased donor.

Pulmonary rehabilitation: Your doctor may recommend PR as part of your treatment plan. PR is a broad program that helps improve the well-being of people who have chronic (ongoing) breathing problems.

PR doesn't replace medical therapy. Instead, it's used with medical therapy and may include the following:

- Exercise training

- Nutritional counseling

- Education on your lung disease or condition and how to manage it

- Energy-conserving techniques

- Breathing strategies

- Psychological counseling and/or group support

PR has many benefits. It can improve your ability to function and your quality of life. The program also may help relieve your breathing problems. Even if you have advanced lung disease, you can still benefit from PR.

What is the treatment for digestive problems?

CF can cause many digestive problems, such as bulky stools, intestinal gas, a swollen belly, severe constipation, and pain or discomfort. Digestive problems also can lead to poor growth and development in children.

Nutritional therapy can improve your strength and ability to stay active. It also can improve growth and development in children. Nutritional therapy also may make you strong enough to resist some lung infections. A nutritionist can help you create a nutritional plan that meets your needs.

In addition to having a well-balanced diet that's rich in calories, fat, and protein, your nutritional therapy may include the following:

- Oral pancreatic enzymes to help you digest fats and proteins and absorb more vitamins.

- Supplements of vitamins A, D, E, and K to replace the fat-soluble vitamins that your intestines can't absorb.

- High-calorie shakes to provide you with extra nutrients.

- A high-salt diet or salt supplements that you take before exercising.

- A feeding tube to give you more calories at night while you're sleeping. The tube may be threaded through your nose and throat and into your stomach. Or, the tube may be placed directly into your stomach through a surgically made hole. Before you go to bed each night, you'll attach a bag with a nutritional solution to the entrance of the tube. It will feed you while you sleep.

Other treatments for digestive problems may include enemas and mucus-thinning medicines to treat intestinal blockages. Sometimes surgery is needed to remove an intestinal blockage.

Your doctor also may prescribe medicines to reduce your stomach acid and help oral pancreatic enzymes work better.

Chapter 16

Endocrine Disorders

Chapter Contents

Section 16.1

Congenital Adrenal Hyperplasia (21-Hydroxylase Deficiency)

"Congenital Adrenal Hyperplasia,"
© 2013 A.D.A.M., Inc. Reprinted with permission.

Congenital adrenal hyperplasia refers to a group of inherited disorders of the adrenal gland.

Causes

People have two adrenal glands, one located on top of each of their kidneys. These glands make hormones, cortisol and aldosterone, that are essential for life. People with congenital adrenal hyperplasia lack an enzyme the adrenal gland needs to make the hormones.

At the same time, the body produces more androgen, a type of male sex hormone. This causes male characteristics to appear early (or inappropriately).

Congenital adrenal hyperplasia can affect both boys and girls. About one in ten thousand to eighteen thousand children are born with congenital adrenal hyperplasia.

Symptoms

Symptoms will vary, depending on the type of congenital adrenal hyperplasia someone has and their age when the disorder is diagnosed:

- Children with milder forms may not have signs or symptoms of congenital adrenal hyperplasia and may not be diagnosed until as late as adolescence.

- Girls with a more severe form often have abnormal genitals at birth and may be diagnosed before symptoms appear.

- Boys will appear normal at birth even if they have a more severe form.

In children with the more severe form of the disorder, symptoms often develop within two or three weeks after birth:

- Poor feeding or vomiting

- Dehydration

- Electrolyte changes (abnormal levels of sodium and potassium in the blood)

- Abnormal heart rhythm

Girls with the milder form will usually have normal female reproductive organs (ovaries, uterus, and fallopian tubes). They may also have the following changes:

- Abnormal menstrual periods or failure to menstruate

- Early appearance of pubic or armpit hair

- Excessive hair growth or facial hair

- Failure to menstruate

- Some enlargement of the clitoris

Boys with the milder form often appear normal at birth. However, they may appear to enter puberty early. Symptoms may include:

- deepening voice;

- early appearance of pubic or armpit hair;

- enlarged penis but normal testes;

- well-developed muscles.

Both boys and girls will be tall as children but much shorter than normal as adults.

Exams and Tests

Your child's doctor will order certain tests. Common blood tests include:

- serum electrolytes;

- aldosterone;

- rennin;

- cortisol.

X-ray of the left hand and wrist may show that the child's bones appear to be those of someone older than their actual age.

Genetic tests can help diagnose or confirm the disorder, but they are rarely needed.

Treatment

The goal of treatment is to return hormone levels to normal, or near normal. This is done by taking a form of cortisol, most often hydrocortisone, three times per day. People may need additional doses of medicine during times of stress, such as severe illness or surgery.

The health care provider will determine the genetic sex of the baby with abnormal genitalia by checking the chromosomes (karyotyping). Girls with male-looking genitals may have surgery during infancy to correct the abnormal appearance.

Steroids used to treat congenital adrenal hyperplasia do not usually cause side effects, such as obesity or week bones, because the doses replace what the child cannot make. It is important for parents to report signs of infection and stress to your child's health care provider because the child may need more medication. Steroids cannot be stopped suddenly because doing so may lead to adrenal insufficiency.

Outlook (Prognosis)

People with this disorder must take medication their entire life. They usually have good health. However, they may be shorter than normal adults, even with treatment.

Congenital adrenal hyperplasia does not usually affect fertility.

Possible Complications

- High blood pressure
- Low blood sugar

Prevention

Parents with a family history of congenital adrenal hyperplasia (of any type) or a child who has the condition should consider genetic counseling.

Prenatal diagnosis is available for some forms of congenital adrenal hyperplasia. Diagnosis is made in the first trimester by chorionic villus sampling. Diagnosis in the second trimester is made by measuring hormones such as 17-hydroxyprogesterone in the amniotic fluid.

A newborn screening test is available for the most common form of congenital adrenal hyperplasia. It can be done on heelstick blood (as part of the routine screenings done on newborns). This test is currently performed in most states.

Alternative Names

Adrenogenital syndrome; 21-hydroxylase deficiency

References

White PC. Congenital adrenal hyperplasia due to 17-hydroxylase deficiency. In: Kliegman RM, Stanton BF, St. Geme J, Schor N, Behrman RE. *Nelson Textbook of Pediatrics. 19th ed.* Philadelphia, Pa: Saunders Elsevier; 2011:chap 570.

Section 16.2

Congenital Hypothyroidism

What is Congenital Hypothyroidism?

This is a disorder that affects infants from birth (congenital), resulting from the loss of thyroid function (hypothyroidism), normally due to failure of the thyroid gland to develop correctly. Sometimes the thyroid gland is absent, or ectopic (in an abnormal location). As a result, the thyroid gland does not produce enough thyroxine/T4 after birth. This may result in abnormal growth and development, as well as slower mental function.

What Is the Thyroid Gland?

The thyroid is a bow tie–shaped gland located in the neck, below the Adam's apple. The thyroid gland is part of the endocrine system.

This gland is responsible for secreting a hormone called thyroxine (T4), which plays a vital role in normal growth and development in children. This gland, like other glands in the endocrine system, is controlled by the pituitary gland. It works very much like a thermostat. The brain senses the amount of T4 and then signals the thyroid with another hormone, thyroid-stimulating hormone (TSH), to produce more or less T4. When the thyroid gland produces enough T4, no extra stimulation is needed and the TSH level remains at a normal level. When there is not enough T4, the TSH rises. These characteristics of the T4 and TSH hormones allow for screening of newborns to assess whether or not they have hypothyroidism (an underactive thyroid gland).

Why Did My Child Develop Congenital Hypothyroidism?

In most hypothyroid babies, there is no specific reason why the thyroid gland did not develop normally, although some of these children have an inherited form of this disorder. Congenital hypothyroidism is present in about one in four thousand infants in North America. There are a small proportion of children who have temporary (transient) congenital hypothyroidism for a period of time after birth. It is impossible to distinguish these transient hypothyroid babies from those with true congenital hypothyroidism and so these infants will be treated as well. Often, after the age of two or three, in children for whom transient or temporary hypothyroidism is suspected, the medication can be gradually discontinued for a short amount of time on a trial basis. The child will be retested to see if they can remain off medicine. This is not the case for true congenital hypothyroidism, where L-thyroxine is necessary throughout your child's life.

Symptoms of Congenital Hypothyroidism

Often these babies appear perfectly normal at birth, which is why screening is so vital. However, some may have one or more of the following symptoms: large, despite having poor feeding habits, increased birth weight; puffy face, swollen tongue; hoarse cry; low muscle tone; cold extremities; persistent constipation, bloated or full to the touch; lack of energy, sleeps most of the time, appears tired even when awake; little to no growth.

Children born with symptoms have a greater risk of developmental delay than children born without symptoms.

Tests for Congenital Hypothyroidism

The usual way to discover congenital hypothyroidism is by a screening process done on all newborns between twenty-four and seventy-two hours old. The reason this is done so early is that infants with congenital hypothyroidism usually appear normal at birth, and many do not show any of the signs or symptoms noted before. For the screening test, blood is obtained from your baby's heel and is placed on a filter paper. At a laboratory the T4 and/or TSH level is measured. If the T4 is low and/or the TSH is elevated, indicating hypothyroidism, your pediatrician is contacted immediately so treatment can begin without delay. It is likely that the blood test will be repeated to confirm the diagnosis. The physicians may also take an x-ray of the legs to look at the ends of the bones. In babies with hypothyroidism, the bones have an immature appearance, which helps to confirm diagnosis of congenital hypothyroidism. A thyroid scan should be done to determine the location or absence of the thyroid gland. These tests, bone age, and thyroid scan can be done at the time of diagnosis.

Treatment for Congenital Hypothyroidism

Treatment for congenital hypothyroidism is replacement of the missing thyroid hormone in pill form. It is extremely important that these pills be taken daily for life because thyroxine/T4 is essential for all the body's functions. In general, the average starting dose for L-thyroxine or levothyroxine (synthetic T4) in a newborn is between 25 and 50 mcg per day, or 10mcg to 15mcg/kg of body weight. This value increases dependent upon the individual needs of the child. The pill can be crushed, then administered in a small amount of water/formula or breast milk while your child is still an infant. Please be aware that L-thyroxine should not be mixed with soy formula, as this product interferes with absorption. Blood tests will be done on a regular basis to ensure that the hormone levels are in a normal range. Thyroid hormone is necessary for normal brain and intellectual development and such development can be delayed when there is a lack of L-thyroxine. With early replacement of adequate thyroid hormone and proper follow-up and care, the outlook for most children with congenital hypothyroidism is excellent.

Medical Attention

Generally, children are seen every two to three months for the first three years, once normal levels have been established. The goal is to maintain the concentration of T4 in the mid to upper half of the normal range (10mg/dL to 16mg/dL) for the first years of life. The TSH level should be maintained within the normal reference range for infants. The treatment for hypothyroidism is safe, simple, and effective. Successful treatment, however, depends on lifelong daily medication with close follow-up of hormone levels. This procedure of taking medication on a routine basis needs to become a part of the lifestyle of you and your child in order to assure optimal growth and development.

Section 16.3

Kallmann Syndrome

"Kallmann Syndrome," Genetics Home Reference (http://ghr.nlm.nih.gov), August 2008. Reviewed by David A. Cooke, M.D., FACP, April 2013.

What is Kallmann syndrome?

Kallmann syndrome is a condition characterized by delayed or absent puberty and an impaired sense of smell.

This disorder is a form of hypogonadotropic hypogonadism (HH), which is a condition affecting the production of hormones that direct sexual development. Males with hypogonadotropic hypogonadism are often born with an unusually small penis (micropenis) and undescended testes (cryptorchidism). At puberty, most affected individuals do not develop secondary sex characteristics, such as the growth of facial hair and deepening of the voice in males. Affected females usually do not begin menstruating at puberty and have little or no breast development. In some people, puberty is incomplete or delayed.

In Kallmann syndrome, the sense of smell is either diminished (hyposmia) or completely absent (anosmia). This feature distinguishes Kallmann syndrome from most other forms of hypogonadotropic hypogonadism, which do not affect the sense of smell. Many people with Kallmann syndrome are not aware that they are unable to detect odors until the impairment is discovered through testing.

The features of Kallmann syndrome vary, even among affected people in the same family. Additional signs and symptoms can include a failure of one kidney to develop (unilateral renal agenesis), a cleft lip with or without an opening in the roof of the mouth (a cleft palate), abnormal eye movements, hearing loss, and abnormalities of tooth development. Some affected individuals have a condition called bimanual synkinesis, in which the movements of one hand are mirrored by the other hand. Bimanual synkinesis can make it difficult to do tasks that require the hands to move separately, such as playing a musical instrument.

Researchers have identified four forms of Kallmann syndrome, designated types 1 through 4, which are distinguished by their genetic cause. The four types are each characterized by hypogonadotropic hypogonadism and an impaired sense of smell. Additional features, such as a cleft palate, seem to occur only in types 1 and 2.

How common is Kallmann syndrome?

Kallmann syndrome is estimated to affect 1 in 10,000 to 86,000 people and occurs more often in males than in females. Kallmann syndrome 1 is the most common form of the disorder.

What genes are related to Kallmann syndrome?

Mutations in the KAL1, FGFR1, PROKR2, and PROK2 genes cause Kallmann syndrome. KAL1 mutations are responsible for Kallmann syndrome 1. Kallmann syndrome 2 results from mutations in the FGFR1 gene. Mutations in the PROKR2 and PROK2 genes cause Kallmann syndrome types 3 and 4, respectively.

The genes associated with Kallmann syndrome play a role in the development of certain areas of the brain before birth. Although some of their specific functions are unclear, these genes appear to be involved in the formation and movement (migration) of a group of nerve cells that are specialized to process smells (olfactory neurons). These nerve cells come together into a bundle called the olfactory bulb, which is critical for the perception of odors. The KAL1, FGFR1, PROKR2, and PROK2 genes also play a role in the migration of neurons that produce a hormone called gonadotropin-releasing hormone (GnRH). GnRH controls the production of several other hormones that direct sexual development before birth and during puberty. These hormones are important for the normal function of the gonads (ovaries in women and testes in men).

Studies suggest that mutations in the KAL1, FGFR1, PROKR2, or PROK2 gene disrupt the migration of olfactory nerve cells and GnRH-producing nerve cells in the developing brain. If olfactory nerve cells do not extend to the olfactory bulb, a person's sense of smell will be impaired or absent. Misplacement of GnRH-producing neurons prevents the production of certain sex hormones, which interferes with normal sexual development and causes the characteristic features of hypogonadotropic hypogonadism. It is unclear how gene mutations lead to the other possible signs and symptoms of Kallmann syndrome. Because the features of this condition vary among individuals, researchers suspect that additional genetic and environmental factors may be involved.

Together, mutations in the KAL1, FGFR1, PROKR2, and PROK2 genes account for 25 percent to 30 percent of all cases of Kallmann syndrome. In cases without an identified mutation in one of these genes, the cause of the condition is unknown. Researchers are looking for other genes that can cause this disorder.

How do people inherit Kallmann syndrome?

Kallmann syndrome 1 (caused by KAL1 mutations) has an X-linked recessive pattern of inheritance. The KAL1 gene is located on the X chromosome, which is one of the two sex chromosomes. In males (who have only one X chromosome), one altered copy of the gene in each cell is sufficient to cause the condition. In females (who have two X chromosomes), a mutation must be present in both copies of the gene to cause the disorder. Males are affected by X-linked recessive disorders much more frequently than females. A characteristic of X-linked inheritance is that fathers cannot pass X-linked traits to their sons.

Most cases of Kallmann syndrome 1 are described as simplex, which means only one person in a family is affected. Some affected people inherit a KAL1 mutation from their mothers, who carry a single mutated copy of the gene in each cell. Other people have the condition as a result of a new mutation in the KAL1 gene.

Other forms of Kallmann syndrome can be inherited in an autosomal dominant pattern, which means one copy of the altered gene in each cell is sufficient to cause the disorder. In some cases, an affected person inherits the mutation from one affected parent. Other cases result from new mutations in the gene and occur in people with no history of the disorder in their family.

In several families, Kallmann syndrome has shown an autosomal recessive pattern of inheritance. Autosomal recessive inheritance means both copies of the gene in each cell have mutations. The parents of an individual with an autosomal recessive condition each carry one copy of the mutated gene, but they typically do not show signs and symptoms of the condition.

Chapter 17

Familial Hypercholesterolemia

What is familial hypercholesterolemia?

Familial hypercholesterolemia is an inherited condition that causes high levels of LDL (low-density lipoprotein) cholesterol levels beginning at birth, and heart attacks at an early age. Cholesterol is a fat-like substance that is found in the cells of the body. Cholesterol is also found in some foods. The body needs some cholesterol to work properly and uses cholesterol to make hormones, vitamin D, and substances that help with food digestion. However, if too much cholesterol is present in the bloodstream, it builds up in the walls of the arteries and increases the risk of heart disease.

Cholesterol is carried in the blood stream in small packages called lipoproteins. These small packages are made up of fat (lipid) on the inside and proteins on the outside. There are two main kinds of lipoprotein that carry cholesterol throughout the body. These are low-density lipoprotein (LDL) and high-density lipoprotein (HDL).

The cholesterol carried by LDL is sometimes called the "bad cholesterol." People who have familial hypercholesterolemia have high levels of LDL cholesterol because they cannot remove the LDL from the bloodstream properly. The organ responsible for the removal of the LDL is the liver. High levels of LDL cholesterol in the blood increase the risk for heart attacks and heart disease.

Excerpted from "Learning about Familial Hypercholesterolemia," National Human Genome Research Institute (www.genome.gov), March 23, 2011.

The cholesterol carried by HDL is sometimes called the "good cholesterol." HDL carries cholesterol from other parts of the body to the liver. The liver removes cholesterol from the body. Higher levels of HDL cholesterol lower a person's chance for getting heart disease.

Men who have familial hypercholesterolemia have heart attacks in their forties to their fifties, and 85 percent of men with the disorder have a heart attack by age sixty. Women who have familial hypercholesterolemia also have an increased risk for heart attack, but it happens ten years later than in men (so in their fifties and sixties).

Familial hypercholesterolemia is inherited in families in an autosomal dominant manner. In autosomal dominant inherited conditions, a parent who carries an altered gene that causes the condition has a one in two (50 percent) chance to pass on that altered gene to each of his or her children.

The altered gene (gene mutation) that causes familial hypercholesterolemia is located on chromosome number 19. It contains the information for a protein called LDL receptor that is responsible for clearing up LDL from the bloodstream. One in five hundred individuals carries one altered gene causing familial hypercholesterolemia. These individuals are called heterozygotes. More rarely, a person inherits the gene mutation from both parents, making them genetically homozygous. Individuals who are homozygous have a much more severe form of hypercholesterolemia, with heart attack and death often occurring before age thirty.

What are the symptoms of familial hypercholesterolemia?

The major symptoms and signs of familial hypercholesterolemia are as follows:

- High levels of total cholesterol and LDL cholesterol.
- A strong family history of high levels of total and LDL cholesterol and/or early heart attack.
- Elevated and therapy-resistant levels of LDL in either or both parents.
- Xanthomas (waxy deposits of cholesterol in the skin or tendons).
- Xanthelasmas (cholesterol deposits in the eyelids).
- Corneal arcus (cholesterol deposit around the cornea of the eye).
- If angina (chest pain) is present, it may be a sign that heart disease is present.

Individuals who have homozygous familial hypercholesterolemia develop xanthomas beneath the skin over their elbows, knees, and buttocks as well as in the tendons at a very early age, sometime in infancy. Heart attacks and death may occur before age thirty.

How is familial hypercholesterolemia diagnosed?

Diagnosis of familial hypercholesterolemia is based on physical examination and laboratory testing. Physical examination may find xanthomas and xanthelasmas (skin lesions caused by cholesterol-rich lipoprotein deposits), and cholesterol deposits in the eye called corneal arcus.

Laboratory testing includes blood testing of cholesterol levels, studies of heart function, and genetic testing. Blood testing of cholesterol levels may show: increased total cholesterol usually above 300 mg/dl (total cholesterol of more than 250 mg/dl in children) and LDL levels usually above 200 mg/dl. Studies of heart function, such as a stress test, may be abnormal. Genetic testing may show an alteration (mutation) in the LDL receptor gene.

What is the treatment for familial hypercholesterolemia?

The overall goal of treatment is to lower the risk for atherosclerotic heart disease by lowering the LDL cholesterol levels in the blood-stream. Atherosclerosis is a condition in which fatty material collects along the walls of arteries. This fatty material thickens, hardens, and may eventually block the arteries. Atherosclerosis happens when fat and cholesterol and other substances build up in the arteries and form a hardened material called plaque. The plaque deposits make the arteries less flexible and make it more difficult for blood to flow, leading to heart attack and stroke.

The first step in treatment for an individual who has heterozygous familial hypercholesterolemia is changing the diet to reduce the total amount of fat eaten to 30 percent of the total daily calories. This can be done by limiting the amount of beef, pork, and lamb in the diet; cutting out butter, whole milk, and fatty cheeses as well as some oils like coconut and palm oils; and eliminating egg yolks, organ meats, and other sources of saturated fat from animals. Dietary counseling is often recommended to help people to make these changes in their eating habits.

Exercise, especially to lose weight, may also help in lowering cholesterol levels.

Drug therapy is usually necessary in combination with diet, weight loss, and exercise, as these interventions may not be able to lower cholesterol levels alone. There are a number of cholesterol-lowering medications that are currently used. The first and more effective choice are drugs called "statins." Other drugs that may be used in combination with or instead of the statins are: bile acid sequestrant resins (for example, cholestyramine), ezetimibe, nicotinic acid (niacin), gemfibrozil, and fenofibrate.

Individuals who have homozygous familial hypercholesterolemia need more aggressive therapies to treat their significantly elevated levels of cholesterol. Often drug therapies are not sufficient to lower LDL cholesterol levels to the desiderated goal, and these individuals may require periodical LDL apheresis, a procedure to "clean up" LDL from the bloodstream, or highly invasive surgery such as a liver transplant.

Is familial hypercholesterolemia inherited?

Familial hypercholesterolemia is inherited in an autosomal dominant manner. This means that to have this condition, it is sufficient that the altered (mutated) gene is present on only one of the person's two number 19 chromosomes. A person who inherits one copy of the gene mutation causing familial hypercholesterolemia from one of his or her parents is said to have heterozygous familial hypercholesterolemia. This person has a one in two (50 percent) chance to pass on the mutated gene to each of his or her children.

A person who inherits a mutated copy of the gene causing familial hypercholesterolemia from both parents is said to have homozygous familial hypercholesterolemia. This is a much more severe form of familial hypercholesterolemia than heterozygous familial hypercholesterolemia. Each of this person's children will inherit one copy of the mutated gene and will have heterozygous familial hypercholesterolemia.

Chapter 18

Growth Disorders

Chapter Contents

Section 18.1

Achondroplasia

Excerpted from "Learning about Achondroplasia,"
National Human Genome Research Institute
(www.genome.gov), May 11, 2012.

What is achondroplasia?

Achondroplasia is a disorder of bone growth. It is the most common form of disproportionate short stature. It occurs in one in every fifteen thousand to one in every forty thousand live births. Achondroplasia is caused by a gene alteration (mutation) in the FGFR3 gene. The FGFR3 gene makes a protein called fibroblast growth factor receptor 3 that is involved in converting cartilage to bone. FGFR3 is the only gene known to be associated with achondroplasia. All people who have only a single copy of the normal FGFR3 gene and a single copy of the FGFR3 gene mutation have achondroplasia.

Most people who have achondroplasia have average-size parents. In this situation, the FGFR3 gene mutation occurs in one parent's egg or sperm cell before conception. Other people with achondroplasia inherit the condition from a parent who has achondroplasia.

What are the symptoms of achondroplasia?

People who have achondroplasia have abnormal bone growth that causes the following clinical symptoms: short stature with disproportionately short arms and legs, short fingers, a large head (macrocephaly), and specific facial features with a prominent forehead (frontal bossing) and mid-face hypoplasia.

The intelligence and life span in individuals with achondroplasia is usually normal.

Infants born with achondroplasia typically have weak muscle tone (hypotonia). Because of the hypotonia, there may be delays in walking and other motor skills. Compression of the spinal cord and/or upper airway obstruction increases the risk of death in infancy.

People with achondroplasia commonly have breathing problems in which breathing stops or slows down for short periods (apnea). Other health issues include obesity and recurrent ear infections. Adults with achondroplasia may develop a pronounced and permanent sway of the lower back (lordosis) and bowed legs. The problems with the lower back can cause back pain, leading to difficulty with walking.

How is achondroplasia diagnosed?

Achondroplasia is diagnosed by characteristic clinical and x-ray findings in most affected individuals. In individuals who may be too young to make a diagnosis with certainty or in individuals who do not have the typical symptoms, genetic testing can be used to identify a mutation in the FGFR3 gene.

Genetic testing can identify mutations in 99 percent of individuals who have achondroplasia. Testing for the FGFR3 gene mutation is available in clinical laboratories.

What is the treatment for achondroplasia?

No specific treatment is available for achondroplasia. Children born with achondroplasia need to have their height, weight, and head circumference monitored using special growth curves standardized for achondroplasia. Measures to avoid obesity at an early age are recommended.

A magnetic resonance imaging (MRI) or CT scan may be needed for further evaluation of severe muscle weakness (hypotonia) or signs of spinal cord compression. To help with breathing, surgical removal of the adenoids and tonsils, continuous positive airway pressure (CPAP) by nasal mask, or a surgical opening in the airway (tracheostomy) may be needed to correct obstructive sleep apnea.

When there are problems with the lower limbs, such as hyperreflexia, clonus, or central hypopnea, then surgery called suboccipital decompression is performed to decrease pressure on the brain.

Children who have achondroplasia need careful monitoring and support for social adjustment.

Is achondroplasia inherited?

Most cases of achondroplasia are not inherited. When achondroplasia is inherited, it is inherited in an autosomal dominant manner.

Over 80 percent of individuals who have achondroplasia have parents with normal stature and are born with achondroplasia as a result of a new (de novo) gene alteration (mutation). These parents have a small chance of having another child with achondroplasia.

A person who has achondroplasia who is planning to have children with a partner who does not have achondroplasia has a 50 percent chance, with each pregnancy, of having a child with achondroplasia. When both parents have achondroplasia, the chance for them, together, to have a child with normal stature is 25 percent. Their chance of having a child with achondroplasia is 50 percent. Their chance for having a child who inherits the gene mutation from both parents (called homozygous achondroplasia—a condition that leads to death) is 25 percent.

Section 18.2

Dwarfism

"Dwarfism," March 2011, reprinted with permission from www.kidshealth .org. This information was provided by KidsHealth®, one of the largest resources online for medically reviewed health information written for parents, kids, and teens. For more articles like this, visit www.KidsHealth .org, or www.TeensHealth.org. Copyright © 1995–2012 The Nemours Foundation. All rights reserved.

There's been a lot of discussion over the years about the proper way to refer to someone with dwarfism. Many people who have the condition prefer the term "little person" or "person of short stature." For some, "dwarf" is acceptable. For most, "midget" definitely is not.

But here's an idea everyone can agree on: Why not simply call a person with dwarfism by his or her name?

Being of short stature is only one of the characteristics that make a little person who he or she is. If you're the parent or loved one of a little person, you know this to be true.

But here are some facts that other people may not realize about dwarfism and those who have it.

Dwarfism:

- is characterized by short stature. Technically, that means an adult height of 4 feet 10 inches or under, according to the advocacy group Little People of America (LPA).

- can be caused by any one of more than three hundred conditions, most of which are genetic. The most common type, accounting for 70 percent of all cases of short stature, is called achondroplasia.

- can and most often does occur in families where both parents are of average height. In fact, four out of five children with achondroplasia are born to average-size parents.

Dwarfism isn't:

- an intellectual disability. A person who has dwarfism is typically of normal intelligence.

- a disease that requires a "cure." Most people with one of these conditions live long, fulfilling lives.

- a reason to assume someone is incapable. Little people go to school, go to work, marry, and raise children, just like their average-size peers.

What Causes Short Stature?

More than three hundred well-described conditions are known to cause short stature in a child. Most are caused by a spontaneous genetic change (mutation) in the egg or sperm cells prior to conception. Others are caused by genetic changes inherited from one or both parents.

Similarly, depending on the type of condition causing the short stature, it is possible for two average-size parents to have a child with short stature, and is also possible for parents who are little people to have an average-size child.

What prompts a gene to mutate is not yet clearly understood. The change is seemingly random and unpreventable, and can occur in any pregnancy. If parents have some form of dwarfism themselves, the odds are much greater that their children will also be little people. A genetic counselor can help determine the likelihood of passing on the condition in these cases.

Dwarfism has other causes, including metabolic or hormonal disorders in infancy or childhood. Chromosomal abnormalities, pituitary gland disorders (which influence growth and metabolism), absorptive problems (when the body can't absorb nutrients adequately), and kidney disease can all lead to short stature if a child fails to grow at a normal rate.

Types of Short Stature

Most types of dwarfism are known as skeletal dysplasias, which are conditions of abnormal bone growth. They're divided into two types: short-trunk and short-limb dysplasias. People with short-trunk dysplasia have a shortened trunk with more average-sized limbs, whereas those with short-limb dysplasia have an average-sized trunk but shortened arms and legs.

By far, the most common skeletal dysplasia is achondroplasia, a short-limb dysplasia that occurs in about one of every fifteen thousand to forty thousand babies born of all races and ethnicities. It can be caused by a spontaneous mutation in a gene called FGFR3, or a child can inherit a change in this gene from a parent who also has achondroplasia.

People with achondroplasia have a relatively long trunk and shortened upper parts of their arms and legs. They may share other features as well, such as a larger head with a prominent forehead, a flattened bridge of the nose, shortened hands and fingers, and reduced muscle tone. The average adult height for someone with achondroplasia is a little over 4 feet.

Diastrophic dysplasia is a different form of short-limb dwarfism. It occurs in about one in one hundred thousand births, and is also sometimes associated with cleft palate, clubfeet, and ears with a cauliflower-like appearance. People who have this diagnosis tend to have shortened forearms and calves (this is known as mesomelic shortening).

Spondyloepiphyseal dysplasias (SED) refers to a group of various short-trunk skeletal conditions that occurs in about one in ninety-five thousand babies. Along with achondroplasia and diastrophic dysplasia, it is one of the most common forms of dwarfism. In some forms, a lack of growth in the trunk area may not become apparent until the child is between five and ten years old; other forms are apparent at birth. Kids with this disorder also might have clubfeet, cleft palate, and a barrel-chested appearance.

In general, dwarfism caused by skeletal dysplasias results in what is known as disproportionate short stature—meaning the limbs and the trunk are not the same proportionally as those of typically statured people.

Metabolic or hormonal disorders typically cause proportionate dwarfism, meaning a person's arms, legs, and trunk are all shortened but remain in proportion to overall body size.

Diagnosis

Some types of dwarfism can be identified through prenatal testing if a doctor suspects a particular condition and tests for it.

But most cases are not identified until after the child is born. In those instances, the doctor makes a diagnosis based on the child's appearance, failure to grow, and x-rays of the bones. Depending on the type of dwarfism the child has, diagnosis often can be made almost immediately after birth.

Once a diagnosis is made, there is no "treatment" for most of the conditions that lead to short stature. Hormonal or metabolic problems may be treated with hormone injections or special diets to spark a child's growth, but skeletal dysplasias cannot be "cured."

People with these types of dwarfism can, however, get medical care for some of the health complications associated with their short stature.

Some forms of dwarfism also involve issues in other body systems— such as vision or hearing—and require careful monitoring.

Possible Complications and Treatments

Short stature is the one quality all people with dwarfism have in common. After that, each of the many conditions that cause dwarfism has its own set of characteristics and possible complications.

Fortunately, many of these complications are treatable, so that people of short stature can lead healthy, active lives.

For example, a small percentage of babies with achondroplasia may experience hydrocephalus (excess fluid around the brain). They may also have a greater risk of developing apnea—a temporary stop in breathing during sleep—because of abnormally small or misshapen anatomy or, more likely, because of airway obstruction by the adenoids or the tonsils. Occasionally, a part of the brain or spinal cord is compressed. With close monitoring by doctors, however, these potentially serious problems can be detected early and surgically corrected.

As a child with dwarfism grows, other issues may also become apparent, including:

- delayed development of some motor skills, such as sitting up and walking;
- a greater susceptibility to ear infections and hearing loss;
- breathing problems caused by small chests;
- weight problems;
- curvature of the spine (scoliosis, kyphosis, and/or lordosis);
- bowed legs;
- trouble with joint flexibility and early arthritis;
- lower back pain or leg numbness;
- crowding of teeth in the jaw.

Proper medical care can alleviate many of these problems. For example, surgery often can bring relief from the pain of joints that wear out under the stress of bearing weight differently with limited flexibility.

Surgery also can be used to improve some of the leg, hip, and spine problems people with short stature sometimes face.

Nonsurgical options may help, too—for instance, excessive weight can worsen many orthopedic problems, so a nutritionist might help develop a healthy plan for shedding extra pounds. And doctors or physical therapists can recommend ways to increase physical activity without putting extra stress on the bones and joints.

Helping Your Child

Although types of dwarfism, and their severity and complications, vary from person to person, in general a child's life span is not affected by dwarfism. Although the Americans with Disabilities Act protects the rights of people with dwarfism, many members of the short-statured community don't feel that they have a disability.

You can help your child with dwarfism lead the best life possible by building his or her sense of independence and self-esteem right from the start.

Here are some tips to keep in mind:

- Treat your child according to his or her age, not size. If you expect a six-year-old to clean up his or her room, don't make an exception simply because your child is small.

- Adapt to your child's limitations. Something as simple as a light switch extender can give a short-statured child a sense of independence around the house.

- Present your child's condition—both to your child and to others—as a difference rather than a hindrance. Your attitude and expectations can have a significant influence on your child's self-esteem.

- Learn to deal with people's reactions, whether it's simple curiosity or outright ignorance, without anger. Address questions or comments as directly as possible, then take a moment to point out something special about your child. If your child is with you, this approach shows that you notice all the other qualities that make him or her unique. It will also help prepare your child for dealing with these situations when you're not there.

- If your child is teased at school, don't overlook it. Talk to teachers and administrators to make sure your child is getting the support he or she needs.

- Encourage your child to find a hobby or activity to enjoy. If sports aren't going to be your child's forte, then maybe music, art, computers, writing, or photography will be.

- Finally, get involved with support associations like the Little People of America. Getting to know other people with dwarfism—both as peers and as mentors—can show your child just how much he or she can achieve.

Section 18.3

Multiple Epiphyseal Dysplasia

Excerpted from "Multiple Epiphyseal Dysplasia,"
Genetics Home Reference (http://ghr.nlm.nih.gov), February 2008.
Revised by David A. Cooke, M.D., FACP, May 2013.

What is multiple epiphyseal dysplasia?

Multiple epiphyseal dysplasia is a disorder of cartilage and bone development primarily affecting the ends of the long bones in the arms and legs (epiphyses). There are six known types of multiple epiphyseal dysplasia, which appear to correlate with different gene mutations. Both dominant and recessive types are known to occur. The most common symptoms are joint pain that most commonly affects the hips and knees, early-onset arthritis, and a waddling walk. Although some people with multiple epiphyseal dysplasia have mild short stature as adults, most are of normal height. The majority of individuals are diagnosed during childhood; however, some mild cases may not be diagnosed until adulthood.

Recessive multiple epiphyseal dysplasia is distinguished from the dominant type by malformations of the hands, feet, and knees and abnormal curvature of the spine (scoliosis). About 50 percent of individuals with recessive multiple epiphyseal dysplasia are born with at least one abnormal feature, including an inward- and upward-turning foot (clubfoot), an opening in the roof of the mouth (cleft palate), an unusual curving of the fingers or toes (clinodactyly), or ear swelling. An abnormality of the kneecap called a double-layered patella is also relatively common.

How common is multiple epiphyseal dysplasia?

The incidence of dominant multiple epiphyseal dysplasia is estimated to be at least one in ten thousand newborns. The incidence of recessive multiple epiphyseal dysplasia is unknown. Both forms of this disorder may actually be more common because some people with mild symptoms are never diagnosed.

What genes are related to multiple epiphyseal dysplasia?

Mutations in the COMP, COL9A1, COL9A2, COL9A3, or MATN3 genes can cause dominant multiple epiphyseal dysplasia. These genes provide instructions for making proteins that are found in the spaces between cartilage-forming cells (chondrocytes). These proteins interact with each other and play an important role in cartilage and bone formation. Cartilage is a tough, flexible tissue that makes up much of the skeleton during early development. Most cartilage is later converted to bone, except for the cartilage that continues to cover and protect the ends of bones and is present in the nose and external ears.

The majority of individuals with dominant multiple epiphyseal dysplasia have mutations in the COMP gene. About 10 percent of affected individuals have mutations in the MATN3 gene. Mutations in the COMP or MATN3 gene prevent the release of the proteins produced from these genes into the spaces between the chondrocytes. The absence of these proteins leads to the formation of abnormal cartilage, which can cause the skeletal problems characteristic of dominant multiple epiphyseal dysplasia.

The COL9A1, COL9A2, and COL9A3 genes provide instructions for making a protein called type IX collagen. Collagens are a family of proteins that strengthen and support connective tissues, such as skin, bone, cartilage, tendons, and ligaments. Mutations in the COL9A1, COL9A2, or COL9A3 gene are found in less than 5 percent of individuals with dominant multiple epiphyseal dysplasia. It is not known how mutations in these genes cause the signs and symptoms of this disorder. Research suggests that mutations in these genes may cause type IX collagen to accumulate inside the cell or interact abnormally with other cartilage components.

Some people with dominant multiple epiphyseal dysplasia do not have a mutation in the COMP, COL9A1, COL9A2, COL9A3, or MATN3 gene. In these cases, the cause of the condition is unknown.

Mutations in the SLC26A2 (also known as DTDSD) gene cause recessive multiple epiphyseal dysplasia. This gene provides instructions for making a protein that is essential for the normal development of cartilage and for its conversion to bone. Mutations in the SLC26A2 gene alter the structure of developing cartilage, preventing bones from forming properly and resulting in the skeletal problems characteristic of recessive multiple epiphyseal dysplasia.

COL9A1 gene mutations have also been reported to cause a recessive form of multiple epiphyseal dysplasia, in addition to the more common dominant variety.

How do people inherit multiple epiphyseal dysplasia?

Multiple epiphyseal dysplasia can have different inheritance patterns.

This condition can be inherited in an autosomal dominant pattern, which means one copy of the altered gene in each cell is sufficient to cause the disorder. In some cases, an affected person inherits the mutation from one affected parent. Other cases may result from new mutations in the gene. These cases occur in people with no history of the disorder in their family.

Multiple epiphyseal dysplasia can also be inherited in an autosomal recessive pattern, which means both copies of the gene in each cell have mutations. Most often, the parents of an individual with an autosomal recessive condition each carry one copy of the mutated gene, but do not show signs and symptoms of the condition.

Section 18.4

Russell-Silver Syndrome

Russell-Silver syndrome is a disorder present at birth involving poor growth. One side of the body also will appear to be larger than the other.

Causes

Up to one in ten children with this syndrome have a problem involving chromosome 7. In other patients, the syndrome may affect chromosome 11.

Most of the time, it occurs in people with no family history of the disease.

The estimated number of people who develop this condition varies greatly. Some say it affects about one in three thousand people. Other reports say it affects one in one hundred thousand people. Males and females are equally affected.

Symptoms

Symptoms can include:

- birthmarks that are the color of coffee with milk (cafe-au-lait marks);

- curving of the pinky toward the ring finger;

- delayed bone age;

- failure to thrive;

- gastroesophageal reflux disease;

- kidney problems, such as:

  - horseshoe kidney;

  - hydronephrosis;

- posterior urethral valves;
- renal tubular acidosis;
- low birth weight;
- large head for body size;
- poor growth;
- short arms;
- short height (stature);
- short, stubby fingers and toes;
- delayed stomach emptying, and constipation;
- wide forehead with a small, triangle-shaped face and small, narrow chin.

Exams and Tests

The condition is usually diagnosed by early childhood. The doctor will perform a physical exam. Signs include:

- pointed chin that is not fully developed;
- thin, wide mouth;
- triangle-shaped face with broad forehead.

There are no specific laboratory tests to diagnose Russell-Silver syndrome. Diagnosis is usually based on the judgment of your child's pediatrician. However, the following tests may be done:

- Blood sugar (some children may have low blood glucose)
- Bone age testing (bone age is often younger than the child's actual age)
- Chromosome testing (may detect a chromosomal problem)
- Growth hormone (some children may have a deficiency)
- Skeletal survey (to rule out other conditions that may mimic Russell-Silver syndrome)

Treatment

Growth hormone replacement may help if this hormone is lacking. Other treatments include:

- making sure the person gets enough calories, to prevent low blood sugar and promote growth;

- physical therapy, to improve muscle tone;

- special education, to address learning disabilities and attention deficit problems the child may have.

Many specialists may be involved in treating this condition:

- A doctor specializing in genetics can help diagnose Russell-Silver syndrome.

- A gastroenterologist or nutritionist can help develop the proper diet to enhance growth.

- An endocrinologist may prescribe growth hormone, if it is needed.

- Genetic counselors and psychologists may also be involved.

Outlook (Prognosis)

Older children and adults do not show typical features as clearly as infants or younger children. Intelligence may be normal, although the patient may have a learning disability.

Possible Complications

- Chewing or speaking difficulty if jaw is very small

- Learning disabilities

When to Contact a Medical Professional

Call your child's health care provider if signs of Russell-Silver syndrome develop. Make sure your child's height and weight are measured during each well child visit. The doctor may refer you to:

- a genetic professional for a full evaluation and chromosome studies

- a pediatric endocrinologist for management of your child's growth problems

Alternative Names

Silver-Russell syndrome; Silver syndrome

Section 18.5

Thanatophoric Dysplasia

Reprinted from "Thanatophoric Dysplasia,"
Genetics Home Reference (http://ghr.nlm.nih.gov), October 2012.

What is thanatophoric dysplasia?

Thanatophoric dysplasia is a severe skeletal disorder characterized by extremely short limbs and folds of extra (redundant) skin on the arms and legs. Other features of this condition include a narrow chest, short ribs, underdeveloped lungs, and an enlarged head with a large forehead and prominent, wide-spaced eyes.

Researchers have described two major forms of thanatophoric dysplasia, type I and type II. Type I thanatophoric dysplasia is distinguished by the presence of curved thigh bones and flattened bones of the spine (platyspondyly). Type II thanatophoric dysplasia is characterized by straight thigh bones and a moderate to severe skull abnormality called a cloverleaf skull.

The term "thanatophoric" is Greek for "death bearing." Infants with thanatophoric dysplasia are usually stillborn or die shortly after birth from respiratory failure; however, a few affected individuals have survived into childhood with extensive medical help.

How common is thanatophoric dysplasia?

This condition occurs in one in twenty thousand to fifty thousand newborns. Type I thanatophoric dysplasia is more common than type II.

What genes are related to thanatophoric dysplasia?

Mutations in the FGFR3 gene cause thanatophoric dysplasia. Both types of this condition result from mutations in the FGFR3 gene. This gene provides instructions for making a protein that is involved in the development and maintenance of bone and brain tissue. Mutations in this gene cause the FGFR3 protein to be overly active, which leads to the severe disturbances in bone growth that are characteristic of thanatophoric dysplasia. It is not known how FGFR3 mutations cause the brain and skin abnormalities associated with this disorder.

How do people inherit thanatophoric dysplasia?

Thanatophoric dysplasia is considered an autosomal dominant disorder because one mutated copy of the FGFR3 gene in each cell is sufficient to cause the condition. Virtually all cases of thanatophoric dysplasia are caused by new mutations in the FGFR3 gene and occur in people with no history of the disorder in their family. No affected individuals are known to have had children; therefore, the disorder has not been passed to the next generation.

Chapter 19

Heart Rhythm Disorders

Chapter Contents

Section 19.1

Brugada Syndrome

Brugada syndrome is an unusual genetic disorder of the heart's electrical system. Although people are born with it, they usually do not know they have it until they reach their thirties or forties. The only symptoms of Brugada syndrome are passing out (called syncope) or sudden cardiac death, but some patients may have heart palpitations, as well.

What causes Brugada syndrome?

Your heart's electrical system requires that electrical signals be sent through specialized electrical tissue and through the heart muscle itself (called the myocardium). These electrical tissues and the myocardium are able to conduct electricity because of special molecules called ion channels, which allow positively and negatively charged particles to pass through the cells' walls.

If you have Brugada syndrome, there is a defect in one of those ion channels. In about one of every three patients with Brugada syndrome, there is a specific ion channel (called the "SCN5A") that has a defect. This defect can lead to a dangerous heart rhythm problem called ventricular fibrillation, which is a much faster, chaotic heartbeat that sometimes reaches three hundred beats a minute. This chaotic heartbeat means very little blood is pumped from the heart to the brain and the body.

What are the risk factors?

Brugada syndrome is usually an inherited condition, which means it is passed down through family members. In about one-third of patients, doctors know which gene is responsible for the condition, but it appears that the remaining number of patients have some genetic defect that has not been identified yet.

In some cases, the signs of Brugada syndrome are mimicked by electrolyte imbalances, certain hormone disorders, or by cocaine use. In these cases, doctors still think that a genetic defect is the cause of Brugada syndrome, but that the defect is not severe enough to cause problems on its own.

Brugada syndrome occurs more often in men than in women. It is usually diagnosed in adults between twenty-five and fifty years old. It is rarely present in young children. Brugada syndrome is found more often in people of Asian descent than in any other race.

What are the signs and symptoms?

Many people who have Brugada syndrome do not have any symptoms, so they do not even know they have it. If people do have symptoms, they may include:

- fainting;

- irregular heartbeats (arrhythmias) or heart palpitations;

- sudden cardiac arrest (SCA).

How is Brugada syndrome diagnosed?

If your doctor thinks you might have Brugada syndrome, he or she may order the following tests:

- An electrocardiogram (ECG or EKG),which helps doctors analyze the electrical currents in your heart and the patterns of your heartbeat. During this test, doctors are looking for a certain kind of arrhythmia called a Brugada sign. A Brugada sign is a pattern of heartbeats that only happens in people with Brugada syndrome. However, not all patients with Brugada syndrome will have a Brugada sign, and the ECG may look completely normal. If this is the case, patients may need to have a number of ECGs at different times. In some cases, doctors may give a medicine that makes the Brugada sign more obvious.

- Electrophysiology studies (EPS), which are usually done in a cardiac catheterization laboratory. Doctors usually perform this test when patients have the Brugada sign but do not have any symptoms. During this test, a long, thin tube called a catheter is inserted into an artery in your leg and guided to your heart. A map of electrical impulses from your heart is sent through the catheter. This map helps doctors find out what kind of arrhythmia you have and where it starts. During this test, doctors may even cause the electrical problems to happen while you are in the safe and controlled environment of the hospital.

How is Brugada syndrome treated?

If your doctor thinks that treatment is needed, the only proven treatment for Brugada syndrome is an implantable cardioverter defibrillator (ICD). This small device monitors your heart rhythm and delivers electrical shocks when needed to control abnormal heartbeats. The ICD, which is about the size of a pager, is implanted beneath the skin, near the collarbone or somewhere at or above the waistline. Special wires, called leads, are placed inside the heart or on its surface and are attached to the ICD.

People with Brugada syndrome can lead normal lives. Whether or not you have an ICD to treat your Brugada syndrome, it is important to have regular check-ups with your doctor, just to make sure that you have the condition under control. Because Brugada syndrome runs in families, it may be a good idea for family members to be screened, as well.

Section 19.2

Familial Atrial Fibrillation

Excerpted from "Familial Atrial Fibrillation,"
Genetics Home Reference (http://ghr.nlm.nih.gov), January 2007.
Revised by David A. Cooke, M.D., FACP, May 2013.

What is familial atrial fibrillation?

Familial atrial fibrillation is an inherited condition that disrupts the heart's normal rhythm. This condition is characterized by uncoordinated electrical activity in the heart's upper chambers (the atria), which causes the heartbeat to become fast and irregular. If untreated, this abnormal heart rhythm can lead to dizziness, chest pain, a sensation of fluttering or pounding in the chest (palpitations), shortness of breath, or fainting (syncope). Atrial fibrillation also increases the risk of stroke and sudden death. Complications of familial atrial fibrillation can occur at any age, although some people with this heart condition never experience any health problems associated with the disorder.

How common is familial atrial fibrillation?

Atrial fibrillation is the most common type of sustained abnormal heart rhythm (arrhythmia), affecting more than three million people in the United States. The risk of developing this irregular heart rhythm increases with age. It is unclear exactly how commonly familial atrial fibrillation occurs, as few patients who develop atrial fibrillation undergo genetic testing. However, recent studies suggest that up to 30 percent of all people with atrial fibrillation may have a history of the condition in their family.

What genes are related to familial atrial fibrillation?

Mutations in at least forty different genes have been reported to cause familial atrial fibrillation. Many of these genes provide instructions for making proteins that act as channels across the cell membrane. These channels transport positively charged atoms (ions) of potassium into and out of cells. In heart (cardiac) muscle, the ion channels produced from the KCNE2, KCNJ2, and KCNQ1 genes play critical roles in maintaining the heart's normal rhythm. Mutations in these genes have been identified in only a few families worldwide. These mutations increase the activity of the channels, which changes the flow of potassium ions between cells. This disruption in ion transport alters the way the heart beats, increasing the risk of syncope, stroke, and sudden death.

Most cases of atrial fibrillation are not caused by mutations in a single gene. This condition is often related to structural abnormalities of the heart or underlying heart disease. Additional risk factors for atrial fibrillation include high blood pressure (hypertension), diabetes mellitus, a previous stroke, or an accumulation of fatty deposits and scar-like tissue in the lining of the arteries (atherosclerosis). Although most cases of atrial fibrillation are not known to run in families, studies suggest that they may arise partly from genetic risk factors. Researchers are working to determine which genetic changes may influence the risk of atrial fibrillation.

How do people inherit familial atrial fibrillation?

Familial atrial fibrillation appears to be inherited in an autosomal dominant pattern, which means one copy of the altered gene in each cell is sufficient to cause the disorder.

Section 19.3

Long QT Syndrome

Excerpted from "What Is Long QT Syndrome?" National
Heart, Lung, and Blood Institute, National Institutes of
Health, September 21, 2011.

What is long QT syndrome?

Long QT syndrome (LQTS) is a disorder of the heart's electrical
activity. It can cause sudden, uncontrollable, dangerous arrhythmias
in response to exercise or stress. Arrhythmias are problems with the
rate or rhythm of the heartbeat.

Overview: On the surface of each heart muscle cell are tiny pores
called ion channels. Ion channels open and close to let electrically
charged sodium, calcium, and potassium atoms (ions) flow into and
out of each cell. This generates the heart's electrical activity.

In people who have LQTS, the ion channels may not work well, or
there may be too few of them. This may disrupt electrical activity in
the heart's ventricles and cause dangerous arrhythmias.

LQTS often is inherited, which means you're born with the condition and have it your whole life.

There are seven known types of inherited LQTS. The most common
ones are LQTS 1, 2, and 3.

In LQTS 1, emotional stress or exercise (especially swimming) can
trigger arrhythmias.

In LQTS 2, extreme emotions, such as surprise, can trigger arrhythmias.

In LQTS 3, a slow heart rate during sleep can trigger arrhythmias.

You also can acquire LQTS. This means you aren't born with the
disorder, but you develop it during your lifetime. Some medicines and
conditions can cause acquired LQTS.

Outlook: More than half of the people who have untreated, inherited types of LQTS die within ten years. However, lifestyle changes
and medicines can help people who have LQTS prevent complications
and live longer.

199

Who is at risk for Long QT syndrome?

Long QT syndrome (LQTS) is a rare disorder. Experts think that about one in seven thousand people has LQTS. But no one knows for sure, because LQTS often goes undiagnosed.

LQTS causes about three thousand to four thousand sudden deaths in children and young adults each year in the United States. Unexplained sudden deaths in children are rare. When they do occur, LQTS often is the cause.

Inherited LQTS usually is first detected during childhood or young adulthood. Half of all people who have LQTS have their first abnormal heart rhythm by the time they're twelve years old, and 90 percent by the time they're forty years old. The condition rarely is diagnosed after age forty.

In boys who have LQTS, the QT interval (which can be seen on an electrocardiogram [EKG] test) often returns toward normal after puberty. If this happens, the risk of LQTS symptoms and complications goes down.

LQTS is more common in women than men. Women who have LQTS are more likely to faint or die suddenly from the disorder during menstruation and shortly after giving birth.

Children who are born deaf also are at increased risk for LQTS. This is because the same genetic problem that affects hearing also affects the function of ion channels in the heart.

Major risk factors: You're at risk of having LQTS if anyone in your family has ever had it. Unexplained fainting or seizures, drowning or near drowning, and unexplained sudden death are all possible signs of LQTS.

You're also at risk for LQTS if you take medicines that make the QT interval longer. Your doctor can tell you whether your prescription or over-the-counter medicines might do this.

You also may develop LQTS if you have excessive vomiting or diarrhea or other conditions that cause low blood levels of potassium or sodium. These conditions include the eating disorders anorexia nervosa and bulimia, as well as some thyroid disorders.

What are the signs and symptoms of long QT syndrome?

Major signs and symptoms: If you have long QT syndrome (LQTS), you can have sudden and dangerous arrhythmias (abnormal heart rhythms). Signs and symptoms of LQTS-related arrhythmias often first occur during childhood and include the following:

- **Unexplained fainting:** This happens because the heart isn't pumping enough blood to the brain. Fainting may occur during physical or emotional stress. Fluttering feelings in the chest may occur before fainting.

- **Unexplained drowning or near drowning:** This may be due to fainting while swimming.

- **Unexplained sudden cardiac arrest (SCA) or death:** SCA is a condition in which the heart suddenly stops beating for no obvious reason. People who have SCA die within minutes unless they receive treatment. In about one out of ten people who have LQTS, SCA or sudden death is the first sign of the disorder.

Other signs and symptoms: Often, people who have LQTS 3 develop an abnormal heart rhythm during sleep. This may cause noisy gasping while sleeping.

Silent long QT syndrome: Sometimes long QT syndrome doesn't cause any signs or symptoms. This is called silent LQTS. For this reason, doctors often advise family members of people who have LQTS to be tested for the disorder, even if they have no symptoms.

Medical and genetic tests may reveal whether these family members have LQTS and what type of the condition they have.

How is long QT syndrome diagnosed?

Cardiologists diagnose and treat long QT syndrome. Cardiologists are doctors who specialize in diagnosing and treating heart diseases and conditions. To diagnose LQTS, your cardiologist will consider the following things:

- Your EKG (electrocardiogram) results

- Your medical history and the results from a physical exam

- Your genetic test results

How is long QT syndrome treated?

The goal of treating long QT syndrome is to prevent life-threatening, abnormal heart rhythms and fainting spells.

Treatment isn't a cure for the disorder and may not restore a normal QT interval on an EKG. However, treatment greatly improves the chances of survival.

Specific types of treatment: People who have LQTS without symptoms may be advised to do the following things:

- Make lifestyle changes that reduce the risk of fainting or SCA. Lifestyle changes may include avoiding certain sports and strenuous exercise, such as swimming, which can cause abnormal heart rhythms.

- Avoid medicines that may trigger abnormal heart rhythms. This may include some medicines used to treat allergies, infections, high blood pressure, high blood cholesterol, depression, and arrhythmias.

- Take medicines such as beta-blockers, which reduce the risk of symptoms by slowing the heart rate.

If your doctor thinks you're at increased risk for LQTS complications, he or she may suggest more aggressive treatments. These treatments may include the following:

- A surgically implanted device, such as a pacemaker or implantable cardioverter defibrillator (ICD). These devices help control abnormal heart rhythms.

- Surgery on the nerves that regulate your heartbeat.

What do people living with long QT syndrome need to remember?

Long QT syndrome usually is a lifelong condition. The risk of having an abnormal heart rhythm that leads to fainting or sudden cardiac arrest may lessen as you age. However, the risk never completely goes away.

You'll need to take certain steps for the rest of your life to prevent abnormal heart rhythms. You can do the following things:

- Avoid things that trigger abnormal heart rhythms.

- Let others know you might faint or your heart might stop beating, and tell them what steps they can take.

- Have a plan in place for how to handle abnormal heart rhythms.

If an abnormal heart rhythm does occur, you'll need to seek treatment right away.

Ongoing health care needs: You should see your cardiologist (heart specialist) regularly. He or she will adjust your treatment as needed.

Chapter 20

Hereditary Deafness

Chapter Contents

Section 20.1

Usher Syndrome

Excerpted from the National Institute on Deafness and Other
Communication Disorders, National Institutes of Health,
NIH Publication No. 98-4291, February 1, 2013.

What is Usher syndrome?

Usher syndrome is the most common condition that affects both
hearing and vision. A syndrome is a disease or disorder that has more
than one feature or symptom. The major symptoms of Usher syndrome
are hearing loss and an eye disorder called retinitis pigmentosa, or
RP. RP causes night-blindness and a loss of peripheral vision (side vision) through the progressive degeneration of the retina. The retina is
a light-sensitive tissue at the back of the eye and is crucial for vision.
As RP progresses, the field of vision narrows—a condition known as
"tunnel vision"—until only central vision (the ability to see straight
ahead) remains. Many people with Usher syndrome also have severe
balance problems.

There are three clinical types of Usher syndrome: type 1, type 2,
and type 3. In the United States, types 1 and 2 are the most common
types. Together, they account for approximately 90 to 95 percent of all
cases of children who have Usher syndrome.

Who is affected by Usher syndrome?

Approximately 3 to 6 percent of all children who are deaf and another 3 to 6 percent of children who are hard of hearing have Usher
syndrome. In developed countries such as the United States, about four
babies in every one hundred thousand births have Usher syndrome.

What causes Usher syndrome?

Usher syndrome is inherited, which means that it is passed from
parents to their children through genes. Genes are located in almost
every cell of the body. Genes contain instructions that tell cells what
to do. Every person inherits two copies of each gene, one from each

parent. Sometimes genes are altered, or mutated. Mutated genes may cause cells to act differently than expected.

Usher syndrome is inherited as an autosomal recessive trait. The term "autosomal" means that the mutated gene is not located on either of the chromosomes that determine a person's sex; in other words, both males and females can have the disorder and can pass it along to a child. The word "recessive" means that, to have Usher syndrome, a person must receive a mutated form of the Usher syndrome gene from each parent. If a child has a mutation in one Usher syndrome gene but the other gene is normal, he or she is predicted to have normal vision and hearing. People with a mutation in a gene that can cause an autosomal recessive disorder are called carriers, because they "carry" the gene with a mutation, but show no symptoms of the disorder. If both parents are carriers of a mutated gene for Usher syndrome, they will have a one-in-four chance of having a child with Usher syndrome with each birth.

Usually, parents who have normal hearing and vision do not know if they are carriers of an Usher syndrome gene mutation. Currently, it is not possible to determine whether a person who does not have a family history of Usher syndrome is a carrier. Scientists at the National Institute on Deafness and Other Communication Disorders (NIDCD) are hoping to change this, however, as they learn more about the genes responsible for Usher syndrome.

What are the characteristics of the three types of Usher syndrome?

Type 1: Children with type 1 Usher syndrome are profoundly deaf at birth and have severe balance problems. Many of these children obtain little or no benefit from hearing aids. Parents should consult their doctor and other hearing health professionals as early as possible to determine the best communication method for their child. Intervention should be introduced early, during the first few years of life, so that the child can take advantage of the unique window of time during which the brain is most receptive to learning language, whether spoken or signed. If a child is diagnosed with type 1 Usher syndrome early on, before he or she loses the ability to see, that child is more likely to benefit from the full spectrum of intervention strategies that can help him or her participate more fully in life's activities.

Because of the balance problems associated with type 1 Usher syndrome, children with this disorder are slow to sit without support and typically don't walk independently before they are eighteen months old.

These children usually begin to develop vision problems in early childhood, almost always by the time they reach age ten. Vision problems most often begin with difficulty seeing at night, but tend to progress rapidly until the person is completely blind.

Type 2: Children with type 2 Usher syndrome are born with moderate to severe hearing loss and normal balance. Although the severity of hearing loss varies, most of these children can benefit from hearing aids and can communicate orally. The vision problems in type 2 Usher syndrome tend to progress more slowly than those in type 1, with the onset of RP often not apparent until the teens.

Type 3: Children with type 3 Usher syndrome have normal hearing at birth. Although most children with the disorder have normal to near-normal balance, some may develop balance problems later on. Hearing and sight worsen over time, but the rate at which they decline can vary from person to person, even within the same family. A person with type 3 Usher syndrome may develop hearing loss by the teens, and he or she will usually require hearing aids by mid- to late adulthood. Night blindness usually begins sometime during puberty. Blind spots appear by the late teens to early adulthood, and, by mid-adulthood, the person is usually legally blind.

How is Usher syndrome diagnosed?

Because Usher syndrome affects hearing, balance, and vision, diagnosis of the disorder usually includes the evaluation of all three senses. Evaluation of the eyes may include a visual field test to measure a person's peripheral vision, an electroretinogram (ERG) to measure the electrical response of the eye's light-sensitive cells, and a retinal examination to observe the retina and other structures in the back of the eye. A hearing (audiologic) evaluation measures how loud sounds at a range of frequencies need to be before a person can hear them. An electronystagmogram (ENG) measures involuntary eye movements that could signify a balance problem.

Early diagnosis of Usher syndrome is very important. The earlier that parents know if their child has Usher syndrome, the sooner that child can begin special educational training programs to manage the loss of hearing and vision.

Is genetic testing for Usher syndrome available?

So far, eleven genetic loci (a segment of chromosome on which a certain gene is located) have been found to cause Usher syndrome, and nine genes have been pinpointed that cause the disorder. They are as follows:

- **Type 1 Usher syndrome:** MY07A, USH1C, CDH23, PCDH15, SANS

- **Type 2 Usher syndrome:** USH2A, VLGR1, WHRN

- **Type 3 Usher syndrome:** USH3A

With so many possible genes involved in Usher syndrome, genetic tests for the disorder are not conducted on a widespread basis. Diagnosis of Usher syndrome is usually performed through hearing, balance, and vision tests. Genetic testing for a few of the identified genes is clinically available.

Table 20.1. Characteristics of Usher Syndrome

	Type 1	Type 2	Type 3
Hearing	Profound deafness in both ears from birth	Moderate to severe hearing loss from birth	Normal at birth; progressive loss in childhood or early teens
Vision	Decreased night vision before age ten	Decreased night vision begins in late childhood or teens	Varies in severity; night vision problems often begin in teens
Vestibular function (balance)	Balance problems from birth	Normal	Normal to near-normal, chance of later problems

How is Usher syndrome treated?

Currently, there is no cure for Usher syndrome. The best treatment involves early identification so that educational programs can begin as soon as possible. The exact nature of these programs will depend on the severity of the hearing and vision loss as well as the age and abilities of the person. Typically, treatment will include hearing aids, assistive listening devices, cochlear implants, or other communication methods such as American Sign Language; orientation and mobility training; and communication services and independent-living training that may include Braille instruction, low-vision services, or auditory training.

Some ophthalmologists believe that a high dose of vitamin A palmitate may slow, but not halt, the progression of retinitis pigmentosa. This belief stems from the results of a long-term clinical trial supported by the National Eye Institute and the Foundation for Fighting

Blindness. Based on these findings, the researchers recommend that most adult patients with the common forms of RP take a daily supplement of 15,000 international units (IU) of vitamin A in the palmitate form under the supervision of their eye care professional. (Because people with type 1 Usher syndrome did not take part in the study, high-dose vitamin A is not recommended for these patients.) People who are considering taking vitamin A should discuss this treatment option with their health care provider before proceeding. Other guidelines regarding this treatment option include the following:

- Do not substitute vitamin A palmitate with a beta-carotene supplement.

- Do not take vitamin A supplements greater than the recommended dose of 15,000 IU or modify your diet to select foods with high levels of vitamin A.

- Women who are considering pregnancy should stop taking the high-dose supplement of vitamin A three months before trying to conceive due to the increased risk of birth defects.

- Women who are pregnant should stop taking the high-dose supplement of vitamin A due to the increased risk of birth defects.

- In addition, according to the same study, people with RP should avoid using supplements of more than 400 IU of vitamin E per day.

What research is being conducted on Usher syndrome?

Researchers are currently trying to identify all of the genes that cause Usher syndrome and determine the function of those genes. This research will lead to improved genetic counseling and early diagnosis, and may eventually expand treatment options.

Scientists also are developing mouse models that have the same characteristics as the human types of Usher syndrome. Mouse models will make it easier to determine the function of the genes involved in Usher syndrome. Other areas of study include the early identification of children with Usher syndrome, treatment strategies such as the use of cochlear implants for hearing loss, and intervention strategies to help slow or stop the progression of RP.

What are some of the latest research findings?

NIDCD researchers, along with collaborators from universities in New York and Israel, pinpointed a mutation, named R245X, of the

PCDH15 gene that accounts for a large percentage of type 1 Usher syndrome in today's Ashkenazi Jewish population. (The term "Ashkenazi" describes Jewish people who originate from Eastern Europe.) Based on this finding, the researchers conclude that Ashkenazi Jewish infants with bilateral, profound hearing loss who lack another known mutation that causes hearing loss should be screened for the R245X mutation.

Section 20.2

Waardenburg Syndrome

Waardenburg syndrome is a group of conditions passed down through families that involve deafness and pale skin, hair, and eye color.

Causes

Waardenburg syndrome is inherited as an autosomal dominant trait, meaning only one parent has to pass on the faulty gene for a child to be affected.

There are four main types of Waardenburg syndrome. The most common are type I and type II.

Type III (Klein-Waardenburg syndrome) and type IV (Waardenburg-Shah syndrome) are more rare.

The multiple types of this syndrome result from defects in different genes. Most people with this disease have a parent with the disease, but the symptoms in the parent can be quite different from those in the child.

Symptoms

Symptoms may include:

- cleft lip (rare);

- constipation;

- deafness (more common in type II disease);

- extremely pale blue eyes or eye colors that don't match (hetero-chromia);

- pale color skin, hair, and eyes (partial albinism);

- difficulty completely straightening joints;

- possible slight decrease in intellectual function;

- wide-set eyes (in type I);

- white patch of hair or early graying of the hair.

Less common types of this disease may cause problems with the arms or intestines.

Exams and Tests

Tests may include:

- audiometry;

- bowel transit time;

- colon biopsy;

- genetic testing.

Treatment

There is no specific treatment. Symptoms will be treated as appropriate. Special diets and medicines to keep the bowel moving are prescribed to those patients who have constipation.

Outlook (Prognosis)

Once hearing problems are corrected, most people with this syndrome should be able to lead a normal life. Those with rarer forms of the syndrome may have other complications.

Possible Complications

- Constipation severe enough to require part of large bowel to be removed

- Hearing loss

- Self-esteem problems, or other problems related to appearance

- Slight decreased intellectual functioning (possible, unusual)

- Slight increased risk for muscle tumor called rhabdomyosarcoma

When to Contact a Medical Professional

Genetic counseling may be helpful if you have a family history of Waardenburg syndrome and plan to have children. Call for a hearing test if you or your child has deafness or decreased hearing.

Alternative Names

Klein-Waardenburg syndrome; Waardenburg-Shah syndrome

References

Morelli JG. Hypopigmented lesions. In: Kliegman RM, Behrman RE, Jenson HB, Stanton BF, eds. *Nelson Textbook of Pediatrics. 18th ed.* Philadelphia, Pa: Saunders Elsevier; 2007:chap 652.

Chapter 21

Huntington Disease

In 1872, the American physician George Huntington wrote about an illness that he called "an heirloom from generations away back in the dim past." He was not the first to describe the disorder, which has been traced back to the Middle Ages at least. One of its earliest names was chorea, which, as in "choreography," is the Greek word for dance. The term chorea describes how people affected with the disorder writhe, twist, and turn in a constant, uncontrollable dance-like motion. Later, other descriptive names evolved. "Hereditary chorea" emphasizes how the disease is passed from parent to child. "Chronic progressive chorea" stresses how symptoms of the disease worsen over time. Today, physicians commonly use the simple term Huntington disease (HD) to describe this highly complex disorder that causes untold suffering for thousands of families.

More than 15,000 Americans have HD. At least 150,000 others have a 50 percent risk of developing the disease and thousands more of their relatives live with the possibility that they, too, might develop HD.

Until recently, scientists understood very little about HD and could only watch as the disease continued to pass from generation to generation. Families saw the disease destroy their loved ones' ability to feel, think, and move. In the last several years, scientists working with support from the National Institute of Neurological Disorders

Excerpted from "Huntington's Disease: Hope Through Research," National Institute of Neurological Disorders and Stroke, National Institutes of Health, April 24, 2013.

and Stroke (NINDS) have made several breakthroughs in the area of HD research. With these advances, our understanding of the disease continues to improve.

What causes Huntington disease?

HD results from genetically programmed degeneration of nerve cells, called neurons, in certain areas of the brain. This degeneration causes uncontrolled movements, loss of intellectual faculties, and emotional disturbance. Specifically affected are cells of the basal ganglia, structures deep within the brain that have many important functions, including coordinating movement. Within the basal ganglia, HD especially targets neurons of the striatum, particularly those in the caudate nuclei and the pallidum. Also affected is the brain's outer surface, or cortex, which controls thought, perception, and memory.

How is HD inherited?

HD is found in every country of the world. It is a familial disease, passed from parent to child through a mutation or misspelling in the normal gene.

A single abnormal gene, the basic biological unit of heredity, produces HD. Genes are composed of deoxyribonucleic acid (DNA), a molecule shaped like a spiral ladder. Each rung of this ladder is composed of two paired chemicals called bases. There are four types of bases—adenine, thymine, cytosine, and guanine—each abbreviated by the first letter of its name: A, T, C, and G. Certain bases always "pair" together, and different combinations of base pairs join to form coded messages. A gene is a long string of this DNA in various combinations of A, T, C, and G. These unique combinations determine the gene's function, much like letters join together to form words. Each person has about thirty thousand genes—a billion base pairs of DNA or bits of information repeated in the nuclei of human cells—which determine individual characteristics or traits.

Genes are arranged in precise locations along twenty-three rod-like pairs of chromosomes. One chromosome from each pair comes from an individual's mother, the other from the father. Each half of a chromosome pair is similar to the other, except for one pair, which determines the sex of the individual. This pair has two X chromosomes in females and one X and one Y chromosome in males. The gene that produces HD lies on chromosome 4, one of the twenty-two non-sex-linked, or "autosomal," pairs of chromosomes, placing men and women at equal risk of acquiring the disease.

The impact of a gene depends partly on whether it is dominant or recessive. If a gene is dominant, then only one of the paired chromosomes is required to produce its called-for effect. If the gene is recessive, both parents must provide chromosomal copies for the trait to be present. HD is called an autosomal dominant disorder because only one copy of the defective gene, inherited from one parent, is necessary to produce the disease.

The genetic defect responsible for HD is a small sequence of DNA on chromosome 4 in which several base pairs are repeated many, many times. The normal gene has three DNA bases, composed of the sequence CAG. In people with HD, the sequence abnormally repeats itself dozens of times. Over time—and with each successive generation—the number of CAG repeats may expand further.

Each parent has two copies of every chromosome but gives only one copy to each child. Each child of an HD parent has a 50-50 chance of inheriting the HD gene. If a child does not inherit the HD gene, he or she will not develop the disease and cannot pass it to subsequent generations. A person who inherits the HD gene, and survives long enough, will sooner or later develop the disease. In some families, all the children may inherit the HD gene; in others, none do. Whether one child inherits the gene has no bearing on whether others will or will not share the same fate.

A small number of cases of HD are sporadic—that is, they occur even though there is no family history of the disorder. These cases are thought to be caused by a new genetic mutation—an alteration in the gene that occurs during sperm development and that brings the number of CAG repeats into the range that causes disease.

What are the major effects of the disease?

Early signs of the disease vary greatly from person to person. A common observation is that the earlier the symptoms appear, the faster the disease progresses.

Family members may first notice that the individual experiences mood swings or becomes uncharacteristically irritable, apathetic, passive, depressed, or angry. These symptoms may lessen as the disease progresses or, in some individuals, may continue and include hostile outbursts or deep bouts of depression.

HD may affect the individual's judgment, memory, and other cognitive functions. Early signs might include having trouble driving, learning new things, remembering a fact, answering a question, or making a decision. Some may even display changes in handwriting. As the disease progresses, concentration on intellectual tasks becomes increasingly difficult.

In some individuals, the disease may begin with uncontrolled movements in the fingers, feet, face, or trunk. These movements—which are signs of chorea—often intensify when the person is anxious. HD can also begin with mild clumsiness or problems with balance. Some people develop choreic movements later, after the disease has progressed. They may stumble or appear uncoordinated. Chorea often creates serious problems with walking, increasing the likelihood of falls.

The disease can reach the point where speech is slurred and vital functions, such as swallowing, eating, speaking, and especially walking, continue to decline. Some individuals cannot recognize other family members. Many, however, remain aware of their environment and are able to express emotions.

Some physicians have employed a recently developed Unified HD Rating Scale, or UHDRS, to assess the clinical features, stages, and course of HD. In general, the duration of the illness ranges from ten to thirty years. The most common causes of death are infection (most often pneumonia), injuries related to a fall, or other complications.

At what age does HD appear?

The rate of disease progression and the age at onset vary from person to person. Adult-onset HD, with its disabling, uncontrolled movements, most often begins in middle age. There are, however, other variations of HD distinguished not just by age at onset but by a distinct array of symptoms. For example, some persons develop the disease as adults, but without chorea. They may appear rigid and move very little, or not at all, a condition called akinesia.

Some individuals develop symptoms of HD when they are very young—before age twenty. The terms "early-onset" or "juvenile" HD are often used to describe HD that appears in a young person. A common sign of HD in a younger individual is a rapid decline in school performance. Symptoms can also include subtle changes in handwriting and slight problems with movement, such as slowness, rigidity, tremor, and rapid muscular twitching, called myoclonus. Several of these symptoms are similar to those seen in Parkinson disease, and they differ from the chorea seen in individuals who develop the disease as adults. These young individuals are said to have "akinetic-rigid" HD or the Westphal variant of HD. People with juvenile HD may also have seizures and mental disabilities. The earlier the onset, the faster the disease seems to progress. The disease progresses most rapidly in individuals with juvenile or early-onset HD, and death often follows within ten years.

Individuals with juvenile HD usually inherit the disease from their fathers. These individuals also tend to have the largest number of CAG repeats. The reason for this may be found in the process of sperm production. Unlike eggs, sperm are produced in the millions. Because DNA is copied millions of times during this process, there is an increased possibility for genetic mistakes to occur. To verify the link between the number of CAG repeats in the HD gene and the age at onset of symptoms, scientists studied a boy who developed HD symptoms at the age of two, one of the youngest and most severe cases ever recorded. They found that he had the largest number of CAG repeats of anyone studied so far—nearly one hundred. The boy's case was central to the identification of the HD gene and at the same time helped confirm that juveniles with HD have the longest segments of CAG repeats, the only proven correlation between repeat length and age at onset.

A few individuals develop HD after age fifty-five. Diagnosis in these people can be very difficult. The symptoms of HD may be masked by other health problems, or the person may not display the severity of symptoms seen in individuals with HD of earlier onset. These individuals may also show symptoms of depression rather than anger or irritability, or they may retain sharp control over their intellectual functions, such as memory, reasoning, and problem solving.

There is also a related disorder called senile chorea. Some elderly individuals display the symptoms of HD, especially choreic movements, but do not become demented, have a normal gene, and lack a family history of the disorder. Some scientists believe that a different gene mutation may account for this small number of cases, but this has not been proven.

How is HD diagnosed?

The great American folk singer and composer Woody Guthrie died on October 3, 1967, after suffering from HD for thirteen years. He had been misdiagnosed, considered an alcoholic, and shuttled in and out of mental institutions and hospitals for years before being properly diagnosed. His case, sadly, is not extraordinary, although the diagnosis can be made easily by experienced neurologists.

A neurologist will interview the individual intensively to obtain the medical history and rule out other conditions. A tool used by physicians to diagnose HD is to take the family history, sometimes called a pedigree or genealogy. It is extremely important for family members to be candid and truthful with a doctor who is taking a family history.

The doctor will also ask about recent intellectual or emotional problems, which may be indications of HD, and will test the person's hearing, eye movements, strength, coordination, involuntary movements (chorea), sensation, reflexes, balance, movement, and mental status, and will probably order a number of laboratory tests as well.

People with HD commonly have impairments in the way the eye follows or fixes on a moving target. Abnormalities of eye movements vary from person to person and differ, depending on the stage and duration of the illness.

The discovery of the HD gene in 1993 resulted in a direct genetic test to make or confirm a diagnosis of HD in an individual who is exhibiting HD-like symptoms. Using a blood sample, the genetic test analyzes DNA for the HD mutation by counting the number of repeats in the HD gene region. Individuals who do not have HD usually have twenty-eight or fewer CAG repeats. Individuals with HD usually have forty or more repeats. A small percentage of individuals, however, have a number of repeats that fall within a borderline region.

The physician may ask the individual to undergo a brain imaging test. Computed tomography (CT) and magnetic resonance imaging (MRI) provide excellent images of brain structures with little if any discomfort. Those with HD may show shrinkage of some parts of the brain—particularly two areas known as the caudate nuclei and putamen—and enlargement of fluid-filled cavities within the brain called ventricles. These changes do not definitely indicate HD, however, because they can also occur in other disorders. In addition, a person can have early symptoms of HD and still have a normal CT scan. When used in conjunction with a family history and record of clinical symptoms, however, CT can be an important diagnostic tool.

What is presymptomatic testing?

Presymptomatic testing is used for people who have a family history of HD but have no symptoms themselves. If either parent had HD, the person's chance would be 50-50. In the past, no laboratory test could positively identify people carrying the HD gene—or those fated to develop HD—before the onset of symptoms. That situation changed in 1983, when a team of scientists supported by NINDS located the first genetic marker for HD—the initial step in developing a laboratory test for the disease.

A marker is a piece of DNA that lies near a gene and is usually inherited with it. Discovery of the first HD marker allowed scientists to locate the HD gene on chromosome 4. The marker discovery quickly led to the development of a presymptomatic test for some individuals, but this test required blood or tissue samples from both affected and unaffected family members in order to identify markers unique to that particular family. For this reason, adopted individuals, orphans, and people who had few living family members were unable to use the test.

Discovery of the HD gene has led to a less expensive, scientifically simpler, and far more accurate presymptomatic test that is applicable to the majority of at-risk people. The new test uses CAG repeat length to detect the presence of the HD mutation in blood.

How is the presymptomatic test conducted?

An individual who wishes to be tested should contact the nearest testing center. (A list of such centers can be obtained from the Huntington Disease Society of America.) The testing process should include several components. Most testing programs include a neurological examination, pretest counseling, and follow up. The purpose of the neurological examination is to determine whether or not the person requesting testing is showing any clinical symptoms of HD. It is important to remember that if an individual is showing even slight symptoms of HD, he or she risks being diagnosed with the disease during the neurological examination, even before the genetic test. During pretest counseling, the individual will learn about HD, and about his or her own level of risk, about the testing procedure. The person will be told about the test's limitations, the accuracy of the test, and possible outcomes. He or she can then weigh the risks and benefits of testing and may even decide at that time against pursuing further testing.

The genetic testing itself involves donating a small sample of blood that is screened in the laboratory for the presence or absence of the HD mutation. Testing may require a sample of DNA from a closely related affected relative, preferably a parent, for the purpose of confirming the diagnosis of HD in the family. This is especially important if the family history for HD is unclear or unusual in some way.

In order to protect the interests of minors, including confidentiality, testing is not recommended for those under the age of eighteen unless there is a compelling medical reason (for example, the child is exhibiting symptoms).

Testing of a fetus (prenatal testing) presents special challenges and risks; in fact some centers do not perform genetic testing on fetuses. Because a positive test result using direct genetic testing means the at-risk parent is also a gene carrier, at-risk individuals who are considering a pregnancy are advised to seek genetic counseling prior to conception.

Some at-risk parents may wish to know the risk to their fetus but not their own. In this situation, parents may opt for prenatal testing using linked DNA markers rather than direct gene testing. In this case, testing does not look for the HD gene itself but instead indicates whether or not the fetus has inherited a chromosome 4 from the affected grandparent or from the unaffected grandparent on the side of the family with HD. If the test shows that the fetus has inherited a chromosome 4 from the affected grandparent, the parents then learn that the fetus's risk is the same as the parent (50-50), but they learn nothing new about the parent's risk. If the test shows that the fetus has inherited a chromosome 4 from the unaffected grandparent, the risk to the fetus is very low (less than 1 percent) in most cases.

Another option open to parents is in vitro fertilization with preimplantation screening. In this procedure, embryos are screened to determine which ones carry the HD mutation. Embryos determined not to have the HD gene mutation are then implanted in the woman's uterus.

How does a person decide whether to be tested?

The anxiety that comes from living with a 50 percent risk for HD can be overwhelming. How does a young person make important choices about long-term education, marriage, and children? How do older parents of adult children cope with their fears about children and grandchildren? How do people come to terms with the ambiguity and uncertainty of living at risk?

Some individuals choose to undergo the test out of a desire for greater certainty about their genetic status. They believe the test will enable them to make more informed decisions about the future. Others choose not to take the test. They are able to make peace with the uncertainty of being at risk, preferring to forgo the emotional consequences of a positive result, as well as possible losses of insurance and employment. There is no right or wrong decision, as each choice is highly individual.

Whatever the results of genetic testing, the at-risk individual and family members can expect powerful and complex emotional responses. The health and happiness of spouses, brothers and sisters, children, parents, and grandparents are affected by a positive test result, as are an individual's friends, work associates, neighbors, and others. Because receiving test results may prove to be devastating, testing guidelines call for continued counseling even after the test is complete and the results are known.

Is there a treatment for HD?

Physicians may prescribe a number of medications to help control emotional and movement problems associated with HD. It is important to remember however, that while medicines may help keep these clinical symptoms under control, there is no treatment to stop or reverse the course of the disease.

In August 2008 the U.S. Food and Drug Administration approved tetrabenazine to treat Huntington chorea, making it the first drug approved for use in the United States to treat the disease. Antipsychotic drugs, such as haloperidol, or other drugs, such as clonazepam, may help to alleviate choreic movements and may also be used to help control hallucinations, delusions, and violent outbursts. Antipsychotic drugs, however, are not prescribed for another form of muscle contraction associated with HD, called dystonia, and may in fact worsen the condition, causing stiffness and rigidity. These medications may also have severe side effects, including sedation, and for that reason should be used in the lowest possible doses.

For depression, physicians may prescribe fluoxetine, sertraline, nortriptyline, or other compounds. Tranquilizers can help control anxiety and lithium may be prescribed to combat pathological excitement and severe mood swings. Medications may also be needed to treat the severe obsessive-compulsive rituals of some individuals with HD.

Most drugs used to treat the symptoms of HD have side effects such as fatigue, restlessness, or hyperexcitability. Sometimes it may be difficult to tell if a particular symptom, such as apathy or incontinence, is a sign of the disease or a reaction to medication.

What kind of care does the individual with HD need?

Although a psychologist or psychiatrist, a genetic counselor, and other specialists may be needed at different stages of the illness, usually the first step in diagnosis and in finding treatment is to see a neurologist. While the family doctor may be able to diagnose HD, and may continue to monitor the individual's status, it is better to consult with a neurologist about management of the varied symptoms.

Problems may arise when individuals try to express complex thoughts in words they can no longer pronounce intelligibly. It can be helpful to repeat words back to the person with HD so that he or she knows that some thoughts are understood. Sometimes people mistakenly assume that if individuals do not talk, they also do not understand. Never isolate individuals by not talking, and try to keep their environment as normal as possible. Speech therapy may improve the individual's ability to communicate.

It is extremely important for the person with HD to maintain physical fitness as much as his or her condition and the course of the disease allows. Individuals who exercise and keep active tend to do better than those who do not. A daily regimen of exercise can help the person feel better physically and mentally. Although their coordination may be poor, individuals should continue walking, with assistance if necessary. Those who want to walk independently should be allowed to do so as long as possible, and careful attention should be given to keeping their environment free of hard, sharp objects. This will help ensure maximal independence while minimizing the risk of injury from a fall. Individuals can also wear special padding during walks to help protect against injury from falls. Some people have found that small weights around the ankles can help stability. Wearing sturdy shoes that fit well can help too, especially shoes without laces that can be slipped on or off easily.

Impaired coordination may make it difficult for people with HD to feed themselves and to swallow. As the disease progresses, persons with HD may even choke. In helping individuals to eat, caregivers should allow plenty of time for meals. Food can be cut into small pieces, softened, or pureed to ease swallowing and prevent choking. While some foods may require the addition of thickeners, other foods may need to be thinned. Dairy products, in particular, tend to increase the secretion of mucus, which in turn increases the risk of choking. Some individuals may benefit from swallowing therapy, which is especially helpful if started before serious problems arise. Suction cups for plates, special tableware designed for people with disabilities, and plastic cups with tops can help prevent spilling. The individual's physician can offer additional advice about diet and about how to handle swallowing difficulties or gastrointestinal problems that might arise, such as incontinence or constipation.

Caregivers should pay attention to proper nutrition so that the individual with HD takes in enough calories to maintain his or her body weight. Sometimes people with HD, who may burn as many as five thousand calories a day without gaining weight, require five meals a day to take in the necessary number of calories. Physicians may recommend vitamins or other nutritional supplements. In a long-term care institution, staff will need to assist with meals in order to ensure that the individual's special caloric and nutritional requirements are met. Some individuals and their families choose to use a feeding tube; others choose not to.

Individuals with HD are at special risk for dehydration and therefore require large quantities of fluids, especially during hot weather. Bendable straws can make drinking easier for the person. In some cases, water may have to be thickened with commercial additives to give it the consistency of syrup or honey.

What research is being done?

Although HD attracted considerable attention from scientists in the early twentieth century, there was little sustained research on the disease until the late 1960s when the Committee to Combat Huntington's Disease and the Huntington's Chorea Foundation, later called the Hereditary Disease Foundation, first began to fund research and to campaign for federal funding. In 1977, Congress established the Commission for the Control of Huntington's Disease and Its Consequences, which made a series of important recommendations. Since then, Congress has provided consistent support for federal research, primarily through the National Institute of Neurological Disorders and Stroke, the government's lead agency for biomedical research on disorders of the brain and nervous system. The effort to combat HD proceeds along the following lines of inquiry, each providing important information about the disease:

- **Basic neurobiology:** Now that the HD gene has been located, investigators in the field of neurobiology—which encompasses the anatomy, physiology, and biochemistry of the nervous system—are continuing to study the HD gene with an eye toward understanding how it causes disease in the human body.

- **Clinical research:** Neurologists, psychologists, psychiatrists, and other investigators are improving our understanding of the symptoms and progression of the disease in patients while attempting to develop new therapeutics.

- **Imaging:** Scientific investigations using positron emission tomography (PET) and other technologies are enabling scientists to see what the defective gene does to various structures in the brain and how it affects the body's chemistry and metabolism.

- **Animal models:** Laboratory animals, such as mice, are being bred in the hope of duplicating the clinical features of HD and can soon be expected to help scientists learn more about the symptoms and progression of the disease.

- **Fetal tissue research:** Investigators are implanting fetal tissue in rodents and nonhuman primates with the hope that success

223

in this area will lead to understanding, restoring, or replacing functions typically lost by neuronal degeneration in individuals with HD.

These areas of research are slowly converging and, in the process, are yielding important clues about the gene's relentless destruction of mind and body. The NINDS supports much of this exciting work.

Molecular genetics: For ten years, scientists focused on a segment of chromosome 4 and, in 1993, finally isolated the HD gene. The process of isolating the responsible gene—motivated by the desire to find a cure—was more difficult than anticipated. Scientists now believe that identifying the location of the HD gene is the first step on the road to a cure.

Finding the HD gene involved an intense molecular genetics research effort with cooperating investigators from around the globe. In early 1993, the collaborating scientists announced they had isolated the unstable triplet repeat DNA sequence that has the HD gene. Investigators relied on the NINDS-supported Research Roster for Huntington's Disease, based at Indiana University in Indianapolis, to accomplish this work. First started in 1979, the roster contains data on many American families with HD, provides statistical and demographic data to scientists, and serves as a liaison between investigators and specific families. It provided the DNA from many families affected by HD to investigators involved in the search for the gene and was an important component in the identification of HD markers.

For several years, NINDS-supported investigators involved in the search for the HD gene made yearly visits to the largest known kindred with HD—fourteen thousand individuals—who live on Lake Maracaibo in Venezuela. The continuing trips enable scientists to study inheritance patterns of several interrelated families.

The HD gene and its product: Although scientists know that certain brain cells die in HD, the cause of their death is still unknown. Recessive diseases are usually thought to result from a gene that fails to produce adequate amounts of a substance essential to normal function. This is known as a loss-of-function gene. Some dominantly inherited disorders, such as HD, are thought to involve a gene that actively interferes with the normal function of the cell. This is known as a gain-of-function gene.

How does the defective HD gene cause harm? The HD gene encodes a protein—which has been named huntingtin—the function of which is as yet unknown. The repeated CAG sequence in the gene causes an abnormal form of huntingtin to be made, in which the amino acid glutamine is repeated. It is the presence of this abnormal form, and not the absence of the normal form, that causes harm in HD. This explains why the disease is dominant and why two copies of the defective gene—one from both the mother and the father—do not cause a more serious case than inheritance from only one parent. With the HD gene isolated, NINDS-supported investigators are now turning their attention toward discovering the normal function of huntingtin and how the altered form causes harm. Scientists hope to reproduce, study, and correct these changes in animal models of the disease.

Huntingtin is found everywhere in the body but only outside the cell's nucleus. Mice called "knockout mice" are bred in the laboratory to produce no huntingtin; they fail to develop past a very early embryo stage and quickly die. Huntingtin, scientists now know, is necessary for life. Investigators hope to learn why the abnormal version of the protein damages only certain parts of the brain. One theory is that cells in these parts of the brain may be supersensitive to this abnormal protein.

Cell death in HD: Although the precise cause of cell death in HD is not yet known, scientists are paying close attention to the process of genetically programmed cell death that occurs deep within the brains of individuals with HD. This process involves a complex series of interlinked events leading to cellular suicide. Related areas of investigation include:

- *Excitotoxicity:* Overstimulation of cells by natural chemicals found in the brain.

- *Defective energy metabolism:* A defect in the power plant of the cell, called mitochondria, where energy is produced.

- *Oxidative stress:* Normal metabolic activity in the brain that produces toxic compounds called free radicals.

- *Trophic factors:* Natural chemical substances found in the human body that may protect against cell death.

Several HD studies are aimed at understanding losses of nerve cells and receptors in HD. Neurons in the striatum are classified both by their size (large, medium, or small) and appearance (spiny or aspiny). Each type of neuron contains combinations of neurotransmitters. Scientists know that the destructive process of HD affects different subsets of neurons to varying degrees. The hallmark of HD, they are learning, is selective degeneration of medium-sized spiny neurons in the striatum. NINDS-supported studies also suggest that losses of certain types of neurons and receptors are responsible for different symptoms and stages of HD.

What do these changes look like? In spiny neurons, investigators have observed two types of changes, each affecting the nerve cells' dendrites. Dendrites, found on every nerve cell, extend out from the cell body and are responsible for receiving messages from other nerve cells. In the intermediate stages of HD, dendrites grow out of control. New, incomplete branches form and other branches become contorted. In advanced, severe stages of HD, degenerative changes cause sections of dendrites to swell, break off, or disappear altogether. Investigators believe that these alterations may be an attempt by the cell to rebuild nerve cell contacts lost early in the disease. As the new dendrites establish connections, however, they may in fact contribute to nerve cell death. Such studies give compelling, visible evidence of the progressive nature of HD and suggest that new experimental therapies must consider the state of cellular degeneration. Scientists do not yet know exactly how these changes affect subsets of nerve cells outside the striatum.

Animal models of HD: As more is learned about cellular degeneration in HD, investigators hope to reproduce these changes in animal models and to find a way to correct or halt the process of nerve cell death. Such models serve the scientific community in general by providing a means to test the safety of new classes of drugs in nonhuman primates. NINDS-supported scientists are currently working to develop both nonhuman primate and mouse models to investigate nerve degeneration in HD and to study the effects of excitotoxicity on nerve cells in the brain.

Investigators are working to build genetic models of HD using transgenic mice. To do this, scientists transfer the altered human HD gene into mouse embryos so that the animals will develop the anatomical and biological characteristics of HD. This genetic model of mouse HD will enable in-depth study of the disease and testing of new therapeutic compounds.

Another idea is to insert into mice a section of DNA containing CAG repeats in the abnormal, disease gene range. This mouse equivalent of HD could allow scientists to explore the basis of CAG instability and its role in the disease process.

Fetal tissue research: A relatively new field in biomedical research involves the use of brain tissue grafts to study, and potentially treat, neurodegenerative disorders. In this technique, tissue that has degenerated is replaced with implants of fresh, fetal tissue, taken at the very early stages of development. Investigators are interested in applying brain tissue implants to HD research. Extensive animal studies will be required to learn if this technique could be of value in patients with HD.

Clinical studies: Scientists are pursuing clinical studies that may one day lead to the development of new drugs or other treatments to halt the disease's progression. Examples of NINDS-supported investigations, using both asymptomatic and symptomatic individuals, include the following:

- Genetic studies on age of onset, inheritance patterns, and markers found within families. These studies may shed additional light on how HD is passed from generation to generation.

- Studies of cognition, intelligence, and movement. Studies of abnormal eye movements, both horizontal and vertical, and tests of patients' skills in a number of learning, memory, neuropsychological, and motor tasks may serve to identify when the various symptoms of HD appear and to characterize their range and severity.

- Clinical trials of drugs. Testing of various drugs may lead to new treatments and at the same time improve our understanding of the disease process in HD. Classes of drugs being tested include those that control symptoms, slow the rate of progression of HD, and block effects of excitotoxins, and those that might correct or replace other metabolic defects contributing to the development and progression of HD.

Imaging: NINDS-supported scientists are using positron emission tomography (PET) to learn how the gene affects the chemical systems of the body. PET visualizes metabolic or chemical abnormalities in the body, and investigators hope to ascertain if PET scans can reveal any abnormalities that signal HD. Investigators conducting HD research are also using PET to characterize neurons that have died and chemicals that are depleted in parts of the brain affected by HD.

Like PET, a form of magnetic resonance imaging (MRI) called functional MRI can measure increases or decreases in certain brain chemicals thought to play a key role in HD. Functional MRI studies are also helping investigators understand how HD kills neurons in different regions of the brain.

Imaging technologies allow investigators to view changes in the volume and structures of the brain and to pinpoint when these changes occur in HD. Scientists know that in brains affected by HD, the basal ganglia, cortex, and ventricles all show atrophy or other alterations.

Chapter 22

Hypohidrotic Ectodermal Dysplasia

What is hypohidrotic ectodermal dysplasia?

Hypohidrotic ectodermal dysplasia is one of about 150 types of ectodermal dysplasia in humans. Before birth, these disorders result in the abnormal development of structures including the skin, hair, nails, teeth, and sweat glands.

Most people with hypohidrotic ectodermal dysplasia have a reduced ability to sweat (hypohidrosis) because they have fewer sweat glands than normal or their sweat glands do not function properly. Sweating is a major way that the body controls its temperature; as sweat evaporates from the skin, it cools the body. An inability to sweat can lead to a dangerously high body temperature (hyperthermia), particularly in hot weather. In some cases, hyperthermia can cause life-threatening medical problems.

Affected individuals tend to have sparse scalp and body hair (hypotrichosis). The hair is often light-colored, brittle, and slow growing. This condition is also characterized by absent teeth (hypodontia) or teeth that are malformed. The teeth that are present are frequently small and pointed.

Hypohidrotic ectodermal dysplasia is associated with distinctive facial features including a prominent forehead, thick lips, and a flattened bridge of the nose. Additional features of this condition include thin,

Excerpted from "Hypohidrotic Ectodermal Dysplasia," Genetics Home Reference (http://ghr.nlm.nih.gov), August 2006. Reviewed by David A. Cooke, M.D., FACP, May 2013.

wrinkled, and dark-colored skin around the eyes; chronic skin problems such as eczema; and a bad-smelling discharge from the nose (ozena).

How common is hypohidrotic ectodermal dysplasia?

Hypohidrotic ectodermal dysplasia is the most common form of ectodermal dysplasia in humans. It is estimated to affect at least one in seventeen thousand people worldwide.

What genes are related to hypohidrotic ectodermal dysplasia?

Mutations in the EDA, EDAR, and EDARADD genes cause hypohidrotic ectodermal dysplasia.

The EDA, EDAR, and EDARADD genes provide instructions for making proteins that work together during embryonic development. These proteins form part of a signaling pathway that is critical for the interaction between two cell layers, the ectoderm and the mesoderm. In the early embryo, these cell layers form the basis for many of the body's organs and tissues. Ectoderm-mesoderm interactions are essential for the formation of several structures that arise from the ectoderm, including the skin, hair, nails, teeth, and sweat glands.

Mutations in the EDA, EDAR, or EDARADD gene prevent normal interactions between the ectoderm and the mesoderm and impair the normal development of hair, sweat glands, and teeth. The improper formation of these ectodermal structures leads to the characteristic features of hypohidrotic ectodermal dysplasia.

How do people inherit hypohidrotic ectodermal dysplasia?

Hypohidrotic ectodermal dysplasia has several different inheritance patterns. Most cases are caused by mutations in the EDA gene, which are inherited in an X-linked recessive pattern. A condition is considered X-linked if the mutated gene that causes the disorder is located on the X chromosome, one of the two sex chromosomes. In males (who have only one X chromosome), one altered copy of the gene in each cell is sufficient to cause the condition. In females (who have two X chromosomes), a mutation must be present in both copies of the gene to cause the disorder. Males are affected by X-linked recessive disorders much more frequently than females. A characteristic of X-linked inheritance is that fathers cannot pass X-linked traits to their sons.

In X-linked recessive inheritance, a female with one altered copy of the gene in each cell is called a carrier. In about 70 percent of cases, carriers of hypohidrotic ectodermal dysplasia experience some features of the condition. These signs and symptoms are usually mild and include a few missing or abnormal teeth, sparse hair, and some problems with sweat gland function. Some carriers, however, have more severe features of this disorder.

Less commonly, hypohidrotic ectodermal dysplasia results from mutations in the EDAR or EDARADD gene. EDAR mutations can have an autosomal dominant or autosomal recessive pattern of inheritance, and EDARADD mutations have an autosomal recessive pattern of inheritance. Autosomal dominant inheritance means one copy of the altered gene in each cell is sufficient to cause the disorder. Autosomal recessive inheritance means two copies of the gene in each cell are altered. Most often, the parents of an individual with an autosomal recessive disorder are carriers of one copy of the altered gene but do not show signs and symptoms of the disorder.

Chapter 23

Inborn Errors of Metabolism

Chapter Contents

Section 23.1

Biotinidase Deficiency

"Biotinidase Deficiency," a Family Fact Sheet from the Minnesota Newborn Screening Program, 601 Robert St. N., St. Paul, MN 55155, Phone: (800) 664-7772, Fax: (651) 201-5471. © 2012 Minnesota Department of Health. Reprinted with permission. For additional information, visit www.health.state.mn.us/newbornscreening.

What is a positive newborn screen?

Newborn screening is done on tiny samples of blood taken from your baby's heel twenty-four to forty-eight hours after birth. Newborn screening tests for rare, hidden disorders that may affect your baby's health and development. The newborn screen suggests your baby might have a disorder called biotinidase deficiency.

A positive newborn screen does not mean your baby has biotinidase deficiency, but it does mean your baby needs more testing to know for sure.

Your baby's doctor will help arrange for more testing with specialists in disorders like biotinidase deficiency.

What is biotinidase deficiency?

Biotinidase deficiency affects an enzyme needed to free biotin (one of the B vitamins) from the food we eat, so it can be used for energy and growth.

A person with biotinidase deficiency doesn't have enough enzyme to free biotin from foods so it can be used by the body.

Biotinidase deficiency is a disorder that is passed on, or inherited, from a child's mother and father. Because biotinidase deficiency is a genetic disease, family members are at risk of having biotinidase deficiency too, even if no one in the family has had it before.

What problems can biotinidase deficiency cause?

Biotinidase deficiency is different for each child. Some children have a mild, partial biotinidase deficiency with few health problems, while other children may have complete biotinidase deficiency with serious complications.

If biotinidase deficiency is not treated, a child might develop:

- muscle weakness;
- hearing loss;
- vision (eye) problems;
- hair loss;
- skin rashes;
- seizures;
- developmental delay.

It is very important to follow the doctor's instructions for testing and treatment.

What is the treatment for biotinidase deficiency?

Biotinidase deficiency can be treated. The treatment is lifelong. Treatment for children with biotinidase deficiency includes:

- daily biotin vitamin pill(s) or liquid.

Children with biotinidase deficiency should see their regular doctor, and a doctor who specializes in biotinidase deficiency.

With prompt and careful treatment, children with biotinidase deficiency have a good chance to live healthy lives with normal growth and development.

Section 23.2

Fructose Intolerance

"Hereditary Fructose Intolerance," © 2013 A.D.A.M., Inc.
Reprinted with permission.

Hereditary fructose intolerance is a disorder in which a person lacks the protein needed to break down fructose. Fructose is a fruit sugar that naturally occurs in the body. Man-made fructose is used as a sweetener in many foods, including baby food and drinks.

Causes

This condition occurs when the body is missing an enzyme called aldolase B. This substance is needed to break down fructose.

If a person without this substance eats fructose and sucrose (cane or beet sugar, table sugar), complicated chemical changes occur in the body. The body cannot change its energy storage material, glycogen, into glucose. As a result, the blood sugar falls and dangerous substances build up in the liver.

Hereditary fructose intolerance is inherited, which means it is passed down through families. If both parents carry an abnormal gene, each of their children has a 25 percent chance of being affected. The condition may be as common as one in twenty thousand people in some European countries.

Symptoms

Symptoms can be seen after a baby starts eating food or formula.

The early symptoms of fructose intolerance are similar to those of galactosemia. Later symptoms relate more to liver disease.

Symptoms may include:

- convulsions;
- excessive sleepiness;
- irritability;
- jaundice;

- poor feeding as a baby;
- problems after eating fruits and fructose/sucrose-containing foods;
- vomiting.

Exams and Tests

Physical examination may show:

- enlarged liver and spleen (hepatosplenomegaly);
- yellow skin or eyes.

Tests that confirm the diagnosis include:

- blood clotting tests;
- blood sugar test;
- enzyme studies;
- genetic testing;
- kidney function tests;
- liver function tests;
- liver biopsy;
- uric acid blood test;
- urinalysis.

Blood sugar will be low, especially after receiving fructose or sucrose. Uric acid levels will be high.

Treatment

Removing fructose and sucrose from the diet is an effective treatment for most patients. Complications are treated. For example, some patients can take medication to lower the level of uric acid in their blood and decrease their risk for gout.

Outlook (Prognosis)

Hereditary fructose intolerance may be mild or severe.
Avoiding fructose and sucrose helps most children with this condition.

A few children with a severe form of the disease will develop severe liver disease. Even removing fructose and sucrose from the diet may not prevent severe liver disease in these children.

How well a person does depends on:

- how soon the diagnosis is made;

- how soon fructose and sucrose can be removed from the diet;

- how well the enzyme works in the body.

Possible Complications

- Avoidance of fructose-containing foods due to their effects

- Bleeding

- Death

- Gout

- Illness from eating foods containing fructose or sucrose

- Liver failure

- Low blood sugar (hypoglycemia)

- Seizures

When to Contact a Medical Professional

Call your health care provider if your child develops symptoms of this condition after feeding starts. If your child has this condition, experts recommend seeing a doctor who specializes in biochemical genetics or metabolism.

Prevention

Couples with a family history of fructose intolerance who wish to have a baby may consider genetic counseling.

Most of the damaging effects of the disease can be prevented by sticking to a fructose-free diet.

Alternative Names

Fructosemia; Fructose intolerance; Fructose aldolase B-deficiency; Fructose 1, 6 bisphosphate aldolase deficiency

References

Steinmann B, Santer R, van den Berghe G. Disorders of Fructose Metabolism. In: Fernandes J, Saudubray JM, van den Berghe G, Walter JH, eds. *Inborn Metabolic Diseases. 4th ed.* New York, NY: Springer; 2006:chap 9.

Section 23.3

Galactosemia

What is galactosemia?

Galactosemia is a rare disorder that affects the body's ability to break down a food sugar called galactose (found in milk and other dairy products).

The body breaks down lactose into galactose and glucose and uses these sugars for energy. Most people with galactosemia are missing an enzyme (called GALT) that helps further break down galactose. Defects in galactose metabolism cause toxic chemicals to build up in cells of the body.

How do people get galactosemia?

The most common form of the disorder, classic galactosemia, is passed down in an autosomal recessive pattern. To get the disorder, a child must inherit one defective gene from each parent. Inheriting one normal gene and one mutated gene makes a person a carrier. A carrier produces less of the GALT enzyme than normal, but is still able to break down galactose and avoid having symptoms of galactosemia. However, carriers can still pass on the mutated gene to their children.

What are the symptoms of galactosemia?

Defects in galactose metabolism can cause several severe symptoms: kidney failure, an enlarged liver, cataracts (clouding of the eye lens), poor growth, and mental retardation.

People can inherit a milder form of the disorder when a different gene, also involved in galactose metabolism, is mutated. These patients often suffer from cataracts, but not the other symptoms associated with classical galactosemia.

How do doctors diagnose galactosemia?

In most states, babies are tested for galactosemia at birth. Using a tiny blood sample taken from the baby's heel, the test checks for low levels of the GALT enzyme. This allows for prompt treatment, which can substantially prevent the serious symptoms of this disorder.

For those families with a history of the disorder, a doctor can determine during a woman's pregnancy whether her baby has galactosemia: (1) by taking a sample of fluid from around the fetus (amniocentesis), or (2) by taking a sample of fetal cells from the placenta (chorionic villus sampling or CVS).

How is galactosemia treated?

The only way to treat galactosemia is through dietary restrictions. People with the disorder must stay away from foods and drinks containing galactose, including milk, cheese, and legumes (dried beans).

Interesting Facts about Galactosemia

- Galactosemia was first discovered in 1908 by the physician Von Ruess.

- Classical galactosemia affects one in every fifty-five thousand newborns.

Section 23.4

Homocystinuria

© 2013 A.D.A.M., Inc. Reprinted with permission.

Homocystinuria is an inherited disorder that affects the metabolism of the amino acid methionine.

Causes

Homocystinuria is inherited in families as an autosomal recessive trait. This means that the child must inherit the nonworking gene from both parents to be seriously affected.

Homocystinuria has several features in common with Marfan syndrome. Unlike Marfan syndrome, in which the joints tend to be "loose," in homocystinuria the joints tend to be "tight."

Symptoms

Newborn infants appear healthy. Early symptoms, if present at all, are not obvious.

Symptoms may occur as mildly delayed development or failure to thrive. Increasing visual problems may lead to diagnosis of this condition.

Other symptoms include:

- chest deformities (pectus carinatum, pectus excavatum);

- flush across the cheeks;

- high arches of the feet;

- intellectual disability;

- knock knees;

- long limbs;

- mental disorders;

- nearsightedness;

- spidery fingers (arachnodactyly);

- tall, thin build.

Exams and Tests

The health care provider may notice that the child is tall and thin (Marfanoid).

Other signs include:

- curved spine (scoliosis);

- deformity of the chest;

- dislocated lens of the eye.

If there is poor or double vision, an ophthalmologist should perform a dilated eye exam to look for dislocation of the lens or nearsightedness.

There may be a history of blood clots. Intellectual disability, slightly low IQ, or mental illness are common.

Tests:

- amino acid screen of blood and urine;

- genetic testing;

- liver biopsy and enzyme assay;

- skeletal x-ray;

- skin biopsy with a fibroblast culture;

- standard ophthalmic exam.

Treatment

There is no cure for homocystinuria. However, just under half of people respond to high doses of vitamin B6 (also known as pyridoxine).

Those who do respond will need to take vitamin B6 supplements for the rest of their lives. Those who do not respond will need to eat a low-methionine diet. Most will need to be treated with trimethylglycine (a medication also known as betaine).

Neither a low-methionine diet nor medication will improve existing intellectual disability. Medication and diet should be closely supervised by a physician who has experience treating homocystinuria.

Taking a folic acid supplement and adding cysteine (an amino acid) to the diet are helpful.

Outlook (Prognosis)

Although no cure exists for homocystinuria, vitamin B6 therapy can help about half of people affected by the condition.

If the diagnosis is made while a patient is young, starting a low-methionine diet quickly can prevent some intellectual disability and other complications of the disease. For this reason, some states screen for homocystinuria in all newborns.

Patients whose blood homocysteine levels continue to rise are at increased risk for blood clots. Clots can cause serious medical problems and shorten lifespan.

Possible Complications

Most serious complications result from blood clots. These episodes can be life threatening.

Dislocated lenses of the eyes can seriously damage vision. Lens replacement surgery should be considered.

Intellectual disability is a serious consequence of the disease. However, it can be reduced if diagnosed early.

When to Contact a Medical Professional

Call your health care provider if you or a family member shows symptoms of this disorder, especially if you have a family history of homocystinuria. Also call if you have a family history and are planning to have children.

Prevention

Genetic counseling is recommended for people with a family history of homocystinuria who want to have children. Intrauterine diagnosis of homocystinuria is available. This involves culturing amniotic cells or chorionic villi to test for cystathionine synthase (the enzyme that is missing in homocystinuria).

If there are known gene mutations in the parents or family, samples from chorionic villus sampling or amniocentesis can be used to test for these mutations.

Alternative Names

Cystathionine beta synthase deficiency

References

Rezvani I, Melvin JJ. Defects in metabolism of amino acids. In: Kliegman RM, Stanton BF, St. Geme J, Schor N, Behrman RE, eds. *Nelson Textbook of Pediatrics. 19th ed.* Philadelphia, Pa: Saunders Elsevier; 2011:chap 79.

Section 23.5

Maple Syrup Urine Disease

What is maple syrup urine disease (MSUD)?

MSUD is a potentially deadly disorder that affects the way the body breaks down three amino acids, leucine, isoleucine, and valine. When they're not being used to build a protein, these three amino acids can be either recycled or broken down and used for energy. They are normally broken down by six proteins that act as a team and form a complex called BCKD (branched-chain alpha-ketoacid dehydrogenase).

People with MSUD have a mutation that results in a deficiency for one of the six proteins that make up this complex. Therefore, they can't break down leucine, isoleucine, and valine. They end up with dangerously high levels of these amino acids in their blood, causing the rapid degeneration of brain cells and death if left untreated.

Defects in any of the six subunits that make up the BCKD protein complex can cause the development of MSUD. The most common defect is caused by a mutation in a gene on chromosome 19 that encodes the alpha subunit of the BCKD complex (BCKDHA).

How do people get MSUD?

MSUD is inherited in an autosomal recessive pattern. For a child to get the disease, he or she must inherit a defective copy of the gene from each parent. If both parents carry the MSUD gene, each of their children has a 25 percent chance of getting the disorder, and a 50 percent chance of being a carrier.

What are the symptoms of MSUD?

There is a classic form of MSUD and several less common forms. Each form varies in its severity and characteristic features. However, all subtypes of the disorder can be caused by mutations in any of the six genes used to build the BCKD protein complex.

A baby who has the disorder may appear normal at birth. But within three to four days, the symptoms appear. These may include: loss of appetite, fussiness, and sweet-smelling urine. The elevated levels of amino acids in the urine generate the smell, which is reminiscent of maple syrup. This is how MSUD got its name. If left untreated, the condition usually worsens. The baby will have seizures, go into a coma, and die within the first few months of life.

How do doctors diagnose MSUD?

In some states, all babies are screened for MSUD within twenty-four hours after birth. A blood sample taken from the baby's heel is analyzed for high leucine levels.

How is MSUD treated?

Treatment involves dietary restriction of the amino acids leucine, isoleucine, and valine. This treatment must begin very early to prevent brain damage. Babies with the disease must eat a special formula that does not contain the amino acids leucine, isoleucine, and valine. As the person grows to adulthood, he or she must always watch his or her diet, avoiding high-protein foods such as meat, eggs, and nuts.

If levels of the three amino acids still get too high, patients can be treated with an intravenous (given through a vein) solution that helps the body use up excess leucine, isoleucine, and valine for protein synthesis.

Gene therapy is also a potential future treatment for patients with MSUD. This would involve replacing the mutated gene with a good copy, allowing the patient's cells to generate a functional BCKD protein complex and break down the excess amino acids.

Interesting Facts about MSUD

MSUD is an extremely rare disorder; only 1 in 180,000 babies is born with MSUD. But in certain populations, the disease is much more common. Among the Mennonites in Pennsylvania, as many as 1 out of every 176 babies is born with the disorder.

Section 23.6

Medium Chain Acyl-Coenzyme A Dehydrogenase Deficiency

"Medium-Chain Acyl-CoA Dehydrogenase Deficiency (MCAD)," a Family Fact Sheet from the Minnesota Newborn Screening Program, 601 Robert St. N., St. Paul, MN 55155, Phone: (800) 664-7772; Fax: (651) 201-5471. © 2012 Minnesota Department of Health. Reprinted with permission. For additional information, visit www.health.state.mn.us/ newbornscreening.

What is a positive newborn screen?

Newborn screening is done on tiny samples of blood taken from your baby's heel twenty-four to forty-eight hours after birth. Newborn screening tests for rare, hidden disorders that may affect your baby's health and development. The newborn screen suggests your baby might have a disorder called MCAD (em-cad).

A positive newborn screen does not mean your baby has MCAD, but it does mean your baby needs more testing to know for sure.

Your baby's doctor will help arrange for more testing by specialists in disorders like MCAD.

What is MCAD?

MCAD affects an enzyme needed to break down fats in the food we eat, so they can be used for energy and growth. In MCAD, an enzyme used to break down fats is missing or not working properly.

A person who has MCAD doesn't have enough enzyme to break down fat into energy. Using stored fat for energy is especially important between meals when the body is not getting new energy from eating food.

MCAD is a disorder that is passed on, or inherited, from a child's mother and father.

Because MCAD is a genetic disease, family members are at risk of having MCAD too, even if no one in the family has had it before.

What problems can MCAD cause?

MCAD is different for each child. Some children with MCAD have only a few health problems, while other children may have serious complications.

If MCAD is not treated, a child might develop:

- serious illness (metabolic crisis);

- sleepiness or little energy;

- behavior changes (such as crying for no reason);

- irritable mood;

- poor appetite;

- seizures;

- coma.

It is very important to follow the doctor's instructions for testing and treatment.

What is the treatment for MCAD?

There are treatments for children with MCAD, which are lifelong. Treatments for children with MCAD can include:

- frequent meals/snacks and low fat/high carb diet—a dietician will help you set up the best diet for your child;

- medications to help the body make energy and get rid of harmful toxins;

- careful treatment for routine illnesses.

Children with MCAD should see their regular doctor, a doctor who specializes in MCAD, and a dietician.

Children with MCAD can benefit from prompt and careful treatment.

Section 23.7

Methylmalonic Acidemia

Methylmalonic acidemia is a disorder, passed down through families, in which the body cannot break down certain proteins and fats. The result is a buildup of a substance called methylmalonic acid in the blood.

It is considered an inborn error of metabolism.

Causes

The disease is usually diagnosed in the first year of life. It is an autosomal recessive disorder, which means the defective gene must be passed onto the child from both parents.

About one in twenty-five thousand to forty-eight thousand babies are born with this condition. However, the actual rate may be higher, because a newborn may die before the condition is ever diagnosed. Methylmalonic acidemia affects boys and girls equally.

Symptoms

The disease can cause seizures and stroke. Babies may appear normal at birth, but develop symptoms once they start eating more protein, which can cause the condition to get worse.

Symptoms include:

- brain disease that gets worse (progressive encephalopathy);
- dehydration;
- developmental delays;
- failure to thrive;
- lethargy;
- repeated yeast infections;
- seizures;
- vomiting.

Exams and Tests

Testing for methylmalonic acidemia is often done as part of a newborn screening exam. The U.S. Department of Health and Human Services recommends screening for this condition at birth because early detection and treatment has been shown to be beneficial.

Tests that may be done to diagnose this condition include:

- ammonia test;
- blood gases;
- complete blood count;
- computed tomography (CT) scan or magnetic resonance imaging (MRI) of the brain;
- electrolyte levels;
- genetic testing;
- methylmalonic acid blood test;
- plasma amino acid test.

Treatment

Treatment consists of cobalamin and carnitine supplements and a low-protein diet. The child's diet must be carefully controlled.

If supplements do not help, the doctor may also recommend a diet that avoids substances called isoleucine, threonine, methionine, and valine.

Liver or kidney transplantation (or both) have been shown to help some patients. These transplants provide the body with new cells that help break down methylmalonic acid normally.

Outlook (Prognosis)

Patients may not survive their first attack.

Possible Complications

- Coma
- Death
- Kidney failure

When to Contact a Medical Professional

Seek immediate medical help if a child is having a seizure for the first time. See a pediatrician if your child has signs of failure to thrive or developmental delays.

Prevention

A low-protein maintenance diet can help to reduce the number of acidemia attacks. Persons with this condition should avoid those who are sick.

Genetic counseling may be helpful for couples with a family history of this disorder who wish to have a baby.

Some places have expanded newborn screening done at birth, which includes screening for methylmalonic acidemia. You can ask your doctor if this was done on your child.

References

Rezvani I. Defects in metabolism of amino acids. In: Kliegman RM, Behrman RE, Jenson HB, Stanton BF, eds. *Nelson Textbook of Pediatrics. 18th ed*. Philadelphia, Pa: Saunders Elsevier; 2007:chap 85.

Section 23.8

Phenylketonuria (PKU)

Excerpted from "Learning about Phenylketonuria (PKU)," National Human Genome Research Institute (www.genome.gov), National Institutes of Health, August 15, 2012.

What is phenylketonuria (PKU)?

Phenylketonuria (PKU) is an inherited disorder of metabolism that causes an increase in the blood of a chemical known as phenylalanine. Phenylalanine comes from a person's diet and is used by the body to make proteins. Phenylalanine is found in all food proteins and in some artificial sweeteners. Without dietary treatment, phenylalanine can build up to harmful levels in the body, causing mental retardation and other serious problems.

Women who have high levels of phenylalanine during pregnancy are at high risk for having babies born with mental retardation, heart problems, small head size (microcephaly), and developmental delay. This is because the babies are exposed to their mother's very high levels of phenylalanine before they are born.

In the United States, PKU occurs in one in ten thousand to one in fifteen thousand newborn babies. Newborn screening has been used to detect PKU since the 1960s. As a result, the severe signs and symptoms of PKU are rarely seen.

What are the symptoms of PKU?

Symptoms of PKU range from mild to severe. Severe PKU is called classic PKU. Infants born with classic PKU appear normal for the first few months after birth. However, without treatment with a low-phenylalanine diet, these infants will develop mental retardation and behavioral problems. Other common symptoms of untreated classic PKU include seizures, developmental delay, and autism. Boys and girls who have classic PKU may also have eczema of the skin and lighter skin and hair than their family members who do not have PKU.

Babies born with less severe forms of PKU (moderate or mild PKU) may have a milder degree of mental retardation unless treated with the special diet. If the baby has only a very slight degree of PKU, often called mild hyperphenylalaninemia, there may be no problems and the special dietary treatment may not be needed.

How is PKU diagnosed?

PKU is usually diagnosed through newborn screening testing that is done shortly after birth on a blood sample (heel stick). However, PKU should be considered at any age in a person who has developmental delays or mental retardation. This is because, rarely, infants are missed by newborn screening programs.

What is the treatment for PKU?

PKU is treated by limiting the amount of protein (that contains phenylalanine) in the diet. Treatment also includes using special medical foods as well as special low-protein foods and taking vitamins and minerals. People who have PKU need to follow this diet for their lifetime. It is especially important for women who have PKU to follow the diet throughout their childbearing years.

Is PKU inherited?

PKU is inherited in families in an autosomal recessive pattern. Autosomal recessive inheritance means that a person has two copies of the gene that is altered. Usually, each parent of an individual who

251

has PKU carries one copy of the altered gene. Since each parent also has a normal gene, they do not show signs or symptoms of PKU.

Gene alterations (mutations) in the PAH gene cause PKU. Mutations in the PAH gene cause low levels of an enzyme called phenylalanine hydroxylase. These low levels mean that phenylalanine from a person's diet cannot be metabolized (changed), so it builds up to toxic levels in the bloodstream and body. Having too much phenylalanine can cause brain damage unless diet treatment is started.

Section 23.9

Tyrosinemia

Excerpted from "Tyrosinemia," Genetics Home Reference (http://ghr.nlm.nih.gov), January 2008. Reviewed by David A. Cooke, M.D., FACP, May 2013.

What is tyrosinemia?

Tyrosinemia is a genetic disorder characterized by elevated blood levels of the amino acid tyrosine, a building block of most proteins. Tyrosinemia is caused by the shortage (deficiency) of one of the enzymes required for the multistep process that breaks down tyrosine. If untreated, tyrosine and its byproducts build up in tissues and organs, which leads to serious medical problems.

There are three types of tyrosinemia. Each has distinctive symptoms and is caused by the deficiency of a different enzyme. Type I tyrosinemia, the most severe form of this disorder, is caused by a shortage of the enzyme fumarylacetoacetate hydrolase. Symptoms usually appear in the first few months of life and include failure to gain weight and grow at the expected rate (failure to thrive), diarrhea, vomiting, yellowing of the skin and whites of the eyes (jaundice), cabbage-like odor, and increased tendency to bleed (particularly nosebleeds). Type I tyrosinemia can lead to liver and kidney failure, problems affecting the nervous system, and an increased risk of liver cancer.

Type II tyrosinemia is caused by a deficiency of the enzyme tyrosine aminotransferase. This form of the disorder can affect the eyes, skin, and mental development. Symptoms often begin in early childhood and include excessive tearing, abnormal sensitivity to light (photophobia), eye pain and redness, and painful skin lesions on the palms and soles. About 50 percent of individuals with type II tyrosinemia have some degree of intellectual disability.

Type III tyrosinemia is a rare disorder caused by a deficiency of the enzyme 4-hydroxyphenylpyruvate dioxygenase. Characteristic features include intellectual disability, seizures, and periodic loss of balance and coordination (intermittent ataxia).

About 10 percent of newborns have temporarily elevated levels of tyrosine. In these cases, the cause is not genetic. The most likely causes are vitamin C deficiency or immature liver enzymes due to premature birth.

How common is tyrosinemia?

Worldwide, type I tyrosinemia affects about 1 person in 100,000. This type of tyrosinemia is much more common in Quebec, Canada. The overall incidence in Quebec is about 1 in 16,000 individuals. In the Saguenay-Lac St. Jean region of Quebec, type I tyrosinemia affects 1 person in 1,846.

Type II tyrosinemia occurs in fewer than 1 in 250,000 individuals. Type III tyrosinemia is very rare; only a few cases have been reported.

What genes are related to tyrosinemia?

Mutations in the FAH, HPD, and TAT genes cause tyrosinemia.

In the liver, enzymes break down tyrosine in a five-step process into harmless molecules that are either excreted by the kidneys or used in reactions that produce energy. Mutations in the FAH, HPD, or TAT gene cause a shortage of one of the enzymes in this multistep process. The resulting enzyme deficiency leads to a toxic accumulation of tyrosine and its byproducts, which can damage the liver, kidneys, nervous system, and other organs and tissues.

How do people inherit tyrosinemia?

This condition is inherited in an autosomal recessive pattern, which means both copies of the gene in each cell have mutations. The parents of an individual with an autosomal recessive condition each carry one copy of the mutated gene, but they typically do not show signs and symptoms of the condition.

Section 23.10

Urea Cycle Defects

Excerpted from "Hereditary Urea Cycle Abnormality,"
© 2013 A.D.A.M., Inc. Reprinted with permission.

Hereditary urea cycle abnormality is an inherited condition that can cause problems with the removal of waste from the body in the urine.

Causes

The urea cycle is a process in which waste (ammonia) is removed from the body. When you eat proteins, the body breaks them down into amino acids. Ammonia is produced from leftover amino acids, and it must be removed from the body.

The liver produces several chemicals (enzymes) that change ammonia into a form called urea, which the body can remove in the urine. If this process is disturbed, ammonia levels begin to rise.

Several inherited conditions can cause problems with this waste-removal process. People with a urea cycle disorder are missing a gene that makes the enzymes needed to break down ammonia in the body.

These diseases include:

- argininosuccinic aciduria;
- arginase deficiency;
- carbamyl phosphate synthetase (CPS) deficiency;
- citrullinemia;
- N-acetyl glutamate synthetase deficiency (NAGS);
- ornithine transcarbamylase deficiency (OTC).

As a group, these disorders occur in one in thirty thousand newborns. Ornithine transcarbamylase deficiency is the most common of these disorders.

Boys are more often affected by ornithine transcarbamylase deficiency than girls. Girls are rarely affected. Those girls who are affected have milder symptoms and develop the disease later in life.

To get the other types of disorders, you need to receive a nonworking copy of the gene from both parents. Sometimes parents don't know they carry the gene until their child gets the disorder.

Symptoms

Typically, the baby begins nursing well and seems normal. However, over time the baby develops poor feeding, vomiting, and sleepiness which may be so deep that the baby is difficult to awaken. This usually occurs within the first week after birth.

Symptoms include:

- confusion;
- decreased food intake;
- disliking protein-containing foods;
- increased sleepiness, difficulty waking up;
- nausea, vomiting.

Exams and Tests

The doctor will often diagnose these disorders when the child is still an infant.

Signs may include:

- abnormal amino acids in blood and urine;
- abnormal level of orotic acid in blood or urine;
- high blood ammonia level;
- normal level of acid in blood.

Tests may include:

- genetic tests;
- liver biopsy;
- magnetic resonance imaging (MRI) or computed tomography (CT) scan.

Treatment

Limiting protein in the diet can help treat these disorders by reducing the amount of nitrogen wastes the body produces. Special low-protein infant and toddler formulas are available.

It is important that a health care provider guide protein intake. The health care provider can balance the amount of protein so that the baby has enough to grow, but not enough to cause symptoms.

It is extremely important for people with these disorders to avoid fasting.

People with urea cycle abnormalities must also be very careful under times of stress, such as when they have infections. Stress, such as a fever, can cause the body to break down its own proteins. These extra proteins can make it difficult for the abnormal urea cycle to remove the byproducts.

Develop a plan with your doctor for when you are sick to avoid all protein, drink high-carbohydrate drinks, and get enough fluids.

Most patients with urea cycle disorders will need to stay in the hospital at some point. During such times, they may be treated with medicines that help the body remove nitrogen-containing wastes. Dialysis may help rid the body of excess ammonia during extreme illness.

Outlook (Prognosis)

How well patients do depends on:

- which urea cycle abnormality they have;
- how severe it is;
- how early it is discovered;
- how closely they follow a protein-restricted diet.

Babies diagnosed in the first week of life and put on a protein-restricted diet right away do well.

Sticking to the diet can lead to normal adult intelligence. Repeatedly not following the diet or having stress-induced symptoms can lead to brain swelling and brain damage.

Major stresses, such as surgery or accidents, can be complicated for these patients. Extreme care is needed to avoid problems during such periods.

Possible Complications

- Coma
- Confusion and eventually disorientation
- Death
- Increases in blood ammonia level

- Swelling of the brain

When to Contact a Medical Professional

If your child has a test that shows increased ammonia in the blood, have the child examined by a genetic or metabolic specialist. If there is a family history of urea cycle disorder, seek genetic counseling before trying to get pregnant.

A dietician is important to help plan and update a protein-restricted diet as the child grows.

Prevention

As with most inherited diseases, there is no way to prevent these disorders. Prenatal testing is available. Genetic testing before an embryo is implanted may be available for those using in vitro fertilization.

Teamwork between parents, the affected child, and doctors can help prevent severe illness.

Alternative Names

Abnormality of the urea cycle—hereditary; Urea cycle—hereditary abnormality

References

Balistreri WF, Carey RG. Metabolic diseases of the liver. In: Kliegman RM, Stanton BF, St. Geme J, Schor N, Behrman RE, eds. *Nelson Textbook of Pediatrics. 19th ed*. Philadelphia, Pa: Saunders Elsevier; 2011:chap 349.

Chapter 24

Kidney and Urinary System Disorders

Chapter Contents

Section 24.1

Cystinuria

"Learn More: Cystinuria," Rare Diseases Clinical Research Network, National Institutes of Health. The full text of this document may be accessed online at http://rarediseasesnetwork.epi.usf.edu/RKSC/cystinuria/; accessed September 12, 2012.

What is cystinuria?

Cystinuria is an inherited disease of amino acid transport affecting the absorption of four structurally similar amino acids from excretory pathways. In all people, cystine, ornithine, lysine, and arginine are filtered from the blood into the urine. Normally, those amino acids are reclaimed from the urine for recirculation in the blood. However, cystinuric patients lack the necessary ability to transport those molecules. As a result, they become concentrated in the urine, where cystine, being uniquely insoluble, tends to crystallize and form cystine stones. The result is recurring stone formation. These stones can pass spontaneously; however, larger stones may become stuck in the urinary tract and require surgical intervention for removal. Frequent stone formation, kidney blockage, surgical procedures, and resulting consequences can impact kidney function over time.

Who gets cystinuria?

Cystinuria is a genetic condition passed from parents to children. It is generally accepted that one in ten thousand people worldwide are cystinuric. However, as with any genetic disease, the prevalence can vary greatly among communities. As a genetic condition, the disease is present from birth and persists for life. However, symptoms, including kidney stone formation, may not occur immediately. While some patients form stones at infancy, others may not be aware of their disease until decades later. Some cystinuric people will never form kidney stones, despite having high urinary cystine concentrations. The underlying cause of why some people seem to be more affected than others is currently unknown.

What causes cystinuria?

When genes responsible for making specific transport proteins are defective, the transport system fails to transport cystine from the urine. These defective gene copies are inherited from parents and cannot be changed. When cystine cannot be absorbed from the urine, it can concentrate to a point where it forms solid crystals that grow into stones in the urinary tract. Ornithine, arginine, and lysine also accumulate in the urine, but are generally soluble even at the elevated concentrations and do not impact the health of the patient.

How is cystinuria diagnosed?

Cystinuria is usually diagnosed when a person goes to the doctor with the symptoms of kidney stones (generally pain called "renal colic"), and those stones are later found through lab analysis to be composed of cystine. Cystine crystals in the urine are also a diagnostic symptom of the disease. In some areas, genetic screening programs have identified cystinuric individuals based directly on finding the defective copies of the cystine transporter gene. Interestingly, not all people genetically identified as cystinuric go on to be stone-forming patients, indicating that not all people with the disease are equally affected by the symptoms.

What is/is there treatment for cystinuria?

As cystinuric is a genetic disease, it cannot be fundamentally cured. Treatment is instead focused on reducing the occurrence of resulting kidney stone formation. All current efforts are aimed at preventing stone formation by decreasing the amount of solid cystine in the urinary tract. Cystine solubility can be improved by increasing urine volume (by consistently drinking large quantities of fluids) or decreasing urinary cystine excretion via dietary changes like reducing salt and protein intake. Cystine becomes more soluble as urinary acidity decreases, and therefore diets (high in vegetables) or medication (bicarbonate or citrate compounds) that promote less-acidic urine are considered powerful in reducing the rate of stone formation. Finally, for the most severely affected patients, medications are available that break apart the cystine and form more soluble complexes. These medications may not be well tolerated by the patient, and therefore careful monitoring is necessary to determine the lowest effective dose necessary.

Section 24.2

Polycystic Kidney Disease

Excerpted from "Polycystic Kidney Disease,"
National Institute of Diabetes and Digestive and Kidney Diseases,
National Institutes of Health, September 2, 2010.

Polycystic kidney disease (PKD) is a genetic disorder characterized by the growth of numerous cysts in the kidneys. The kidneys are two organs, each about the size of a fist, located in the upper part of a person's abdomen, toward the back. The kidneys filter wastes and extra fluid from the blood to form urine. They also regulate amounts of certain vital substances in the body. When cysts form in the kidneys, they are filled with fluid. PKD cysts can profoundly enlarge the kidneys while replacing much of the normal structure, resulting in reduced kidney function and leading to kidney failure.

When PKD causes kidneys to fail—which usually happens after many years—the patient requires dialysis or kidney transplantation. About one-half of people with the most common type of PKD progress to kidney failure, also called end-stage renal disease (ESRD).

PKD can also cause cysts in the liver and problems in other organs, such as blood vessels in the brain and heart. The number of cysts as well as the complications they cause help doctors distinguish PKD from the usually harmless "simple" cysts that often form in the kidneys in later years of life.

In the United States, about six hundred thousand people have PKD, and cystic disease is the fourth leading cause of kidney failure.[1] Two major inherited forms of PKD exist:

- Autosomal dominant PKD is the most common inherited form. Symptoms usually develop between the ages of 30 and 40, but they can begin earlier, even in childhood. About 90 percent of all PKD cases are autosomal dominant PKD.

- Autosomal recessive PKD is a rare inherited form. Symptoms of autosomal recessive PKD begin in the earliest months of life, even in the womb.

Autosomal Dominant PKD

What is autosomal dominant PKD?

Autosomal dominant PKD is the most common inherited disorder of the kidneys. The phrase "autosomal dominant" means that if one parent has the disease, there is a 50 percent chance that the disease gene will pass to a child. In some cases—perhaps 10 percent—autosomal dominant PKD occurs spontaneously in patients. In these cases, neither of the parents carries a copy of the disease gene.

Many people with autosomal dominant PKD live for several decades without developing symptoms. For this reason, autosomal dominant PKD is often called "adult polycystic kidney disease." Yet, in some cases, cysts may form earlier in life and grow quickly, causing symptoms in childhood.

The cysts grow out of nephrons, the tiny filtering units inside the kidneys. The cysts eventually separate from the nephrons and continue to enlarge. The kidneys enlarge along with the cysts—which can number in the thousands—while roughly retaining their kidney shape. In fully developed autosomal dominant PKD, a cyst-filled kidney can weigh as much as twenty to thirty pounds. High blood pressure is common and develops in most patients by age twenty or thirty.

What are the symptoms of autosomal dominant PKD?

The most common symptoms are pain in the back and the sides—between the ribs and the hips—and headaches. The pain can be temporary or persistent, mild or severe.

People with autosomal dominant PKD also can experience the following complications:

- Urinary tract infections—specifically, in the kidney cysts

- Hematuria—blood in the urine

- Liver and pancreatic cysts

- Abnormal heart valves

- High blood pressure

- Kidney stones

- Aneurysms—bulges in the walls of blood vessels—in the brain

- Diverticulosis—small pouches bulge outward through the colon

How is autosomal dominant PKD diagnosed?

Autosomal dominant PKD is usually diagnosed by kidney imaging studies. The most common form of diagnostic kidney imaging is ultrasound, but more precise studies, such as computerized tomography (CT) scans or magnetic resonance imaging (MRI) are also widely used. In autosomal dominant PKD, the onset of kidney damage and how quickly the disease progresses can vary. Kidney imaging findings can also vary considerably, depending on a patient's age. Younger patients usually have both fewer and smaller cysts. Doctors have therefore developed specific criteria for diagnosing the disease with kidney imaging findings, depending on patient age. For example, the presence of at least two cysts in each kidney by age thirty in a patient with a family history of the disease can confirm the diagnosis of autosomal dominant PKD. If there is any question about the diagnosis, a family history of autosomal dominant PKD and cysts found in other organs make the diagnosis more likely.

In most cases of autosomal dominant PKD, patients have no symptoms and their physical condition appears normal for many years, so the disease can go unnoticed. Physical checkups and blood and urine tests may not lead to early diagnosis. Because of the slow, undetected progression of cyst growth, some people live for many years without knowing they have autosomal dominant PKD.

Once cysts have grown to about one-half inch, however, diagnosis is possible with imaging technology. Ultrasound, which passes sound waves through the body to create a picture of the kidneys, is used most often. Ultrasound imaging does not use any injected dyes or radiation and is safe for all patients, including pregnant women. It can also detect cysts in the kidneys of a fetus, but large cyst growth this early in life is uncommon in autosomal dominant PKD.

More powerful and expensive imaging procedures such as CT scans and MRI also can detect cysts. Recently, MRI has been used to measure kidney and cyst volume and monitor kidney and cyst growth, which may serve as a way to track progression of the disease.

Diagnosis can also be made with a genetic test that detects mutations in the autosomal dominant PKD genes, called PKD1 and PKD2. Although this test can detect the presence of the autosomal dominant PKD mutations before large cysts develop, its usefulness is limited by two factors: detection of a disease gene cannot predict the onset of symptoms or ultimate severity of the disease, and if a disease gene is detected, no specific prevention or cure for the disease exists. However, a young person who knows of a PKD gene mutation may be able to forestall the loss of kidney function through diet and blood pressure control. The genetic test may also be used to determine whether a young member of a PKD family can safely donate a kidney to a family member with the disease. Individuals with a family history of PKD who are of childbearing age might also want to know whether they have the potential of passing a PKD gene to a child. Anyone considering genetic testing should receive counseling to understand all the implications of the test.

How is autosomal dominant PKD treated?

Although a cure for autosomal dominant PKD is not available, treatment can ease symptoms and prolong life.

Pain: Pain in the area of the kidneys can be caused by cyst infection, bleeding into cysts, kidney stones, or stretching of the fibrous tissue around the kidney with cyst growth. A doctor will first evaluate which of these causes are contributing to the pain to guide treatment. If it is determined to be chronic pain due to cyst expansion, the doctor may initially suggest over-the-counter pain medications, such as aspirin or acetaminophen (Tylenol). Consult your doctor before taking any over-the-counter medication because some may be harmful to the kidneys. For most but not all cases of severe pain due to cyst expansion, surgery to shrink cysts can relieve pain in the back and sides. However, surgery provides only temporary relief and does not slow the disease's progression toward kidney failure.

Headaches that are severe or that seem to feel different from other headaches might be caused by aneurysms—blood vessels that balloon out in spots—in the brain. These aneurysms could rupture, which can have severe consequences. Headaches also can be caused by high blood pressure. People with autosomal dominant PKD should see a doctor if they have severe or recurring headaches—even before considering over-the-counter pain medications.

Urinary tract infections: People with autosomal dominant PKD tend to have frequent urinary tract infections, which can be treated with antibiotics. People with the disease should seek treatment for urinary tract infections immediately because infection can spread from the urinary tract to the cysts in the kidneys. Cyst infections are difficult to treat because many antibiotics do not penetrate the cysts.

High blood pressure: Keeping blood pressure under control can slow the effects of autosomal dominant PKD. Lifestyle changes and various medications can lower high blood pressure. Patients should ask their doctors about such treatments. Sometimes proper diet and exercise are enough to keep blood pressure controlled.

End-stage renal disease (ESRD): After many years, PKD can cause the kidneys to fail. Because kidneys are essential for life, people with ESRD must seek one of two options for replacing kidney functions: dialysis or transplantation. In hemodialysis, blood is circulated into an external filter, where it is cleaned before reentering the body; in peritoneal dialysis, a fluid is introduced into the abdomen, where it absorbs wastes and is then removed. Transplantation of healthy kidneys into ESRD patients has become a common and successful procedure. Healthy non-PKD kidneys transplanted into PKD patients do not develop cysts.

Autosomal Recessive PKD

What is autosomal recessive PKD?

Autosomal recessive PKD is caused by a mutation in the autosomal recessive PKD gene, called PKHD1. Other genes for the disease might exist but have not yet been discovered by scientists. We all carry two copies of every gene. Parents who do not have PKD can have a child with the disease if both parents carry one copy of the abnormal gene and both pass that gene copy to their baby. The chance of the child having autosomal recessive PKD when both parents carry the abnormal gene is 25 percent. If only one parent carries the abnormal gene, the baby cannot get autosomal recessive PKD but could ultimately pass the abnormal gene to his or her children.

The signs of autosomal recessive PKD frequently begin before birth, so it is often called "infantile PKD." Children born with autosomal recessive PKD often, but not always, develop kidney failure before reaching adulthood. Severity of the disease varies. Babies with the worst cases die hours or days after birth due to respiratory difficulties or respiratory failure.

Some people with autosomal recessive PKD do not develop symptoms until later in childhood or even adulthood. Liver scarring occurs in all patients with autosomal recessive PKD and tends to become more of a medical concern with increasing age.

What are the symptoms of autosomal recessive PKD?

Children with autosomal recessive PKD experience high blood pressure, urinary tract infections, and frequent urination. The disease usually affects the liver and spleen, resulting in low blood cell counts, varicose veins, and hemorrhoids. Because kidney function is crucial for early physical development, children with autosomal recessive PKD and decreased kidney function are usually smaller than average size. Recent studies suggest that growth problems may be a primary feature of autosomal recessive PKD.

How is autosomal recessive PKD diagnosed?

Ultrasound imaging of the fetus or newborn reveals enlarged kidneys with an abnormal appearance, but large cysts such as those in autosomal dominant PKD are rarely seen. Because autosomal recessive PKD tends to scar the liver, ultrasound imaging of the liver also aids in diagnosis.

How is autosomal recessive PKD treated?

Medicines can control high blood pressure in autosomal recessive PKD, and antibiotics can control urinary tract infections. Eating increased amounts of nutritious food improves growth in children with autosomal recessive PKD. In some cases, growth hormones are used. In response to kidney failure, autosomal recessive PKD patients must receive dialysis or transplantation. If serious liver disease develops, some people can undergo combined liver and kidney transplantation.

Hope through Research

Scientists have begun to identify the processes that trigger formation of PKD cysts. Advances in the field of genetics have increased our understanding of the abnormal genes responsible for autosomal dominant and autosomal recessive PKD. Scientists have located two genes associated with autosomal dominant PKD. The first was located in 1985 on chromosome 16 and labeled PKD1. PKD2 was localized to chromosome 4 in 1993. Within three years, scientists had isolated the proteins these two genes produce—polycystin-1 and polycystin-2.

When both the PKD1 and PKD2 genes are normal, the proteins they produce work together to foster normal kidney development and inhibit cyst formation. A mutation in either of the genes can lead to cyst formation, but evidence suggests that disease development also requires other factors, in addition to the mutation in one of the PKD genes.

Genetic analyses of most families with PKD confirm mutations in either the PKD1 or PKD2 gene. In about 10 to 15 percent of cases, however, families with autosomal dominant PKD do not show obvious abnormalities or mutations in the PKD1 and PKD2 genes, using current testing methods.

Researchers have also recently identified the autosomal recessive PKD gene, called PKHD1, on chromosome 6. Genetic testing for autosomal recessive PKD to detect mutations in PKHD1 is now offered by a limited number of molecular genetic diagnostics laboratories in the United States.

Researchers have bred rodents with a genetic disease that parallels both inherited forms of human PKD. Studying these mice will lead to greater understanding of the genetic and nongenetic mechanisms involved in cyst formation. In recent years, researchers have discovered several compounds that appear to inhibit cyst formation in mice with the PKD gene. Some of these compounds are in clinical testing in humans. Scientists hope further testing will lead to safe and effective treatments for humans with the disease.

Recent clinical studies of autosomal dominant PKD are exploring new imaging methods for tracking progression of cystic kidney disease. These methods, using MRI, are helping scientists design better clinical trials for new treatments of autosomal dominant PKD.

References

1. Grantham JJ, Nair V, Winklhoffer F. Cystic diseases of the kidney. In: Brenner BM, ed. *Brenner & Rector's The Kidney. Vol. 2. 6th ed*. Philadelphia: WB Saunders Company; 2000: 1699–1730.

Chapter 25

Leukodystrophies

The leukodystrophies are a group of rare genetic disorders that affect the central nervous system by disrupting the growth or maintenance of the myelin sheath that insulates nerve cells. These disorders are progressive, meaning that they tend to get worse throughout the life of the patient. Below we describe the source of the disorders in more detail.

What is the nervous system?

In order to understand the leukodystrophies, we need to discuss some basic facts about the nervous system. The nervous system is made up of two main components: the central nervous system (CNS) and the peripheral nervous system (PNS). Together, these two systems interact to carry and receive signals that are responsible for nearly everything we do, including involuntary functions such as our heartbeat, and voluntary functions such as walking.

The CNS consists of the brain and the spinal cord, and contains billions of specialized cells known as neurons. Neurons have specialized projections called dendrites and axons that contribute to their unique function of transmitting signals throughout the body. Dendrites carry electrical signals to the neuron, while axons carry them away from the neuron.

The PNS consists of the rest of the neurons in the body. These include the sensory neurons, which detect any sensory stimuli and alert the CNS of their presence, and motor neurons, which connect the CNS to the muscles and carry out instructions from the CNS for movement.

What is myelin?

Myelin, sometimes referred to as "white matter" because of its white, fatty appearance, protects and insulates the axons. It consists of a protective sheath of many different molecules that include both lipids (fatty molecules) and proteins. This protective sheath acts in a manner very similar to that of the protective insulation that surrounds an electric wire; that is, it is necessary for the rapid transmission of electrical signals between neurons. It does this primarily by containing the electrical molecules within the axon so that they are all properly transmitted to the next neuron. With the protective myelin coat, neurons can transmit signals at speeds up to sixty meters per second. When the coat is damaged, the maximum speed can decrease by tenfold or more, since some of the signal is lost during transmission. This decrease in speed of signal transmission leads to significant disruption in the proper functioning of the nervous system.

What is a leukodystrophy?

The word leukodystrophy comes from the Greek words *leuko* (meaning white), trophy (meaning growth), and *dys* (meaning ill). If you put these words together, the word leukodystrophy describes a set of diseases that affect the growth or maintenance of the white matter (myelin).

How are the leukodystrophies different from one another?

All leukodystrophies are a result of problems with the growth or maintenance of the myelin sheath. However, there are many genes that are important in this process. For example, some genes are involved with the synthesis of the proteins needed for the myelin, while others are required for the proper transport of these proteins to their final location in the myelin sheath that covers the axons. Defects in any of the genes (called a mutation) may lead to a leukodystrophy. However, the symptoms of the individual leukodystrophies may vary because of the differences in their genetic cause.

How do you get leukodystrophy?

Leukodystrophies are mostly inherited disorders, meaning that they are passed on from parent to child. They may be inherited in a recessive, dominant, or X-linked manner, depending on the type of leukodystrophy.

There are some leukodystrophies that do not appear to be inherited, but rather arise spontaneously. They are still caused by a mutation in a particular gene, but it just means that the mutation was not inherited. In this case, the birth of one child with the disease does not necessarily increase the likelihood of a second child having the disease.

Are the leukodystrophies related to multiple sclerosis?

The leukodystrophies do share some common features with multiple sclerosis (MS). Like the leukodystrophies, MS is caused by the loss of myelin from the axons. However, the cause is different; whereas leukodystrophies are generally caused by a defect in one of the genes involved with the growth or maintenance of the myelin, MS is thought to be caused by an attack on the myelin by the body's own immune system.

Chapter 26

Lipid Storage Diseases

Chapter Contents

Section 26.1

Batten Disease

Excerpted from "Batten Disease Fact Sheet,"
National Institute of Neurological Disorders and Stroke,
National Institutes of Health, October 18, 2012.

What is Batten disease?

Batten disease is a fatal, inherited disorder of the nervous system that typically begins in childhood. Early symptoms of this disorder usually appear between the ages of five and ten years, when parents or physicians may notice a previously normal child has begun to develop vision problems or seizures. In some cases the early signs are subtle, taking the form of personality and behavior changes, slow learning, clumsiness, or stumbling. Over time, affected children suffer mental impairment, worsening seizures, and progressive loss of sight and motor skills. Eventually, children with Batten disease become blind, bedridden, and demented. Batten disease is often fatal by the late teens or twenties.

Batten disease is named after the British pediatrician who first described it in 1903. Also known as Spielmeyer-Vogt-Sjögren-Batten disease, it is the most common form of a group of disorders called the neuronal ceroid lipofuscinoses, or NCLs. Although Batten disease originally referred specifically to the juvenile form of NCL (JNCL), the term Batten disease is increasingly used by pediatricians to describe all forms of NCL.

What are the other forms of NCL?

There are four other main types of NCL, including three forms that begin earlier in childhood and a very rare form that strikes adults. The symptoms of these childhood types are similar to those caused by Batten disease, but they become apparent at different ages and progress at different rates:

- Congenital NCL is a very rare and severe form of NCL. Babies have abnormally small heads (microcephaly) and seizures, and die soon after birth.

- Infantile NCL (INCL or Santavuori-Haltia disease) begins between about ages six months and two years and progresses rapidly. Affected children fail to thrive and have microcephaly. Also typical are short, sharp muscle contractions called myoclonic jerks. These children usually die before age five, although some have survived in a vegetative state a few years longer.

- Late infantile NCL (LINCL, or Jansky-Bielschowsky disease) begins between ages two and four. The typical early signs are loss of muscle coordination (ataxia) and seizures that do not respond to drugs. This form progresses rapidly and ends in death between ages eight and twelve.

- Adult NCL (also known as Kufs disease, Parry disease, and ANCL) generally begins before age forty, causes milder symptoms that progress slowly, and does not cause blindness. Although age of death varies among affected individuals, this form does shorten life expectancy.

There are also "variant" forms of late-infantile NCL (vLINCL) that do not precisely conform to classical late-infantile NCL.

How many people have these disorders?

Batten disease and other forms of NCL are relatively rare, occurring in an estimated two to four of every one hundred thousand live births in the United States. These disorders appear to be more common in Finland, Sweden, other parts of northern Europe, and Newfoundland, Canada. Although NCLs are classified as rare diseases, they often strike more than one person in families that carry the defective genes.

How are NCLs inherited?

Childhood NCLs are autosomal recessive disorders; that is, they occur only when a child inherits two copies of the defective gene, one from each parent. When both parents carry one defective gene, each of their children faces a one in four chance of developing NCL. At the same time, each child also faces a one in two chance of inheriting just one copy of the defective gene. Individuals who have only one defective gene are known as carriers, meaning they do not develop the disease, but they can pass the gene on to their own children. Because the mutated genes that are involved in certain forms of Batten disease are known, carrier detection is possible in some instances.

Adult NCL may be inherited as an autosomal recessive or, less often, as an autosomal dominant disorder. In autosomal dominant inheritance, all people who inherit a single copy of the disease gene develop the disease. As a result, there are no unaffected carriers of the gene.

What causes these diseases?

Symptoms of Batten disease and other NCLs are linked to a buildup of substances called lipofuscins (lipopigments) in the body's tissues. These lipopigments are made up of fats and proteins. Their name comes from the technical word lipo, which is short for "lipid" or fat, and from the term pigment, used because they take on a greenish-yellow color when viewed under an ultraviolet light microscope. The lipopigments build up in cells of the brain and the eye as well as in skin, muscle, and many other tissues. The substances are found inside a part of cells called lysosomes. Lysosomes are responsible for getting rid of things that become damaged or are no longer needed and must be cleared from inside the cell. The accumulated lipopigments in Batten disease and the other NCLs form distinctive shapes that can be seen under an electron microscope. Some look like half-moons, others like fingerprints. These deposits are what doctors look for when they examine a skin sample to diagnose Batten disease. The specific appearance of the lipopigment deposits can be useful in guiding further diagnostic tests that may identify the specific gene defect.

To date, eight genes have been linked to the varying forms of NCL. Mutations of other genes in NCL are likely since some individuals do not have mutations in any of the known genes. More than one gene may be associated with a particular form of NCL. The known NCL genes are:

- CLN1, also known as PPT1, encodes an enzyme called palmitoyl-protein thioesterase 1 that is insufficiently active in infantile NCL.

- CLN 2, or TPP1, produces an enzyme called tripeptidyl peptidase 1—an acid protease that degrades proteins. The enzyme is insufficiently active in late infantile NCL (also referred to as CLN2).

- CLN3 mutation is the major cause of juvenile NCL. The gene codes for a protein called CLN3 or battenin, which is found in the membranes of the cell (most predominantly in lysosomes and in related structures called endosomes). The protein's function is currently unknown.

- CLN5, which causes variant late infantile NCL (vLINCL, also referred to as CLN5), produces a lysosomal protein called CLN5, whose function has not been identified.

- CLN6, which also causes late infantile NCL, encodes a protein called CLN6. The protein is found in the membranes of the cell (most predominantly in a structure called the endoplasmic reticulum). Its function has not been identified.

- MFSD8, seen in variant late infantile NCL (also referred to as CLN7), encodes the MFSD8 protein that is a member of a protein family called the major facilitator superfamily. This superfamily is involved with transporting substances across the cell membranes. The precise function of MFSD8 has not been identified.

- CLN8 causes progressive epilepsy with mental retardation. The gene encodes a protein also called CLN8, which is found in the membranes of the cell—most predominantly in the endoplasmic reticulum. The protein's function has not been identified.

- CTSD, involved with congenital NCL (also referred to as CLN10), encodes cathepsin D, a lysosomal enzyme that breaks apart other proteins. A deficiency of cathepsin D causes the disorder.

How are these disorders diagnosed?

Because vision loss is often an early sign, Batten disease may be first suspected during an eye exam. An eye doctor can detect a loss of cells within the eye that occurs in the childhood forms of NCL. However, because such cell loss occurs in other eye diseases, the disorder cannot be diagnosed by this sign alone. Often an eye specialist or other physician who suspects NCL may refer the child to a neurologist for additional testing.

In order to diagnose NCL, the neurologist needs the individual's medical and family history and information from various laboratory tests. Diagnostic tests used for NCLs include:

- **Blood or urine tests:** These tests can detect abnormalities that may indicate Batten disease. For example, elevated levels of a chemical called dolichol are found in the urine of many individuals with NCL. The presence of vacuolated lymphocytes—white blood cells that contain holes or cavities (observed by microscopic analysis of blood smears)—when combined with other findings that indicate NCL, is suggestive for the juvenile form caused by CLN3 mutations.

- **Skin or tissue sampling:** The doctor can examine a small piece of tissue under an electron microscope. The powerful magnification of the microscope helps the doctor spot typical NCL deposits. These deposits are common in skin cells, especially those from sweat glands.

- **Electroencephalogram or EEG:** An EEG uses special patches placed on the scalp to record electrical currents inside the brain. This helps doctors see telltale patterns in the brain's electrical activity that suggest an individual has seizures.

- **Electrical studies of the eyes:** These tests, which include visual-evoked responses and electroretinograms, can detect various eye problems common in childhood NCLs.

- **Diagnostic imaging using computed tomography (CT) or magnetic resonance imaging (MRI):** Diagnostic imaging can help doctors look for changes in the brain's appearance. CT uses x-rays and a computer to create a sophisticated picture of the brain's tissues and structures, and may reveal brain areas that are decaying, or "atrophic," in persons with NCL. MRI uses a combination of magnetic fields and radio waves, instead of radiation, to create a picture of the brain.

- **Measurement of enzyme activity:** Measurement of the activity of palmitoyl-protein thioesterase involved in CLN1, the acid protease involved in CLN2, and, though more rare, cathepsin D activity involved in CLN10, in white blood cells or cultured skin fibroblasts (cells that strengthen skin and give it elasticity) can be used to confirm or rule out these diagnoses.

- **DNA analysis:** In families where the mutation in the gene for CLN3 is known, DNA analysis can be used to confirm the diagnosis or for the prenatal diagnosis of this form of Batten disease. When the mutation is known, DNA analysis can also be used to detect unaffected carriers of this condition for genetic counseling. If a family mutation has not previously been identified or if the common mutations are not present, recent molecular advances have made it possible to sequence all of the known NCL genes, increasing the chances of finding the responsible mutation(s).

Is there any treatment?

As yet, no specific treatment is known that can halt or reverse the symptoms of Batten disease or other NCLs. However, seizures can sometimes be reduced or controlled with anticonvulsant drugs, and other medical problems can be treated appropriately as they arise. At the same time, physical and occupational therapy may help patients retain function as long as possible.

Some reports have described a slowing of the disease in children with Batten disease who were treated with vitamins C and E and with diets low in vitamin A. However, these treatments did not prevent the fatal outcome of the disease.

Support and encouragement can help patients and families cope with the profound disability and dementia caused by NCLs. Often, support groups enable affected children, adults, and families to share common concerns and experiences.

Meanwhile, scientists pursue medical research that could someday yield an effective treatment.

What research is being done?

The National Institute of Neurological Disorders and Stroke, a part of the National Institutes of Health, is the federal government's leading supporter of biomedical research on the brain and central nervous system. As part of its mission, the NINDS conducts research and supports studies through grants to major medical institutions across the country. Through the work of several scientific teams, the search for the molecular basis of the NCLs is gathering speed.

Studying the lipopigment deposits that contain fats and proteins, one NINDS-supported scientist, using animal models of NCL, found that a large portion of this built-up material is a protein called subunit c. This protein is normally found inside the cell's mitochondria, small structures that produce the energy cells need to do their jobs. Scientists are now working to understand what role this protein may play in NCL, including how this protein accumulates inside diseased cells and whether its accumulation—or the accumulation of other components in the storage material—is harmful to the cell. An important aspect of these studies is looking at how the different gene mutations lead to the lipoprotein deposits, which may involve the same processes.

In addition, research scientists are working with NCL animal models to improve understanding and treatment of these disorders. These include naturally occurring sheep and dog models, and genetically engineered mouse models. Simpler models in lower organisms (such as yeast, zebrafish, and the fruit fly) are useful tools that are being implemented by scientists to study the function of the NCL proteins, most of which remain unknown. Research suggests that many of the NCL genes have conserved functions in the lower organisms; in other words, they work the same way in yeast, fly, or zebrafish cells as they do in humans. Because mice and lower organisms breed or propagate quickly and can be genetically manipulated, their use can speed NCL research.

More recently, advances in human cell research will assist the translation of findings in the model organisms to individuals with NCL disorders. Skin or other cell types taken from those with an NCL disorder can now be manipulated in the laboratory to become "pluripotent," meaning they can be made into cells that have the potential to become any cell type—including brain cells. This process—known as cellular reprogramming—is used to establish patient-derived induced pluripotent stem cells (iPS cells).

Although no therapies are currently available for NCL disorders, a number of NINDS-funded science teams are working toward developing therapies and identifying therapy targets for NCL. The approaches undertaken by scientists include:

- gene therapy (for example, in CLN1 and CLN2);

- enzyme replacement therapy (CLN1 and CLN2);

- stem cell therapy;

- identification of the normal protein functions that are lost as a result of the gene mutations;

- testing candidate drugs that modify known disease abnormalities (for example, immune suppression to eliminate the observed autoimmunity in JNCL/CLN3); and

- screening to identify drugs or other factors that normalize cellular abnormalities in the NCL disease models.

Section 26.2

Fabry Disease

"Fabry Disease Information Page," National Institute of Neurological Disorders and Stroke, National Institutes of Health, October 6, 2011.

What is Fabry disease?

Fabry disease is caused by the lack of or faulty enzyme needed to metabolize lipids, fat-like substances that include oils, waxes, and fatty acids. The disease is also called alpha-galactosidase-A deficiency. A mutation in the gene that controls this enzyme causes insufficient breakdown of lipids, which build up to harmful levels in the eyes, kidneys, autonomic nervous system, and cardiovascular system. Fabry disease is one of several lipid storage disorders and the only X-linked lipid storage disease. Since the gene that is altered is carried on a mother's X chromosome, her sons have a 50 percent chance of inheriting the disorder and her daughters have a 50 percent chance of being a carrier. A milder form is common in females, and occasionally some affected females may have severe manifestations similar to males with the disorder. Symptoms usually begin during childhood or adolescence and include burning sensations in the hands that get worse with exercise and hot weather and small, noncancerous, raised reddish-purple blemishes on the skin. Some boys will also have eye manifestations, especially cloudiness of the cornea. Lipid storage may lead to impaired arterial circulation and increased risk of heart attack or stroke. The heart may also become enlarged and the kidneys may become progressively involved. Other signs include decreased sweating, fever, and gastrointestinal difficulties.

Is there any treatment?

Enzyme replacement therapy has been approved by the U.S. Food and Drug Administration for the treatment of Fabry disease. Enzyme replacement therapy can reduce lipid storage, ease pain, and improve organ function. The pain that accompanies the disease may be treated with anticonvulsants such as phenytoin and carbamazepine. Gastrointestinal hyperactivity may be treated with metoclopramide. Some individuals may require dialysis or kidney transplantation.

What is the prognosis?

Patients with Fabry disease often die prematurely of complications from strokes, heart disease, or renal failure.

What research is being done?

The National Institute of Neurological Disorders and Stroke (NINDS), a component of the National Institutes of Health, supports research to find ways to treat and prevent lipid storage diseases such as Fabry disease.

Section 26.3

Gaucher Disease

Excerpted from "Learning about Gaucher Disease," National Human Genome Research Institute (www.genome.gov), January 4, 2012.

What is Gaucher disease?

Gaucher disease is an autosomal recessive inherited disorder of metabolism where a type of fat (lipid) called glucocerebroside cannot be adequately degraded. Normally, the body makes an enzyme called glucocerebrosidase that breaks down and recycles glucocerebroside—a normal part of the cell membrane. People who have Gaucher disease do not make enough glucocerebrosidase. This causes the specific lipid to build up in the liver, spleen, bone marrow, and nervous system, interfering with normal functioning.

There are three recognized types of Gaucher disease and each has a wide range of symptoms. Type 1 is the most common, does not affect the nervous system, and may appear early in life or adulthood. Many people with Type 1 Gaucher disease have findings that are so mild that they never have any problems from the disorder. Type 2 and 3 do affect the nervous system. Type 2 causes serious medical problems beginning in infancy, while Type 3 progresses more slowly than Type 2.There are also other, more unusual, forms that are hard to categorize within the three types.

Gaucher disease is caused by changes (mutations) in a single gene called GBA. Mutations in the GBA gene cause very low levels of gluco-cerebrosidase. A person who has Gaucher disease inherits a mutated copy of the GBA gene from each of his or her parents.

Gaucher disease occurs in about one in fifty thousand to one in one hundred thousand individuals in the general population. Type 1 is found more frequently among individuals who are of Ashkenazi Jewish ancestry. Type 1 Gaucher disease is present one in five hundred to one in one thousand people of Ashkenazi Jewish ancestry, and approximately one in fourteen Ashkenazi Jews is a carrier. Type 2 and Type 3 Gaucher disease are not as common.

What are the symptoms of Gaucher disease?

Symptoms of Gaucher disease vary greatly among those who have the disorder. The major clinical symptoms include the following:

- Enlargement of the liver and spleen (hepatosplenomegaly)

- A low number of red blood cells (anemia)

- Easy bruising caused, in part, by a low level of platelets (thrombocytopenia)

- Bone disease (bone pain and fractures)

Other symptoms, depending on the type of Gaucher disease, include heart, lung, and nervous system problems.

The symptoms of Type 1 Gaucher disease include bone disease, hepatosplenomegaly, anemia and thrombocytopenia, and lung disease.

The symptoms in Type 2 and Type 3 Gaucher disease include those of Type 1 and other problems involving the nervous system, such as eye problems, seizures, and brain damage. In Type 2 Gaucher disease, severe medical problems begin in infancy. These individuals usually do not live beyond age two. There are also some patients with Type 2 Gaucher disease that die in the newborn period, often with severe skin problems or excessive fluid accumulation (hydrops). Individuals with Type 3 Gaucher disease may have symptoms before they are two years old, but often have a more slowly progressive disease process and the extent of brain involvement is quite variable. They usually have slowing of their horizontal eye movements.

Recently it has been observed that both patients with Gaucher disease and Gaucher carriers have an increased risk of developing Parkinson disease and related disorders.

How is Gaucher disease diagnosed?

The diagnosis of Gaucher disease is based on clinical symptoms and laboratory testing. A diagnosis of Gaucher disease is suspected in individuals who have bone problems, enlarged liver and spleen (hepatosplenomegaly), changes in red blood cell levels, easy bleeding and bruising from low platelets, or signs of nervous system problems.

Laboratory testing involves a blood test to measure the activity level of the enzyme glucocerebrosidase. Individuals who have Gaucher disease have very low levels of this enzyme activity. A second type of laboratory test involves DNA analysis of the GBA gene for the four most common GBA mutations. Both enzyme and DNA testing can be done prenatally. A bone marrow or liver biopsy is not necessary to establish the diagnosis.

When the specific gene mutation causing Gaucher disease is known in a family, DNA testing can be used to accurately identify carriers. However it is often not possible to predict the patient's clinical course based upon DNA testing.

What is the treatment for Gaucher disease?

Enzyme replacement therapy is now available as an effective treatment for individuals who have symptoms from Gaucher disease. The treatment involves giving a modified form of the enzyme glucocerebrosidase by intravenous infusion every two weeks. Enzyme replacement therapy helps to stop progression and often reverse many of the symptoms of Gaucher disease, but does not affect the nervous system involvement.

Several other therapies, including oral treatments, are in various stages of development.

Other treatments that have been required include: removal of the spleen (splenectomy); blood transfusions; pain medications; and joint replacement surgery.

Is Gaucher disease inherited?

Gaucher disease is inherited in families in an autosomal recessive manner. Normally, a person has two copies of the genes that provide instructions for making the enzyme glucocerebrosidase. For most individuals, both genes work properly. When one of the two genes is not functioning properly, the person is a carrier. Carriers do not have Gaucher disease because they have one normally functioning gene that makes enough of the enzyme to carry out normal body functions.

When an individual inherits an altered gene from each carrier parent, he or she has Gaucher disease.

Carrier parents have, with each pregnancy, a one in four (25 percent) chance to have a baby born with Gaucher disease; a one in two (50 percent) chance to have a child who is a carrier like themselves; and a one in four (25 percent) chance to have a child who is neither affected nor a carrier.

Section 26.4

Niemann-Pick Disease

"Niemann-Pick Disease Information Page," National Institute of Neurological Disorders and Stroke, National Institutes of Health, October 6, 2011.

What is Niemann-Pick disease?

Niemann-Pick disease (NP) refers to a group of inherited metabolic disorders known as lipid storage diseases. Lipids (fatty materials such as waxes, fatty acids, oils, and cholesterol) and proteins are usually broken down into smaller components to provide energy for the body. In Niemann-Pick disease, harmful quantities of lipids accumulate in the spleen, liver, lungs, bone marrow, and the brain. Symptoms may include lack of muscle coordination, brain degeneration, eye paralysis, learning problems, loss of muscle tone, increased sensitivity to touch, spasticity, feeding and swallowing difficulties, slurred speech, and an enlarged liver and spleen. There may be clouding of the cornea, and a characteristic cherry-red halo develops around the center of the retina. The disease has four related types. Type A, the most severe form, occurs in early infancy. It is characterized by an enlarged liver and spleen, swollen lymph nodes, and profound brain damage by six months of age. Children with this type rarely live beyond eighteen months. Type B involves an enlarged liver and spleen, which usually occurs in the pre-teen years. The brain is not affected. In types A and B, insufficient activity of an enzyme called sphingomyelinase causes the buildup of toxic amounts of sphingomyelin, a fatty substance present in every cell of the body. Types C and D may appear early in life or develop in the teen or adult years. Affected individuals have only moderate en-largement of the spleen and liver, but brain damage may be extensive and cause an inability to look up and down, difficulty in walking and swallowing, and progressive loss of vision and hearing. Types C and D are characterized by a defect that disrupts the transport of cholesterol between brain cells. Type D usually occurs in people with an ancestral background in Nova Scotia. Types C and D are caused by a lack of the NPC1 or NPC 2 proteins.

Is there any treatment?

There is currently no cure for Niemann-Pick disease. Children usu-ally die from infection or progressive neurological loss. There is cur-rently no effective treatment for persons with type A. Bone marrow transplantation has been attempted in a few patients with type B, and encouraging results have been reported. The development of enzyme replacement and gene therapies might also be helpful for those with type B. Individuals with types C and D are frequently placed on a low-cholesterol diet and/or cholesterol-lowering drugs, but research has not shown these interventions to change the abnormal cholesterol metabolism or halt disease progression.

What is the prognosis?

Infants with type A die in infancy. Children with Type B may live a comparatively long time, but may require supplemental oxygen be-cause of lung impairment. The life expectancy of persons with types C and D varies: some individuals die in childhood while others, who appear to be less severely affected, can live into adulthood.

What research is being done?

The National Institute of Neurological Disorders and Stroke (NINDS), a part of the National Institutes of Health (NIH), conducts research about Niemann-Pick disease in laboratories at the NIH and also supports additional research through grants to major research institutions across the country. Investigators at the NINDS have iden-tified two different genes that, when defective, contribute to Niemann-Pick disease types C and D.

Section 26.5

Sandhoff Disease

"Sandhoff Disease Information Page," National Institute of Neurological Disorders and Stroke, National Institutes of Health, October 6, 2011.

What is Sandhoff disease?

Sandhoff disease is a rare, genetic, lipid storage disorder resulting in the progressive deterioration of the central nervous system. It is caused by a deficiency of the enzyme beta-hexosaminidase, which results in the accumulation of certain fats (lipids) in the brain and other organs of the body. Sandhoff disease is a severe form of Tay-Sachs disease—which is prevalent primarily in people of Eastern European and Ashkenazi Jewish descent—but it is not limited to any ethnic group. Onset of the disorder usually occurs at six months of age. Neurological symptoms may include motor weakness, startle reaction to sound, early blindness, progressive mental and motor deterioration, macrocephaly (an abnormally enlarged head), cherry-red spots in the eyes, seizures, and myoclonus (shock-like contractions of a muscle). Other symptoms may include frequent respiratory infections, doll-like facial appearance, and an enlarged liver and spleen.

Is there any treatment?

There is no specific treatment for Sandhoff disease. Supportive treatment includes proper nutrition and hydration and keeping the airway open. Anticonvulsants may initially control seizures. In other ongoing studies, a small number of children have received an experimental treatment using transplants of stem cells from umbilical cord blood. Although these limited trials have not yet produced a treatment or cure, scientists continue to study these and other investigational approaches.

What is the prognosis?

The prognosis for individuals with Sandhoff disease is poor. Death usually occurs by age three and is generally caused by respiratory infections.

What research is being done?

The National Institute of Neurological Disorders and Stroke (NINDS), a component of the National Institutes of Health (NIH), conducts research about lipid storage diseases in laboratories at the NIH and also supports additional research through grants to major medical institutions across the country.

Section 26.6

Tay-Sachs Disease

Healthy babies develop vision, movement, hearing, and other vital functions in part because enzymes clear out fatty protein and other unwanted material that can interfere with growth.

But a baby with Tay-Sachs disease is born without one of those important enzymes, hexosaminidase A (Hex A). So, as those fatty proteins build up in the brain, they hurt the baby's sight, hearing, movement, and mental development.

A child can only get Tay-Sachs by inheriting it. The genetic trait is relatively common among certain ethnic groups, such as Ashkenazi Jews. Tay-Sachs can be detected before birth, so couples in at-risk ethnic groups who are thinking of having children may want to get a blood test to find out whether their child would be likely to have it.

Who Is at Risk for Tay-Sachs?

Each year, about sixteen cases of Tay-Sachs are diagnosed in the United States. Although Ashkenazi Jews (Jews of central and eastern European descent) are at the highest risk, it is now also prevalent in non-Jewish populations, including people of French-Canadian/Cajun heritage.

Some people carry the genetic mutation that causes Tay-Sachs, but do not develop the full-blown disease. Among Ashkenazi Jews, 1 in 27 people are carriers; in the general population, 1 in 250 people are.

A child can have Tay-Sachs disease only if both parents are carriers of the gene. When two carriers have a child together, there's a:

- 50 percent chance that their child will be a carrier, but not have the disease;

- 25 percent chance that their child will not be a carrier and not have the disease;

- 25 percent chance that their child will have the disease.

Screening

Couples who are considering having children—or are already expecting—can get screened for the Tay-Sachs gene with a simple blood test. If both the mother and father carry the Tay-Sachs gene, an obstetrician/gynecologist may refer the couple to a genetic counselor for more information.

Prenatal Diagnosis

Pregnant mothers can have their unborn babies tested for the Hex A deficit that causes Tay-Sachs disease. (If the tests do not detect Hex A, the infant will have Tay-Sachs disease. If the tests do detect Hex A, the infant won't have it.)

Between the tenth and twelfth weeks of pregnancy, an expectant mother can get a chorionic villus sampling, or CVS, in which a small sample of the placenta is drawn into a needle or a small tube for analysis.

Between the fifteenth and eighteenth weeks of pregnancy, the mother can have an amniocentesis to test for the Tay-Sachs gene. In this test, a needle is inserted into the mother's belly to draw a sample of the amniotic fluid that surrounds the fetus.

Signs and Symptoms

Kids are usually tested for Tay-Sachs after having hearing, sight, and movement problems. A doctor can identify the disease with a physical exam and blood tests.

A baby born with Tay-Sachs develops normally in the first three to six months of life. During the next months—or even years—the baby will progressively lose the ability to see, hear, and move. A red spot will develop in the back of the child's eyes. The child will stop smiling, crawling, turning over, and reaching out for things. By the age of two, the child may have seizures and become completely disabled. Death usually occurs by the time the child is five years old.

In rare forms of the disease, a child may have the Hex A enzyme, but not enough of it to prevent developmental problems. In one of these forms, called juvenile Hex A deficiency, those problems may not appear until the child is two to five years old. The disease progresses more slowly, but death usually occurs by the time the child is fifteen years old.

In another, milder form of Tay-Sachs, the disease causes muscle weakness and slurred speech, but sight, hearing, and mental capabilities remain intact.

Helping a Child with Tay-Sachs

There is no cure for any form of Tay-Sachs disease. But doctors may be able to help a child with Tay-Sachs cope with the symptoms of the disease by prescribing medication to relieve pain, manage seizures, and control muscle spasticity.

Researchers are studying ways to improve treatment for Tay-Sachs disease and screening methods for the disease.

If your child has been diagnosed with Tay-Sachs or both you and your partner are carriers of the gene, talk to your doctor or a genetic counselor about ongoing research. You also might seek support from a group such as the National Tay-Sachs and Allied Diseases Foundation or the March of Dimes Birth Defects Foundation.

Chapter 27

Mitochondrial Diseases

Chapter Contents

Section 27.1

Basic Facts about Mitochondrial Diseases

"Overview of Mitochondrial Diseases," Rare Diseases Clinical Research Network, National Institutes of Health. The complete text of this document is available online at http://rarediseasesnetwork.epi.usf.edu/NAMD/learnmore/index.htm; accessed September 12, 2012.

What are mitochondrial diseases?

Mitochondrial diseases are very diverse conditions due to dysfunction of mitochondria, specialized compartments (organelles) in virtually every cell of the body (only red blood cells lack mitochondria). Mitochondria generate more than 90 percent of the energy required by the body.

Mitochondrial dysfunction depletes cells of energy, causing cell damage and even cell death.

Due to the high energy requirements of brain and muscle, mitochondrial disease typically affects these parts of the body, causing encephalomyopathies (brain and muscle disease). Other organs are frequently affected, including the eye, ear (the hearing organ called the cochlea), heart, liver, gastrointestinal tract, liver, kidney, endocrine organs (such as the thyroid gland and insulin-producing cells in the pancreas), and blood.

Who gets mitochondrial diseases?

The diseases predominantly affect children, but adult-onset disorders are being recognized with increasing frequency.

What causes mitochondrial disease?

Mitochondria are unique organelles because they are the products of their own genetic material (mitochondrial deoxyribonucleic acid [DNA] or mtDNA) and nuclear DNA. Therefore, mitochondrial diseases are caused by mutations in either mtDNA or nuclear DNA.

292

How are mitochondrial diseases diagnosed?

Mitochondrial diseases are often difficult to diagnose, and therefore it is important for patients to be evaluated at a medical center with appropriate expertise. In some cases, symptoms and signs may suggest a particular mitochondrial disease. Physical examination and laboratory tests are necessary to characterize involvement of various organs and to reach the correct diagnosis. Laboratory studies typically include: blood tests, brain magnetic resonance imaging (MRI) or computed tomography (CT) scans, heart tests (electrocardiogram and echocardiograms), ophthalmological and neurological evaluations, and hearing tests. Elevated lactic acid (lactate) or lactate to pyruvate ratio (>20:1) in blood or cerebrospinal fluid is a common sign of mitochondrial dysfunction. Muscle biopsy is the gold standard for the diagnosis of many mitochondrial diseases and requires specialized microscopic analyses and biochemical tests (such as measurements of mitochondrial respiratory chain enzyme activities). Finally, genetic testing of blood, urine, or muscle is performed to pinpoint the exact mutation responsible for a specific disease.

What is the treatment for mitochondrial disease?

Treatment of mitochondrial diseases is limited. Therapies to treat specific symptoms and signs of mitochondrial diseases are very important. For example, in mitochondrial patients, epilepsy typically responds to anticonvulsant drugs while insulin and other standard treatments are effective for diabetes mellitus. Nutritional supplements such as vitamins and co-factors are often taken by patients with mitochondrial diseases and are most useful in patients with specific deficiencies (e.g., coenzyme Q10 [CoQ10] supplementation is particularly effective in patients with CoQ10 deficiencies).

Section 27.2

Treatments and Therapies for Mitochondrial Diseases

The management of mitochondrial disease is largely supportive,[1] as there is no way of simply increasing the capacity of the cell to generate energy.[2] Treatment therefore involves optimizing energy production, reducing energy losses, meeting lifestyle needs such as education, and monitoring for complications.[2]

Optimizing Energy Production

Adequate nutrition: Adequate calories and nutrition can dramatically improve a patient's overall clinical state and slow the progression of the illness.[2] Special diets may benefit some patients, such as high-fat diets with restriction of simple carbohydrates, fructose restriction, and/or high complex carbohydrate intake.[3] Eating smaller meals more regularly and avoidance of fasting, particularly prolonged fasting, is also extremely important in optimizing mitochondrial function.

Adequate sleep: Improving sleep is a correctable component of fatigue. Therefore, issues like sleep apnea need to be managed. Central sleep apnea can occur in more advanced disease, whereas obstructive sleep apnea (due to muscle hypotonia or weakness) is more common.[2]

Promoting activity: Regular exercise not only improves stamina, it also improves mitochondrial function.[4,5] To maximize energy production, mitochondrial patients must remain active, though exhaustion should be avoided and achieving a "normal" level of endurance is unrealistic.[2]

Supplementation with certain vitamins and cofactors: It is considered standard care to use a cocktail of vitamin and cofactor supplementation for patients with mitochondrial disorders, although there are a large variety of studies with even a larger variety of answers regarding their efficacy. At present, there are no cures for these disorders except in very rare and specific disorders such as primary carnitine deficiency or primary coenzyme Q10 deficiency.[3] The goals of supplementation are to improve symptoms and to halt the progression of the illness. The effectiveness of treatment varies with each patient but it will not reverse any damage that has already occurred.[6]

There is no standard vitamin cocktail, commonly known as the "mito cocktail." Ideally, vitamins should be started one at a time to allow observation of any benefit or adverse reaction.

Reducing Energy Losses

Prevention of infections: Patients with mitochondrial disease frequently do not tolerate infections well and they may cause prolonged, debilitating fatigue and weakness, and possibly even death. As a result, their vaccinations should be kept up-to-date, including the seasonal vaccinations (e.g., influenza), and antibiotics should be considered early in any infective illness.

Avoiding excessive physical activity: "Overdoing it" produces no benefit and can leave a patient exhausted, in pain, nauseous, and miserable.

Treating emotional distress: Frequent or persistent anxiety, depression, or obsessive-compulsive behaviors are very energy demanding.

Maintaining a suitable ambient temperature: Patients with mitochondrial disease often don't tolerate extremes of temperature.

Avoidance of Toxins

Alcohol and smoking have been known to hasten the progression of some conditions, so should be avoided. Monosodium glutamate (MSG) can trigger migraine headaches in healthy people, so the potential is to do the same in those susceptible with mitochondrial disease.[7] Iron can increase free radical production, so although excessive amounts should be avoided, a normal diet containing iron is encouraged.[6,7]

Antiretroviral medications are toxic to mitochondria, so azidothymidine (AZT) and other nucleoside drugs such as Fialuridine (FIAU) should be avoided. Similarly, doxorubicin, a chemotherapy medication can cause a cardiomyopathy through mitochondrial damage so it should also be avoided.

Sodium valproate, statins, erythromycin, aspirin and other NSAIDS, amphotericin and propofol are best avoided but are not absolute contraindications. Other amino-glycosides antibiotics such as gentamicin, streptomycin, and tobramycin can induce hearing loss by damaging mitochondria, so alternatives should be sought.

In the anesthetic situation, intravenous (IV) solutions that contain lactic acid (e.g., lactated Ringer's solution) should be avoided while some patients are more sensitive to volatile anesthetics, so lower doses are required.

Educational Needs

The majority of children with mitochondrial disease show learning and/or behavioral problems that are typically unique to each child, so an educational plan should be tailored to each child, not based on his or her diagnosis. However, a medical plan is frequently needed as well to create an optimal learning environment.

Points to consider include:

- pacing the child to match their fatigability;
- never forget they have "good and bad" days;
- a comfortable classroom temperature;
- avoidance of infective illnesses;
- avoidance of unnecessary emotional distress.[2]

Monitoring Complications

The caring physician must have a thorough knowledge of the potential complications of mitochondrial disorders in order to prevent unnecessary morbidity and mortality. This includes the early diagnosis and/or management of diabetes mellitus, seizures, cardiac pacing, ptosis correction, and intraocular lens replacement for cataracts.

Unless a patient has a very specific disease with a predictable phenotype, routine monitoring of the following organs is generally on a one- to two-year schedule.

Blood and Urine Testing

1. Bone marrow involvement: Full blood count (FBC), white blood cell count (WBC) differential, platelets.

2. Liver involvement: Aspartate aminotransferase (AST), alanine aminotransferase (ALT), bilirubin.

3. Kidney involvement: Blood urea nitrogen (BUN), creatinine (blood), urinalysis, urine amino acids (quantitative).

4. Muscle involvement: Creatine kinase (CK).

5. Endocrine involvement: thyroid functions, calcium, phosphorus. Adrenal insufficiency is also a possibility.

6. Metabolic status: lactate and pyruvate, carnitine and acylcarnitines, leukocyte coenzyme Q10, urine organic acid analysis.

Other Testing

1. Ophthalmological evaluation and especially screening for visual function if concerned

2. Audiology testing

3. Cardiac evaluation, including electrocardiogram (ECG), echocardiogram

4. Developmental or neuropsychological testing according to the patient's needs.[2]

References

1. Epidemiology and treatment of mitochondrial disorders. Chinnery PF, Turnbull DM. *Am J Med Genet*. 2001; 106: 94–101.

2. *A Clinician's Guide to the Management of Mitochondrial Disease: A Manual for Primary Care Providers* developed by Margaret Klehm, Mark Korson, and mitoaction.org, 2008: www .mitoaction.org.

3. *A Primary Care Physician's Guide, the Spectrum of Mitochondrial Disease*. Robert K. Naviaux, MD, PhD. United Mitochondrial Disease Foundation at www.umdf.org.

4. Mahoney, 2002: *A Clinician's Guide to the Management of Mitochondrial Disease: A Manual for Primary Care Providers* developed by Margaret Klehm, Mark Korson, and mitoaction.org, 2008: www.mitoaction.org.

5. Jeppesen 2006: *A Clinician's Guide to the Management of Mitochondrial Disease: A Manual for Primary Care Providers* developed by Margaret Klehm, Mark Korson, and mitoaction.org, 2008: www.mitoaction.org.

6. Diagnosis and Treatment of Childhood Mitochondrial Diseases. Andrea L. Gropman, MD. *Current Neurology and Neuroscience Reports* 2001, 1:185–94.

7. United Mitochondrial Disease Foundation, www.umdf.org.

Chapter 28

Neurofibromatosis

What is neurofibromatosis?

Neurofibromatosis (NF) is a genetic neurological disorder that can affect the brain, spinal cord, nerves, and skin. Tumors, or neurofibromas, grow along the body's nerves or on or underneath the skin. Scientists have classified NF into two distinct types: neurofibromatosis type 1 (NF1) and NF2. NF1, formerly known as von Recklinghausen NF, is the more common of the types. It occurs in approximately one in four thousand births. NF2, also referred to as bilateral acoustic NF, central NF, or vestibular NF, occurs less frequently—in one in forty thousand births. Occurrences of NF1 and NF2 are present among all racial groups and affect both sexes equally. The tumors arise from changes in the nerve cells and skin cells. Tumors also may press on the body's vital areas as their size increases. NF may lead to developmental abnormalities and/ or increased chances of having learning disabilities. Other forms of NF, where the symptoms are not consistent with that of NF1 or NF2, have been observed. A rare form of NF is schwannomatosis. However, the genetic cause of this form of NF has not been found.

What are the symptoms of neurofibromatosis?

Symptoms for neurofibromatosis type 1 include the following:

Excerpted from "Learning about Neurofibromatosis," National Human Genome Research Institute (www.genome.gov), September 16, 2010.

- Presence of light brown spots (café-au-lait) on the skin.

- Appearance of two or more neurofibromas (pea-sized bumps) that can grow either on the nerve tissue, under the skin, or on many nerve tissues.

- Manifestation of freckles under the armpits or in the groin areas.

- Appearance of tiny tan clumps of pigment in the iris of the eyes (Lisch nodules).

- Tumors along the optic nerve of the eye (optic glioma).

- Severe curvature of the spine (scoliosis).

- Enlargement or malformation of other bones in the skeletal system.

Symptoms for NF1 vary for each individual. Those that are skin-related are often present at birth, during infancy, and by a child's tenth birthday. From ages ten to fifteen, neurofibromas may become apparent. Symptoms such as café-au-lait spots, freckling, and Lisch nodules pose minimal or no health risk to a person. Though neurofibromas are generally a cosmetic concern for those with NF1, they can sometimes be psychologically distressing. For 15 percent of individuals with NF1, the symptoms can be severely debilitating. Neurofibromas can grow inside the body and may affect organ systems. Hormonal changes at puberty and/or even pregnancy may increase the size of neurofibromas. Nearly 50 percent of children with NF1 have speech problems, learning disabilities, seizures, and hyperactivity. Less than 1 percent of those affected with NF1 may have malignant tumors and may require treatment.

Symptoms for neurofibromatosis type 2 include:

- Tumors along the eighth cranial nerve (schwannomas).

- Meningiomas and other brain tumors.

- Ringing noises inside the ear (tinnitus), hearing loss, and/or deafness.

- Cataracts at a young age.

- Spinal tumors.

- Balance problems.

- Wasting of muscles (atrophy).

Individuals with NF2 develop tumors that grow on the eighth cranial nerves and on the vestibular nerves. These tumors often cause pressure on the acoustic nerves, which results in hearing loss. Hearing loss may begin as early as an individual's teenage years. Tinnitus, dizziness, facial numbness, balance problems, and chronic headaches may also surface during the teenage years. Numbness may also occur in other parts of the body, due to spinal cord tumors.

The rare form of NF, schwannomatosis, which was recently identified, does not develop on the eighth cranial nerves, and does not cause hearing loss. It causes pain primarily, and in any part of the body. Though schwannomatosis may also lead to numbness, weakness, or balance problems like NF1 or NF2, the symptoms are less severe.

How is neurofibromatosis diagnosed?

Neurofibromatosis is diagnosed from a combination of findings. For children to be diagnosed with NF1, they must show at least two of the aforementioned symptoms associated with NF1. A physical examination by a doctor familiar with the disorder is usually performed. Doctors may use special lamps to examine the skin for café-au-lait spots. Doctors may also rely on magnetic resonance imaging (MRI), x-rays, computerized tomography (CT scan), and blood tests to detect defects in the NF1 gene.

For NF2, doctors will pay close attention to hearing loss. Hearing tests as well as imaging tests are used to look for tumors in and around the auditory nerves, the spinal cord, or the brain. Audiometry and brainstem auditory evoked response tests can help determine whether the eighth cranial nerve is functioning properly. Family history of NF2 is also a key focal area for diagnosis.

Genetic testing is also used to diagnose NF1 and NF2. Testing conducted before birth (prenatal) is helpful to identify individuals who have a family history of the disorder, but do not yet have the symptoms. Still, gene tests have no way of predicting the severity of NF1 or NF2. Genetic testing is performed by either direct gene mutation analysis and/or linkage analysis. Mutation analysis looks to identify the particular gene changes that cause NF. A linkage analysis is useful if the mutation analysis does not provide enough conclusive information. With a linkage analysis, blood tests from multiple family members are taken to track the chromosome that carry the disease-causing gene through two or more generations. Linkage testing is around 90 percent accurate in determining whether individuals have NF. Mutation analysis is 95 percent accurate in finding a mutation for NF1, and 65 percent accurate for NF2.

How is neurofibromatosis treated?

Though there is no cure for either NF1 or NF2, there are ways to treat the effects of the disease. Surgery may be helpful in removing tumors, though there is a risk of the tumors regenerating. For optic gliomas, treatment may include surgery and/or radiation. For scoliosis, treatment may include surgery or back braces. For symptoms associated with NF2, surgery may be a viable option, however not without complications that could result in additional loss of hearing or deafness. Hearing aids are ineffective when parts of the auditory nerve are removed. A breakthrough in treatment became available recently to NF2 patients, when the Food and Drug Administration approved an auditory brainstem implant for those who have parts of their auditory nerve removed and have suffered from subsequent hearing loss. The implant transmits sound signals to the brain directly and allows people to hear certain sounds and speech. Radiation treatment may also help relieve symptoms associated with NF2.

What do we know about heredity and neurofibromatosis?

Neurofibromatosis can either be an inherited disorder or the product of a gene mutation. Both NF1 and NF2 are caused by two separate abnormal genes and may be inherited from parents who have NF or may be the result of a mutation in the sperm or egg cells. NF is considered an autosomal dominant disorder because the gene is located on one of the 22 chromosome pairs, called autosomes. The gene for NF1 is located on chromosome 17. The gene for NF2 is located on chromosome 22. Children have a 50 percent chance of inheriting the genes that cause NF if the parent has NF. The type of NF the child inherits will be the same as that of the parent. Therefore, if the parent has NF1, there will be a 50 percent chance the child will have NF1. If the parent has NF2, there will be a 50 percent chance the child will have NF2. The only difference between the child and the parent in these circumstances is the severity of NF and the appearance of symptoms. The presence of only one changed or affected gene can cause the disorder to appear. However, the action of the unaffected gene that is paired with the dominant gene does not prevent the disorder from appearing. People with NF can make two different kinds of reproductive cells: one that can cause a child to have NF and the other that will produce an unaffected child, if that is the gene that happens to be used. When an unaffected individual conceives a child with a person with NF, there are four possible cell combinations—two combinations that will yield a child with NF and the other two that will yield an unaffected child.

Chapter 29

Neuromuscular Disorders

Chapter Contents

Section 29.1

Charcot-Marie-Tooth Disease

"Charcot-Marie-Tooth Disease Information Page," National
Institute of Neurological Disorders and Stroke, National
Institutes of Health, February 15, 2011.

What is Charcot-Marie-Tooth disease?

Charcot-Marie-Tooth disease (CMT) is one of the most common inherited neurological disorders, affecting approximately 1 in 2,500 people in the United States. CMT, also known as hereditary motor and sensory neuropathy (HMSN) or peroneal muscular atrophy, comprises a group of disorders caused by mutations in genes that affect the normal function of the peripheral nerves. The peripheral nerves lie outside the brain and spinal cord and supply the muscles and sensory organs in the limbs. A typical feature includes weakness of the foot and lower leg muscles, which may result in foot drop and a high-stepped gait with frequent tripping or falls. Foot deformities, such as high arches and hammertoes (a condition in which the middle joint of a toe bends upwards), are also characteristic due to weakness of the small muscles in the feet. In addition, the lower legs may take on an "inverted champagne bottle" appearance due to the loss of muscle bulk. Later in the disease, weakness and muscle atrophy may occur in the hands, resulting in difficulty with fine motor skills. Some patients experience pain, which can range from mild to severe.

Is there any treatment?

There is no cure for CMT, but physical therapy, occupational therapy, braces and other orthopedic devices, and orthopedic surgery can help patients cope with the disabling symptoms of the disease. In addition, pain-killing drugs can be prescribed for patients who have severe pain.

What is the prognosis?

Onset of symptoms of CMT is most often in adolescence or early adulthood, however presentation may be delayed until mid-adulthood.

Progression of symptoms is very gradual. The degeneration of motor nerves results in muscle weakness and atrophy in the extremities (arms, legs, hands, or feet), and the degeneration of sensory nerves results in a reduced ability to feel heat, cold, and pain. There are many forms of CMT disease. The severity of symptoms is quite variable in different patients, and some people may never realize they have the disorder. CMT is not fatal, and people with most forms of CMT have a normal life expectancy.

What research is being done?

The National Institute of Neurological Disorders and Stroke (NINDS) conducts CMT research in its laboratories at the National Institutes of Health (NIH) and also supports CMT research through grants to major medical institutions across the country. Ongoing research includes efforts to identify more of the mutant genes and proteins that cause the various disease subtypes. This research includes studies in the laboratory to discover the mechanisms of nerve degeneration and muscle atrophy, and clinical studies to find therapies to slow down or even reverse nerve degeneration and muscle atrophy.

Section 29.2

Early-Onset Primary Dystonia

Excerpted from "Early Onset Primary Dystonia,"
Genetics Home Reference (http://ghr.nlm.nih.gov), May 2008.
Revised by David A. Cooke, M.D., FACP, May 2013.

What is early-onset primary dystonia?

Early-onset primary dystonia is a condition characterized by progressive problems with movement, typically beginning in childhood. Dystonia is a movement disorder that involves involuntary tensing of the muscles (muscle contractions), twisting of specific body parts such as an arm or a leg, rhythmic shaking (tremors), and other uncontrolled movements. A primary dystonia is one that occurs without other neurological symptoms, such as seizures or a loss of intellectual function (dementia). Early-onset primary dystonia does not affect a person's intelligence.

On average, the signs and symptoms of early-onset primary dystonia appear around age twelve. Abnormal muscle spasms in an arm or a leg are usually the first sign. These unusual movements initially occur while a person is doing a specific action, such as writing or walking. In some affected people, dystonia later spreads to other parts of the body and may occur at rest. The abnormal movements persist throughout life, but they do not usually cause pain.

The signs and symptoms of early-onset primary dystonia vary from person to person, even among affected members of the same family. The mildest cases affect only a single part of the body, causing isolated problems such as a writer's cramp in the hand. Severe cases involve abnormal movements affecting many regions of the body.

How common is early-onset primary dystonia?

Early-onset primary dystonia is among the most common forms of childhood dystonia. This disorder occurs most frequently in people of Ashkenazi (central and eastern European) Jewish heritage, affecting one in three thousand to nine thousand people in this population. The condition is less common among people with other backgrounds; it is estimated to affect one in ten thousand to thirty thousand non-Jewish people worldwide.

What genes are related to early-onset primary dystonia?

A particular mutation in the TOR1A gene (also known as DYT1) is responsible for most cases of early-onset primary dystonia. The TOR1A gene provides instructions for making a protein called torsinA. Although little is known about its function, this protein may help process and transport other proteins within cells. It appears to be critical for the normal development and function of nerve cells in the brain.

A mutation in the TOR1A gene alters the structure of torsinA. The altered protein's effect on the function of nerve cells in the brain is unclear. People with early-onset primary dystonia do not have a loss of nerve cells or obvious changes in the structure of the brain that would explain the abnormal muscle contractions. However, functional brain studies in people with primary dystonia show abnormal metabolism in portions of the midbrain. Microscopic studies of brain tissue from affected individuals show abnormal protein accumulations in certain nerve cells in the midbrain. Researchers are working to determine how a change in the torsinA protein leads to the characteristic features of this disorder.

How do people inherit early-onset primary dystonia?

Mutations in the TOR1A gene are inherited in an autosomal dominant pattern, which means one of the two copies of the gene is altered in each cell. Many people who have a mutation in this gene are not affected by the disorder and may never know they have the mutation. Only 30 to 40 percent of people who inherit a TOR1A mutation will ever develop signs and symptoms of early-onset primary dystonia.

Everyone who has been diagnosed with early-onset primary dystonia has inherited a TOR1A mutation from one parent. The parent may or may not have signs and symptoms of the condition, and other family members may or may not be affected.

Section 29.3

Friedreich Ataxia

"Friedreich's Ataxia Information Page,"
National Institute of Neurological Disorders and Stroke,
National Institutes of Health, August 16, 2011.

What is Friedreich ataxia?

Friedreich ataxia is an inherited disease that causes progressive damage to the nervous system, resulting in symptoms ranging from muscle weakness and speech problems to heart disease. Ataxia results from the degeneration of nerve tissue in the spinal cord and of nerves that control muscle movement in the arms and legs. Symptoms usually begin between the ages of five and fifteen but can appear as early as eighteen months or as late as thirty years of age. The first symptom is usually difficulty in walking. The ataxia gradually worsens and slowly spreads to the arms and then the trunk. Foot deformities such as clubfoot, flexion (involuntary bending) of the toes, hammer toes, or foot inversion (turning in) may be early signs. Rapid, rhythmic, involuntary movements of the eyeball are common. Most people with Friedreich ataxia develop scoliosis (a curving of the spine to one side), which, if severe, may impair breathing. Other symptoms include chest pain, shortness of breath, and heart palpitations. Some individuals may develop diabetes. Doctors diagnose Friedreich ataxia by performing a careful clinical examination, which includes a medical history and a thorough physical examination. Several tests may be performed, including electromyogram (EMG) and genetic testing.

Is there any treatment?

There is currently no effective cure or treatment for Friedreich ataxia. However, many of the symptoms and accompanying complications can be treated to help patients maintain optimal functioning as long as possible. Diabetes and heart problems can be treated with medications. Orthopedic problems such as foot deformities and scoliosis can be treated with braces or surgery. Physical therapy may prolong use of the arms and legs.

What is the prognosis?

Generally, within fifteen to twenty years after the appearance of the first symptoms, the person is confined to a wheelchair, and in later stages of the disease, individuals become completely incapacitated. Most people with Friedreich ataxia die in early adulthood if there is significant heart disease, the most common cause of death. Some people with less severe symptoms live much longer.

What research is being done?

Studies have revealed that frataxin, a protein that should normally be present in the nervous system, the heart, and the pancreas, is severely reduced in patients with Friedreich ataxia. Studies have shown that patients have abnormally high levels of iron in their heart tissue. It is believed that the nervous system, heart, and pancreas may be particularly susceptible to damage from free radicals (produced when the excess iron reacts with oxygen) because once certain cells in these tissues are destroyed by free radicals they cannot be replaced. Nerve and muscle cells also have metabolic needs that may make them particularly vulnerable to free radical damage. The discovery of the genetic mutation that causes Friedreich ataxia has added new impetus to research efforts on this disease.

Section 29.4

Hereditary Spastic Paraplegia

What is HSP?

Hereditary spastic paraplegia (HSP) is a group of rare, inherited neurological disorders. Their primary symptoms are progressive spasticity and weakness of the leg and hip muscles. Researchers estimate that some thirty different types of HSP exist; the genetic causes are known for eleven. The HSP incidence rate in the United States is twenty thousand people.

The condition is characterized by insidiously progressive lower extremity weakness and spasticity. HSP is classified as uncomplicated or pure if neurological impairment is limited to the lower body. HSP is classified as complicated or complex if other systems are involved or if there are other neurological findings such as seizures, dementia, amyotrophy, extrapyramidal disturbance, or peripheral neuropathy in the absence of other disorders such as diabetes mellitus.

Many different names are used for HSP. The most common are hereditary spastic paraplegia (or paraparesis), familial spastic paraparesis (or paraplegia), and Strümpell-Lorrain disease. Others are spastic paraplegia, hereditary Charcot disease, spastic spinal paralysis, diplegia spinalis progressiva, French settlement disease, Troyer syndrome, and Silver syndrome.

The disorder was first identified in the late 1800s by A. Strümpell, a neurologist in Heidelberg, Germany. He observed two brothers and their father, all of whom had gait disorders and spasticity in their legs. After the death of the brothers, Strümpell showed through autopsy the degeneration of the nerve fibers leading through the spinal cord. HSP was originally named after Strümpell, and later after two Frenchmen, Lorrain and Charcot, who provided more information.

What is (apparently sporadic) spastic paraplegia?

Many individuals with all the signs and symptoms of HSP do not appear to have similarly affected family members. Without proof of a hereditary link, some neurologists call the condition spastic paraplegia or apparently sporadic spastic paraplegia. Other clinicians may diagnosis the same condition as primary lateral sclerosis (PLS), which mimics HSP in how it affects the lower body. However, current research indicates that PLS eventually affects the arms and speech and swallowing muscles as well as the leg muscles.

There are many reasons why someone with HSP may not have a family history. Recessive and X-linked forms skip generations, which means the disorder may pass silently for generations and then suddenly appear. In addition, the age of onset, progression rate, and severity vary widely, so that the disease could have gone undiagnosed in previous generations or an affected individual may have died before symptom onset. Mistaken parentage or new genetic mutations are also possible.

What are the symptoms?

The hallmark of HSP is progressive difficulty walking due to increasingly weak and stiff (spastic) muscles. Symptoms appear in most people between the second and fourth decade of life, but they can start at any age.

Initial symptoms are typically difficulty with balance, stubbing the toe, or stumbling. Changes begin so gradually that other people often notice the change first. As the disease progresses, canes, walkers, and eventually wheelchairs may become needed, although some people never require assistive devices.

Other common symptoms of HSP are urinary urgency and frequency, hyperactive reflexes, difficulty with balance, clonus, Babinski sign, diminished vibration sense in the feet, muscle spasms, and congenital foot problems such as pes cavus (high arched foot). Some people may experience problems with their arms or fine motor control of their fingers, but for most people, this is not significant.

Most people with HSP have uncomplicated HSP. There are also rare, complicated forms, which have additional symptoms, such as peripheral neuropathy, ichthyosis (a skin disorder), epilepsy, ataxia, optic neuropathy, retinopathy, dementia, mental retardation, deafness, or problems with speech, swallowing, or breathing. These symptoms may have other causes, though, unrelated to HSP. For example, someone with uncomplicated HSP may have peripheral neuropathy caused by diabetes.

Why are my symptoms different from others in my family?

As noted above, the severity of symptoms and age of onset can vary widely, even within the same family. One reason is that HSP is a group of genetically different disorders, not a single disorder. Some differences may be due to genetic mutations. A child may show symptoms before a parent, and it's possible for some family members to have very mild symptoms while others have more severe symptoms. This may be due to other genes, environment, nutrition, general health, or factors not yet understood.

In some families, symptoms tend to start at younger ages with each generation. Although rare, HSP sometimes shows "incomplete penetrance." This means that occasionally, an individual may have the gene mutation, but for unknown reasons never develop symptoms of HSP. Such individuals can still pass HSP to their children.

How does HSP cause symptoms?

HSP is caused by degeneration of the upper motor neurons in the brain and spinal cord. Upper motor neurons control voluntary movement.

The cell bodies of these neurons are located in the motor cortex area of the brain. They have long, hair-like processes called axons that travel to the brainstem and down the spinal cord. Axons relay the messages to move to lower motor neurons that are located all along the brainstem and spinal cord. Lower motor neurons then carry the messages out to the muscles.

When upper motor neurons degenerate, the correct messages cannot reach the lower motor neurons, and the lower motor neurons cannot transmit the correct messages to the muscles. As the degeneration continues, spasticity and weakness increase. The legs are affected because degeneration occurs primarily at the ends of the longest nerves in the spinal cord, which control the legs. In some cases, the upper body can be minimally affected as well, leading to problems with the arms or speech and swallowing muscles.

How severe will my symptoms get?

There is no way to predict rate of progression or severity of symptoms. Generally, once symptoms begin, progression continues slowly throughout life. For some childhood-onset forms, symptoms become apparent, gradually worsen during childhood, and then stabilize after adolescence. HSP rarely results in complete loss of lower limb mobility.

How is HSP diagnosed?

HSP is diagnosed via a careful clinical examination, by excluding other disorders that cause spasticity and weakness in the legs, and by an observation period to see if other symptoms develop that indicate another condition, such as PLS. Disorders that can be ruled out with testing are amyotrophic lateral sclerosis (ALS), tropical spastic paraparesis (TSP), vitamin deficiencies (B12 or E), thoracic spine herniated disks, and spinal cord tumors or injuries and multiple sclerosis. HSP can resemble cerebral palsy, however, HSP is degenerative and thereby causes increasing spasticity and weakness of the muscles. Two other disorders with spastic paraplegia symptoms termed lathyrism and konzo are caused by toxins in the plants *Lathyrus sativus* and cassava.

HSP is hereditary, and examining family history is important in diagnosing HSP. However, many individuals with all the signs and symptoms of HSP do not have a family history.

What genetic testing is available?

Athena Diagnostics offers testing for five different types of HSP out of the thirty or more different forms of HSP. As more genes are discovered, it is hopeful that such information will lead to greater availability of testing.

Genetic counselors can be found at many major medical centers or by contacting the National Society of Genetic Counselors. Gene tests can be used for prenatal testing.

What is the treatment?

No treatments are currently available to prevent, stop, or reverse HSP. Treatment is focused on symptom relief, such as medication to reduce spasticity; physical therapy and exercise to help maintain flexibility, strength, and range of motion; assistive devices and communications aids; and supportive therapy and other modalities.

What is the life expectancy?

Life expectancy is normal. However, complications arising from falls or immobility caused by the symptoms of HSP may inadvertently shorten a person's life.

What is the risk of getting HSP?

There are some thirty different forms of HSP, with three different modes of inheritance: autosomal dominant, autosomal recessive, and

X-linked. Each mode has a different risk factor, which ranges from almost none to 50 percent.

What other conditions cause spasticity and weakness of muscles?

Muscle spasticity and weakness can also be caused by other conditions, including (but not limited to) primary lateral sclerosis, spinal cord injury or tumors, cerebral palsy, multiple sclerosis, amyotrophic lateral sclerosis, vitamin absorption, and thoracic spine herniated disks.

There is a virus-caused disease called tropical spastic paraparesis and conditions called lathyrism and konzo caused by toxins in the plants *Lathyrus sativus* and cassava that also cause muscle spasticity and weakness.

Other Questions

Does stress affect symptoms?

Many people find the tightness in their muscles worsens when they are angry, stressed, or upset. This may make it more difficult to walk and speak. It is unknown exactly how emotions affect muscle tone, but it may involve adrenalin levels. Most people also report increased stiffness in cold weather.

Is depression normal?

Periods of feeling down about having HSP are normal and expected. It is not uncommon for people to also experience periods of clinical depression.

Do people with HSP experience memory loss?

Memory disturbance has been reported in some individuals with HSP due to spastin gene mutations. In general, it was mild.

Before attributing memory disturbance to HSP, it is important to consider other causes: stress, anxiety, depression, lack of sleep, medications (including Baclofen), other health conditions including vitamin B12 deficiency.

If memory disturbance is significant, a cause of concern, or worsening, it would be important to discuss this with your primary physician and neurologist.

Are foot problems common?

Yes. Here are a few examples:

- **High arched feet (pes cavus):** High arches occur because there is more weakness in the foot muscles that extend the foot backward and flatten the arch than in the muscles that flex the foot downward.

- **Shortened Achilles tendons:** Achilles tendons are often short, and generally shorten further as HSP progresses.

- **Jumping feet (clonus):** Clonus is an uncontrollable, repetitive jerking of muscles that makes the foot jump rapidly up and down. It occurs when the foot is in a position that causes a disruption of the signals from the brain, leading to an automatic stretch reflex.

- **Hammer toes or bunions:** These may occur due to imbalances in the strength and tone of muscles that maintain proper alignment of joints in the feet.

- **Cold feet and/or foot swelling:** This is most likely caused by poor circulation. Normally, muscle contractions in the legs help pump blood from the legs back to the heart. If the muscles are weakened, or if the person is relatively inactive, the blood flow from the legs may be decreased, and fluids may accumulate. This can cause swelling, or a sensation of "cold feet."

Can my arms be affected?

Some people may experience problems with their arms or fine motor control of their fingers. The degeneration in nerves that supply the arms is mild compared to that which occurs in the nerves that supply the legs. For most people, this is not significant.

Can HSP affect sexual function?

The short answer appears to be "yes," although it is important to remember that sexual desire and/or function can be affected by many other factors such as age, stress, depression, fatigue, and medical disorders or medications.

Some people report that stiffness, spasms, and cramps that are part of HSP may either inhibit (or intensify) orgasm, or that orgasm may bring on leg stiffness, spasms, or clonus. Stiffness of the legs or arms may cause difficulty using certain positions for intercourse.

315

Is HSP an ataxia?

No. The group of disorders known as ataxias (such as Friedreich ataxia) are spinocerebellar disorders in which there is a disturbance either in the part of the brain known as the cerebellum or in the connections to it. HSP does not involve the cerebellum. Ataxias can be hereditary or sporadic.

The term "ataxia" means without coordination, and can also refer to a symptom in which there is a lack of muscle control resulting in a jerky or unsteady movement. People with HSP may have incoordination as a symptom. This does not mean they have ataxia.

Can I donate blood?

HSP cannot be passed to others through donation of blood. There is no medical reason why a person with HSP cannot donate blood.

When was HSP identified?

In the late 1800's, A. Strümpell, a neurologist in Heidelberg Germany, described this disorder. He observed two brothers and their father, who had gait disorders and spasticity in their legs. After the death of the brothers, Strümpell was able to show through autopsy the degeneration of the nerve fibers leading through the spinal cord. The disorder was originally named after Strümpell, and after two Frenchmen who later provided more information about the disorder, Lorrain and Charcot.

Is HSP more prevalent in certain ethnic groups?

There is no evidence that HSP is more prevalent in one ethnic group than another.

Section 29.5

Muscular Dystrophy

About MD

Muscular dystrophy (MD) is a genetic disorder that gradually weakens the body's muscles. It's caused by incorrect or missing genetic information that prevents the body from making the proteins needed to build and maintain healthy muscles.

A child who is diagnosed with MD gradually loses the ability to do things like walk, sit upright, breathe easily, and move the arms and hands. This increasing weakness can lead to other health problems.

There are several major forms of muscular dystrophy, which can affect the muscles to varying degrees. In some cases, MD starts causing muscle problems in infancy; in others, symptoms don't appear until adulthood.

There is no cure for MD, but researchers are quickly learning more about how to prevent and treat it. Doctors are also working on improving muscle and joint function and slowing muscle deterioration so that those with MD can live as actively and independently as possible.

First Symptoms

Many kids with muscular dystrophy follow a normal pattern of development during their first few years of life. But in time common symptoms begin to appear. A child who has MD may start to stumble, waddle, have difficulty going up stairs, and toe walk (walk on the toes without the heels hitting the floor). A child may start to struggle to get up from a sitting position or have a hard time pushing things, like a wagon or a tricycle.

Kids with MD often develop enlarged calf muscles (called calf pseudohypertrophy) as muscle tissue is destroyed and replaced by fat.

Diagnosis

When first suspecting that a child has muscular dystrophy, a doctor will do a physical exam, take a family history, and ask about any problems—particularly those affecting the muscles—that the child might be having.

In addition, the doctor may perform tests to determine what type of MD is involved and to rule out other diseases that could cause the problem. These might include a blood test to measure levels of serum creatine kinase, an enzyme that's released into the bloodstream when muscle fibers are deteriorating. Elevated levels indicate that something is causing muscle damage.

The doctor also may do a blood test to check the deoxyribonucleic acid (DNA) for gene abnormalities or a muscle biopsy to look for patterns of deterioration and abnormal levels of dystrophin, a protein that helps muscle cells keep their shape and length.

Types of Muscular Dystrophy

The different types of muscular dystrophy affect different sets of muscles and result in different degrees of muscle weakness.

Duchenne muscular dystrophy is the most common and the most severe form of MD. It affects about 1 out of every 3,500 boys. (Girls can carry the gene that causes the disease, but they usually have no symptoms.) This form occurs because of a problem with the gene that makes dystrophin. Without this protein, the muscles break down and a child becomes weaker.

In cases of Duchenne MD, symptoms usually appear around age five, as the pelvic muscles begin to weaken. Most kids with this form need to use a wheelchair by age twelve. Over time, their muscles weaken in the shoulders, back, arms, and legs.

Eventually, the respiratory muscles are affected, and a ventilator is required to assist breathing. Kids who have Duchenne MD typically have a life span of about twenty years.

Although most kids with Duchenne MD have average intelligence, about a third experience learning disabilities and a small number are intellectually disabled.

While the incidence of Duchenne is known, it's unclear how common other forms of MD are because the symptoms can vary so widely between individuals. In fact, in some people the symptoms are so mild that the disease goes undiagnosed.

Becker muscular dystrophy is similar to Duchenne, but is less common and progresses more slowly. This form of MD, which affects approximately 1 in 30,000 boys, is caused by insufficient production of dystrophin, too.

Symptoms begin during the teen years, then follow a pattern similar to Duchenne MD. Muscle weakness first begins in the pelvic muscles, then moves into the shoulders and back. Many children with Becker MD have a normal life span and can lead long, active lives without the use of a wheelchair.

Myotonic dystrophy, also known as Steinert disease, is the most common adult form of MD, although half of all cases are diagnosed in people under twenty years old. It is caused by a portion of a particular gene that is larger than it should be. The symptoms can appear at any time during a child's life.

The main symptoms include muscle weakness, myotonia (in which the muscles have trouble relaxing once they contract), and muscle wasting (when the muscles shrink over time). Kids with myotonic dystrophy also can experience cataracts and heart problems.

Limb-girdle muscular dystrophy affects boys and girls equally. Symptoms usually start when kids are between eight and fifteen years old. This form progresses slowly, affecting the pelvic, shoulder, and back muscles. The severity of muscle weakness varies—some kids have only mild weakness while others develop severe disabilities and as adults need to use a wheelchair.

Facioscapulohumeral muscular dystrophy can affect both boys and girls, and the symptoms usually first appear during the teen years. It tends to progress slowly.

Muscle weakness first develops in the face, making it difficult for a child to close the eyes, whistle, or puff out the cheeks. The shoulder and back muscles gradually become weak, and kids have difficulty lifting objects or raising their hands overhead. Over time, the legs and pelvic muscles also may lose strength.

Other types of MD, which are rare, include distal, ocular, oculopharyngeal, and Emery-Dreifuss.

Caring for a Child with MD

Though there's no cure for MD yet, doctors are working to improve muscle and joint function, and slow muscle deterioration.

If your child is diagnosed with MD, a team of medical specialists will work with you and your family, including: a neurologist, orthopedist, pulmonologist, physical and occupational therapist, nurse practitioner, cardiologist, registered dietician, and a social worker.

Muscular dystrophy is often degenerative, so kids may pass through different stages as it progresses and require different kinds of treatment. During the early stages, physical therapy, joint bracing, and medications are often used.

During the later stages, doctors may use assistive devices such as:

- physical therapy and bracing to improve flexibility;

- power wheelchairs and scooters to improve mobility;

- a ventilator to support breathing;

- robotics to help your child perform routine daily tasks.

Physical Therapy and Bracing

Physical therapy can help a child maintain muscle tone and reduce the severity of joint contractures with exercises that keep the muscles strong and the joints flexible.

A physical therapist also uses bracing to help prevent joint contractures, a stiffening of the muscles near the joints that can make it harder to move and can lock the joints in painful positions. By providing extra support in just the right places, bracing can extend the time that a child with MD can walk independently.

Prednisone

If a child has Duchenne muscular dystrophy, the doctor may prescribe the steroid prednisone to help slow the rate of muscle deterioration. By doing so, the child may be able to walk longer and live a more active life.

There is some debate over the best time to begin prednisone treatment, but most doctors prescribe it when a child is five or six years old or when the child's strength begins to significantly decline. Prednisone does have side effects, though. It can cause weight gain, which can put even greater strain on already weak muscles. It also can cause a loss of bone density and, possibly, lead to fractures. If prescribing prednisone, your doctor will closely monitor your child.

Spinal Fusion

Many children with the Duchenne and Becker forms of MD develop severe scoliosis—an S- or C-shaped curvature of the spine caused by back muscles that are too weak to hold the spine erect.

Some kids with severe cases undergo spinal fusion, a surgery that can reduce pain, lessen the severity of the curvature so that a child can sit upright and comfortably in a chair, and ensure that the spine curvature doesn't have an effect on breathing. Usually, spinal fusion surgery only requires a short hospital stay.

Respiratory Care

Many kids with MD also have weakened heart and respiratory muscles. As a result, they can't cough out phlegm and sometimes develop respiratory infections that can quickly become serious. Good general health care and regular vaccinations are especially important for children with muscular dystrophy to help prevent these infections.

Assistive Devices

A variety of new technologies can provide independence and mobility for kids with muscular dystrophy.

Some kids with Duchenne MD might use a manual wheelchair once it becomes difficult to walk. Others go directly to a motorized wheelchair, which can be equipped to meet their needs as muscle deterioration advances.

Robotic technologies also are under development to help kids move their arms and perform activities of daily living.

If your child would benefit from an assistive technological device, contact your local chapter of the Muscular Dystrophy Association to ask about financial assistance that might be available. In some cases, health insurers cover the cost of these devices.

The Search for a Cure

Researchers are quickly learning more about what causes the genetic disorder that leads to muscular dystrophy, and about possible treatments for the disease.

To learn more about the most current research on MD, contact the local chapter of the Muscular Dystrophy Association or talk to your doctor, who also can tell you about clinical trials on MD.

Section 29.6

Spinal Muscular Atrophy

Excerpted from "Learning about Spinal Muscular Atrophy,"
National Human Genome Research Institute www.genome.gov),
February 19, 2012.

What is spinal muscular atrophy?

Spinal muscular atrophy is a group of inherited disorders that cause progressive muscle degeneration and weakness. Spinal muscular atrophy (SMA) is the second leading cause of neuromuscular disease. It is usually inherited as an autosomal recessive trait (a person must get the defective gene from both parents to be affected).

There are several types of SMA called subtypes. Each of the subtypes is based on the severity of the disorder and the age at which symptoms begin. There are three types of SMA that affect children before the age of one year. There are two types of SMA, type IV and Finkel type, that occur in adulthood, usually after age thirty. Symptoms of adult-onset spinal muscular atrophy are usually mild to moderate and include muscle weakness, tremor, and twitching.

The prognosis for individuals with SMA varies depending on the type of SMA and the degree of respiratory function. The patient's condition tends to deteriorate over time, depending on the severity of the symptoms.

Spinal muscular atrophy affects one in six thousand to one in ten thousand people.

What are the symptoms of spinal muscular atrophy?

Three types of SMA affect children before age one year. Type 0 is the most severe form of spinal muscular atrophy and begins before birth. Usually, the first symptom of type 0 is reduced movement of the fetus that is first seen between thirty and thirty-six weeks of the pregnancy. After birth, these newborns have little movement and have difficulties with swallowing and breathing.

Type I spinal muscular atrophy (called Werdnig-Hoffman disease) is another severe form of SMA. Symptoms of type 1 may be present at birth or within the first few months of life. These infants usually have difficulty breathing and swallowing, and they are unable to sit without support.

Children with type II SMA usually develop muscle weakness between ages six and twelve months. They cannot stand or walk without help.

Type III SMA (called Kugelberg-Welander disease or juvenile type) is a milder form of SMA than types 0, I or II. Symptoms appear between early childhood (older than age one year) and early adulthood. Individuals with type III SMA are able to stand and walk without help. They usually lose their ability to stand and walk later in life. There are two other types of spinal muscular atrophy, type IV and Finkel type, that occur in adulthood, usually after age thirty. Symptoms of adult-onset SMA are usually mild to moderate and include muscle weakness, tremor, and twitching.

How is spinal muscular atrophy diagnosed?

To make a diagnosis of SMA, symptoms need to be present. When symptoms are present, diagnosis can be made by genetic testing. Gene alterations (mutations) in the SMN1 and VAPB genes cause SMA. Having extra copies of the SMN2 gene can modify the course of SMA.

Genetic testing on a blood or tissue sample is done to identify whether there is at least one copy of the SMN1 gene by looking for its special makeup. Mutations in the SMN1 gene cause types 0, I, II, III, and IV. Some people who have SMA type II, III, or IV have three or more copies of the SMN2 gene. Having these extra copies can modify the course of SMA. The more copies of SMN2 gene a person has, the less severe his or her symptoms.

Genetic testing for a mutation in the VAPB gene is done to diagnose the Finkel type SMA.

In some situations other tests such as an electromyography (EMG) or muscle biopsy may be needed because it is not possible to conduct the SMN gene tests or no abnormality is identified.

What is the treatment for spinal muscular atrophy?

There is currently no specific cure for SMA. Infants who have a severe form of SMA frequently die of respiratory failure due to weakness of the muscles that help with breathing. Children who have milder forms of SMA will live much longer but they may need extensive medical support.

The current treatment for SMA involves prevention and management of the secondary effect of muscle weakness and loss.

Today, much can be done for SMA patients in terms of medical and in particular respiratory, nutritional, and rehabilitation care. In addition, several drugs have been identified in laboratory experiments that may help patients. Some of the drugs that are currently being investigated include: Butyrates, valproic acid, hydroxyurea, and riluzole.

At present gene therapy—replacing the altered genes with a normal version—is being tested in animals. Researchers believe that gene replacement for SMA will take many more years of research before it can be used in humans. Other approaches to developing better treatment include searching for drugs that increase SMN levels, enhance residual SMN function, or compensate for its loss.

Is spinal muscular atrophy inherited?

SMA types 0, I, II, III, and IV are inherited in an autosomal recessive pattern in families. In autosomal recessive inheritance, a person who has SMA has inherited two altered (mutated) copies of the SMN1 gene from his or her parents. The parents of an individual with an autosomal recessive inherited disorder such as SMA are carriers of one copy of the altered gene. Since they carry a normal version of the gene, they do not have signs or symptoms of the disorder.

Finkel type SMA is inherited in an autosomal dominant pattern. This means that the person has one copy of the altered gene in each cell that causes the disorder.

Chapter 30

Noonan Syndrome

What is Noonan syndrome?

Noonan syndrome is a disorder that involves unusual facial characteristics, short stature, heart defects present at birth, bleeding problems, developmental delays, and malformations of the bones of the rib cage.

Noonan syndrome is caused by changes in one of several autosomal dominant genes. A person who has Noonan syndrome may have inherited an altered (mutated) gene from one of his or her parents, or the gene change may be a new change due to an error carried by the egg or sperm or occurring at conception. Alterations in four genes—PTPN11, SOS1, RAF1, and KRAS—have been identified to date.

Noonan syndrome is present in about 1 in 1,000 to 1 in 2,500 people.

What are the symptoms of Noonan syndrome?

Symptoms of Noonan syndrome may include the following:

- A characteristic facial appearance

- Short stature

- Heart defect present at birth (congenital heart defect)

- A broad or webbed neck

Excerpted from "Learning about Noonan Syndrome," National Human Genome Research Institute (www.genome.gov), September 26, 2011.

- Minor eye problems such as strabismus in up to 95 percent of individuals

- Bleeding problems such as a history of abnormal bleeding or bruising

- An unusual chest shape with widely spaced and low-set nipples

- Developmental delay of varying degrees, but usually mild

- In males, undescended testes (cryptorchidism)

How is Noonan syndrome diagnosed?

The diagnosis of Noonan syndrome is based on the person's clinical symptoms and signs. The specialist examines the person, looking for the specific features of Noonan syndrome.

Individuals who have Noonan syndrome have normal chromosome studies. Four genes—PTPN11, SOS1, RAF1, and KRAS—are the only genes that are known to be associated with Noonan syndrome. Approximately 50 percent of individuals with Noonan syndrome have mutations in the PTPN11 gene. Twenty percent of those with Noonan syndrome have mutations in the SOS1. Mutations in the RAF1 gene account for between 10 and 15 percent of Noonan syndrome cases. About 5 percent of people with Noonan syndrome have mutations in the KRAS gene and usually have a more severe or atypical form of the disorder. The cause of Noonan syndrome in the remaining 10 to 15 percent of people with this disorder is not yet known.

What is the treatment for Noonan syndrome?

Treatment for individuals who have Noonan syndrome is based on their particular symptoms. Heart problems are treated in the same way that they are for individuals in the general population. Early intervention programs are used to help with developmental disabilities, when present. Bleeding problems that can be present in Noonan syndrome may have a variety of causes and are treated according to their cause. Growth problems may be caused by lack of growth hormone and may be treated with growth hormone treatment. Symptoms such as heart problems are followed on a regular basis.

Is Noonan syndrome inherited?

Noonan syndrome is inherited in families in an autosomal dominant pattern. This means that a person who has Noonan syndrome has one copy of an altered gene that causes the disorder. In about one-third to two-thirds of families one of the parents also has Noonan syndrome. The parent who has Noonan syndrome has a one in two (50 percent) chance to pass on the altered gene to a child who will be affected; and a one in two (50 percent) chance to pass on the normal version of the gene to a child who will not have Noonan syndrome. In many individuals who have Noonan syndrome, the altered gene happens for the first time in them, and neither of the parents has Noonan syndrome. This is called a de novo mutation. The chance for these parents to have another child with Noonan syndrome is very small (less than 1 percent).

Chapter 31

Porphyria

What is porphyria?

The porphyrias are a group of different diseases, each caused by a specific abnormality in the heme production process. Heme is a chemical compound that contains iron and gives blood its red color. The essential functions of heme depend on its ability to bind oxygen. Heme is incorporated into hemoglobin, a protein that enables red blood cells to carry oxygen from the lungs to all parts of the body. Heme also plays a role in the liver, where it assists in breaking down chemicals (including some drugs and hormones) so that they are easily removed from the body.

Heme is produced in the bone marrow and liver through a complex process controlled by eight different enzymes. As this production process of heme progresses, several different intermediate compounds (heme precursors) are created and modified. If one of the essential enzymes in heme production is deficient, certain precursors may accumulate in tissues (especially in the bone marrow or liver), appear in excess in the blood, and get excreted in the urine or stool. The specific precursors that accumulate depend on which enzyme is deficient. Porphyria results in a deficiency or inactivity of a specific enzyme in the heme production process, with resulting accumulation of heme precursors.

Excerpted from "Learning about Porphyria," National Human Genome Research Institute (www.genome.gov), December 29, 2010.

What are the signs and symptoms of porphyria?

The signs and symptoms of porphyria vary among types. Some types of porphyria (called cutaneous porphyria) cause the skin to become overly sensitive to sunlight. Areas of the skin exposed to the sun develop redness, blistering, and often scarring.

The symptoms of other types of porphyria (called acute porphyrias) affect the nervous system. These symptoms include chest and abdominal pain, emotional and mental disorders, seizures, and muscle weakness. These symptoms often appear quickly and last from days to weeks. Some porphyrias have a combination of acute symptoms and symptoms that affect the skin.

Environmental factors can trigger the signs and symptoms of porphyria. These include the following:

- Alcohol
- Smoking
- Certain drugs, hormones
- Exposure to sunlight
- Stress
- Dieting and fasting

How is porphyria diagnosed?

Porphyria is diagnosed through blood, urine, and stool tests, especially at or near the time of symptoms. Diagnosis may be difficult because the range of symptoms is common to many disorders and interpretation of the tests may be complex. A large number of tests are available, however, but results among laboratories are not always reliable.

How is porphyria treated?

Each form of porphyria is treated differently. Treatment may involve treating with heme, giving medicines to relieve the symptoms, or drawing blood. People who have severe attacks may need to be hospitalized.

What do we know about porphyria and heredity?

Most of the porphyrias are inherited conditions. The genes for all the enzymes in the heme pathway have been identified. Some forms of porphyria result from inheriting one altered gene from one parent (autosomal dominant). Other forms result from inheriting two altered genes, one from each parent (autosomal recessive). Each type of porphyria carries a different risk that individuals in an affected family will have the disease or transmit it to their children.

Porphyria cutanea tarda (PCT) is a type of porphyria that is most often not inherited. Eighty percent of individuals with PCT have an acquired disease that becomes active when factors such as iron, alcohol, hepatitis C virus (HCV), human immunodeficiency virus (HIV), estrogens (such as those used in oral contraceptives and prostate cancer treatment), and possibly smoking, combine to cause an enzyme deficiency in the liver. Hemochromatosis, an iron overload disorder, can also predispose individuals to PCT. Twenty percent of individuals with PCT have an inherited form of the disease. Many individuals with the inherited form of PCT never develop symptoms.

What triggers a porphyria attack?

Porphyria can be triggered by drugs (barbiturates, tranquilizers, birth control pills, sedatives), chemicals, fasting, smoking, drinking alcohol, infections, emotional and physical stress, menstrual hormones, and exposure to the sun. Attacks of porphyria can develop over hours or days and last for days or weeks.

What are the cutaneous porphyrias?

The cutaneous porphyrias affect the skin. People with cutaneous porphyria develop blisters, itching, and swelling of their skin when it is exposed to sunlight. The cutaneous porphyrias include the following types:

- **Congenital erythropoietic porphyria:** Also called congenital porphyria. This is a rare disorder that mainly affects the skin. It results from low levels of the enzyme responsible for the fourth step in heme production. It is inherited in an autosomal recessive pattern.

- **Erythropoietic protoporphyria:** An uncommon disorder that mainly affects the skin. It results from reduced levels of the enzyme responsible for the eighth and final step in heme production. The inheritance of this condition is not fully understood. Most cases are probably inherited in an autosomal dominant pattern, however, it shows autosomal recessive inheritance in a small number of families.

• **Hepatoerythropoietic porphyria:** A rare disorder that mainly affects the skin. It results from very low levels of the enzyme responsible for the fifth step in heme production. It is inherited in an autosomal recessive pattern.

• **Hereditary coproporphyria:** A rare disorder that can have symptoms of acute porphyria and symptoms that affect the skin. It results from low levels of the enzyme responsible for the sixth step in heme production. It is inherited in an autosomal dominant pattern.

• **Porphyria cutanea tarda:** The most common type of porphyria. It occurs in an estimated one in twenty-five thousand people, including both inherited and sporadic (noninherited) cases. An estimated 80 percent of porphyria cutanea tarda cases are sporadic. It results from low levels of the enzyme responsible for the fifth step in heme production. When this condition is inherited, it occurs in an autosomal dominant pattern.

• **Variegate porphyria:** A disorder that can have symptoms of acute porphyria and symptoms that affect the skin. It results from low levels of the enzyme responsible for the seventh step in heme production. It is inherited in an autosomal dominant pattern.

What are the acute porphyrias?

The acute porphyrias affect the nervous system. Symptoms of acute porphyria include pain in the chest, abdomen, limbs, or back; muscle numbness, tingling, paralysis, or cramping; vomiting; constipation; and personality changes or mental disorders. These symptoms appear intermittently. The acute porphyrias include the following types:

• **Acute intermittent porphyria:** This is probably the most common porphyria with acute (severe but usually not long-lasting) symptoms. It results from low levels of the enzyme responsible for the third step in heme production. It is inherited in an autosomal dominant pattern.

• **Aminolevulinate dehydratase (ALAD) deficiency porphyria:** A very rare disorder that results from low levels of the enzyme responsible for the second step in heme production. It is inherited in an autosomal recessive pattern.

Chapter 32

Retinoblastoma

Retinoblastoma is a cancerous tumor that grows in the retina, a layer of nerve tissue in the back of the eye that senses light and sends images to the brain.

A cancer of early childhood, retinoblastoma can affect developing fetuses in the womb, as well as newborns, babies, toddlers, and children up to five years old.

Many parents first see signs of retinoblastoma after noticing that their child's pupil (the dark circular area in the middle of the iris, the colored part of the eye) appears whitish in bright light. Some parents notice this effect in photographs. This happens because the pupil is translucent; so, retinal tumors that lie behind it may be noticeable.

While the majority of kids who develop retinoblastoma are born with it, most are not diagnosed at birth. The average age at diagnosis is between twelve and eighteen months. When diagnosed, most kids are treated successfully and able to preserve their sight while maintaining good vision.

"Retinoblastoma," March 2012, reprinted with permission from www.kidshealth .org. This information was provided by KidsHealth®, one of the largest resources online for medically reviewed health information written for parents, kids, and teens. For more articles like this, visit www.KidsHealth.org, or www.TeensHealth.org. Copyright © 1995–2012 The Nemours Foundation. All rights reserved.

Causes

Like other forms of cancer, there is a genetic component to retinoblastoma. Kids who carry the genetic mutation (from either a parent or grandparent) usually get more than one tumor and are likely to develop the disease in both eyes. It also usually occurs at a younger age than in kids without the mutation. This is called hereditary retinoblastoma.

The remainder of kids who develop the condition about 60 percent have no family history of the disease, and will usually get it in just one eye, with much less risk of developing retinoblastoma in the other eye. This is called unilateral retinoblastoma.

Kids with hereditary retinoblastoma in one eye could develop it later in the other eye, so regular checkups of the healthy eye should be done every two to four months for at least twenty-eight months. After treatment is completed, follow-up exams should continue until a child is five years old.

Signs and Symptoms

A cloudy white pupil, which might look silvery white or yellow in bright light, is often the first sign of retinoblastoma. This is called leukocoria, or "cat's eye reflex." Other symptoms include:

- poorly aligned or "wandering" eye, known as strabismus;
- reddish pupil, often with pain;
- larger-than-normal pupil;
- different-colored irises;
- poor vision or decreased vision.

Many of these symptoms are common side effects of other eye conditions, and don't necessarily mean a child has retinoblastoma. If your child has any of these symptoms, contact your doctor right away.

Diagnosis

If retinoblastoma is suspected, the doctor will refer your child to a pediatric ophthalmologist, an eye doctor who will examine the retina by dilating the eye, sometimes under general anesthesia. He or she might also order imaging tests, like an ultrasound of the eye, a computerized tomography (CT) scan, or magnetic resonance imaging (MRI), as well as blood tests.

If retinoblastoma is diagnosed, a pediatric oncologist (cancer doctor) will test to see if cancer is anywhere else in the child's body. He or she might perform blood tests, a spinal tap, or bone marrow biopsy. Live tissue samples, or biopsies, are rarely used to diagnose retinoblastoma because they can cause cancer cells to spread beyond the eye.

Staging

Once doctors have made a diagnosis of retinoblastoma, they use detailed staging systems including the St. Jude's Children's Research Hospital and Reese-Ellsworth staging systems to determine the extent of the cancer and whether it has spread to other parts of the body. Knowing the stage of the disease helps doctors decide how to treat it.

Staging categorizes retinoblastoma that is either intraocular (within the eye) or extraocular (outside the eye):

- Intraocular retinoblastoma is found in one or both eyes but does not extend beyond the eye.

- Extraocular retinoblastoma means the cancer has spread beyond the eye to tissues around the eye or to other parts of the body, such as the brain, spinal cord, bone marrow, or lymph nodes.

Under the St. Jude's staging system, intraocular retinoblastoma is classified into four stages:

1. **Stage I:** the tumor is confined to the retina.

2. **Stage II:** It is confined to the eyeball.

3. **Stage III:** The cancer has spread to areas in the region around the eye.

4. **Stage IV:** The cancer has spread through the optic nerve to the brain, or through the blood to soft tissues, bone, or lymph nodes.

The Reese-Ellsworth staging system (an older model of staging developed in the 1960s) classifies retinoblastoma from Group I (cases that are considered the most favorable for saving the eye) to Group V (these cases are unlikely to be controlled with chemotherapy or radiation).

Recently, the National Childhood Cancer Foundation's Children's Oncology Group adopted a more modern staging system that considers a child's disease severity and predicts what type of treatment will be most effective while still preserving the eye.

Treatment

A pediatric ophthalmologist, pediatric oncologist, and radiation therapist will work together to treat a child with retinoblastoma. This team will individualize a plan for each patient based on the extent of the disease within the eye, whether it is in one or both eyes, and whether it has spread beyond the eye.

There are many forms of treatment for retinoblastoma all targeted at killing cancer cells. The following treatments, or a combination of treatments, may be recommended:

- **Chemotherapy:** Tumor-killing medications are given orally, through injection, or intravenously (in a vein).

- **Intra-arterial chemotherapy:** In some cases, doctors are now injecting chemotherapy drugs into the blood vessel that feeds the eye to get the medication to the tumor more directly.

- **External beam radiation:** Beams of radiation are carefully focused onto the tumor to kill cancer cells.

- **Brachytherapy:** Radioactive material (little rods or pellets) is placed within the tumor to deliver beams of radiation to specific areas. This form of treatment minimizes the damage to surrounding healthy tissue.

- **Radioactive plaques:** A disk is implanted in the eye with a dose of radiation applied directly to the tumor site.

- **Cryotherapy:** Liquid nitrogen or argon gases two extremely cold substances are used to freeze and destroy diseased tissue.

- **Transpupillary thermotherapy:** Laser energy (through the use of infrared light) heats up cancer cells and surrounding blood vessels, which kills the cells.

- **Photocoagulation:** Laser energy is delivered to blood vessels surrounding the tumor, causing blood clots and depriving the cancer cells of nutrients.

- **Enucleation:** In severe cases of retinoblastoma, the entire eyeball is removed to prevent the spread of cancerous cells to other areas of the body.

During treatment for retinoblastoma, a child will need periodic examinations of the eyes (usually under anesthesia) to confirm the effectiveness of treatment.

Recurrent retinoblastoma is cancer that has returned or continues to grow after treatment. It may occur in the eye, tissues around the eye, or elsewhere in the body. Kids with hereditary cases of retinoblastoma are more likely to develop new tumors years after treatment. Therefore, close follow-up exams are important for these children, who also are at risk for other types of cancer later in life.

Caring for Your Child

Kids treated with chemotherapy might develop flu-like symptoms afterward. Some might feel nauseated, weak, or dizzy after treatment, or run a fever. Those who undergo radiation therapy might feel more tired than usual. Their skin can become reddened or dry in the area being treated. During this time, the doctor may prescribe pain relievers for your child.

Once treatment is over, kids can get back to normal activities if they feel well enough and if the doctor allows. Recovery periods vary, depending on the treatment and the child.

In many cases, kids with retinoblastoma retain the use of both eyes. Children with one eye removed have good vision and receive a prosthetic eye to replace the missing eye. Prosthetic eyes are of such good quality that most people can't tell which eye is natural and which is prosthetic.

The majority of children treated for retinoblastoma survive and go on to lead normal lives in fact, more than 80 percent of them will retain 20/20 vision. Still, because those with hereditary retinoblastoma have a significant risk of developing secondary cancers, frequent checkups are vital.

Chapter 33

Rett Syndrome

What is Rett syndrome?

Rett syndrome is a neurological and developmental disorder that mostly occurs in females. Infants with Rett syndrome seem to grow and develop normally at first, but then stop developing and even lose skills and abilities.

For instance, they stop talking even though they used to say certain words. They lose their ability to walk properly. They stop using their hands to do things and often develop stereotyped hand movements, such as wringing, clapping, or patting their hands.

Rett syndrome is considered one of the autism spectrum disorders. Most cases of Rett syndrome are caused by a mutation on the MECP2 gene, which is found on the X chromosome.

What are the symptoms of Rett syndrome?

Beginning between three months and three years of age, most children with Rett syndrome start to show some of the following symptoms:

- Loss of purposeful hand movements, such as grasping with fingers, reaching for things, or touching things on purpose

- Loss of speech

Reprinted from "Rett Syndrome," National Institute of Child Health and Human Development, National Institutes of Health, August 2, 2010.

- Balance and coordination problems, including losing the ability to walk in many cases

- Stereotypic hand movements, such as hand wringing

- Breathing problems, such as hyperventilation and breath holding, or apnea when awake

- Anxiety and social-behavioral problems

- Intellectual and developmental disabilities

There are a number of other problems common among those who have Rett syndrome. But having these problems is not necessary to get a diagnosis of Rett syndrome. These problems can include the following:

- Scoliosis, a curving of the spine that occurs in approximately 80 percent of girls with Rett syndrome

- Seizures

- Constipation and gastroesophageal reflux

- Cardiac or heart problems, specifically problems with the rhythm of their heartbeat

- Problems feeding themselves, trouble swallowing and chewing

- Problems with sleep, specifically disrupted sleep patterns at night and an increase in total and daytime sleep

What is the usual course of Rett syndrome?

Health care providers view the onset of Rett syndrome symptoms in four stages:

- **Early onset phase:** Development stalls or stops.

- **Rapid destructive phase:** The child loses skills (regresses) quickly. Purposeful hand movements and speech are usually the first skills lost.

- **Plateau phase:** Regression slows, and other problems may seem to lessen or improve. Most people with Rett syndrome spend most of their lives in stage 3.

- **Late motor deterioration phase:** Individuals may become stiff or lose muscle tone; some may become immobile.

Most girls with Rett syndrome live until adulthood. They will usually need care and assistance throughout their lives.

What is the treatment for Rett syndrome?

There is currently no cure for Rett syndrome. However, girls can be treated for some of the problems associated with the condition. These treatments generally aim to slow the loss of abilities, improve or preserve movement, and encourage communication and social contact.

People with Rett syndrome often benefit from a team approach to care, in which many kinds of health care providers play a role, along with family members. Members of this team may include the following:

- Physical therapists, who can help patients improve or maintain mobility and balance and reduce misshapen back and limbs

- Occupational therapists, who can help patients improve or maintain use of their hands and reduce stereotypic hand movements

- Speech-language therapists, who can help patients use nonverbal ways of communication and improve social interaction

Other options, such as medication (such as for constipation or heart problems) or surgery (to correct spine curvature or correct heart defects) are also effective for treating some of the symptoms of Rett syndrome.

Chapter 34

Tuberous Sclerosis

What is tuberous sclerosis?

Tuberous sclerosis—also called tuberous sclerosis complex (TSC)[1]—is a rare, multisystem genetic disease that causes benign tumors to grow in the brain and on other vital organs such as the kidneys, heart, eyes, lungs, and skin. It usually affects the central nervous system and results in a combination of symptoms including seizures, developmental delay, behavioral problems, skin abnormalities, and kidney disease.

The disorder affects as many as twenty-five thousand to forty thousand individuals in the United States and about one to two million individuals worldwide, with an estimated prevalence of one in six thousand newborns. TSC occurs in all races and ethnic groups, and in both genders.

The name tuberous sclerosis comes from the characteristic tuber or potato-like nodules in the brain, which calcify with age and become hard or sclerotic. The disorder—once known as epiloia or Bourneville disease—was first identified by a French physician more than one hundred years ago.

Many TSC patients show evidence of the disorder in the first year of life. However, clinical features can be subtle initially, and many signs and symptoms take years to develop. As a result, TSC can be unrecognized or misdiagnosed for years.

Excerpted from "Tuberous Sclerosis Fact Sheet," National Institute of Neurological Disorders and Stroke, National Institutes of Health, February 7, 2012.

What causes tuberous sclerosis?

TSC is caused by defects, or mutations, on two genes—TSC1 and TSC2. Only one of the genes needs to be affected for TSC to be present. The TSC1 gene, discovered in 1997, is on chromosome 9 and produces a protein called hamartin. The TSC2 gene, discovered in 1993, is on chromosome 16 and produces the protein tuberin. Scientists believe these proteins act in a complex as growth suppressors by inhibiting the activation of a master, evolutionarily conserved kinase called mTOR. Loss of regulation of mTOR occurs in cells lacking either hamartin or tuberin, and this leads to abnormal differentiation and development, and to the generation of enlarged cells, as are seen in TSC brain lesions.

Is TSC inherited?

Although some individuals inherit the disorder from a parent with TSC, most cases occur as sporadic cases due to new, spontaneous mutations in TSC1 or TSC2. In this situation, neither parent has the disorder or the faulty gene(s). Instead, a faulty gene first occurs in the affected individual.

In familial cases, TSC is an autosomal dominant disorder, which means that the disorder can be transmitted directly from parent to child. In those cases, only one parent needs to have the faulty gene in order to pass it on to a child. If a parent has TSC, each offspring has a 50 percent chance of developing the disorder. Children who inherit TSC may not have the same symptoms as their parent and they may have either a milder or a more severe form of the disorder.

Rarely, individuals acquire TSC through a process called gonadal mosaicism. These patients have parents with no apparent defects in the two genes that cause the disorder. Yet these parents can have a child with TSC because a portion of one of the parent's reproductive cells (sperm or eggs) can contain the genetic mutation without the other cells of the body being involved. In cases of gonadal mosaicism, genetic testing of a blood sample might not reveal the potential for passing the disease to offspring.

What are the signs and symptoms of TSC?

TSC can affect many different systems of the body, causing a variety of signs and symptoms. Signs of the disorder vary depending on which system and which organs are involved. The natural course of TSC varies from individual to individual, with symptoms ranging from very mild to quite severe. In addition to the benign tumors that frequently occur in TSC, other common symptoms include seizures, mental retardation, behavior problems, and skin abnormalities. Tumors can grow in nearly any organ, but they most commonly occur in the brain, kidneys, heart, lungs, and skin. Malignant tumors are rare in TSC. Those that do occur primarily affect the kidneys.

Brain involvement in TSC: Three types of brain lesions are seen in TSC: cortical tubers, for which the disease is named, generally form on the surface of the brain but may also appear in the deep areas of the brain; subependymal nodules (SEN), which form in the walls of the ventricles—the fluid-filled cavities of the brain; and subependymal giant-cell astrocytomas (SEGA), which develop from SEN and grow such that they may block the flow of fluid within the brain, causing a buildup of fluid and pressure and leading to headaches and blurred vision.

TSC usually causes the greatest problems for those affected and their family members through effects on brain function. Most individuals with TSC will have seizures at some point during their life. Seizures of all types may occur, including infantile spasms; tonic-clonic seizures (also known as grand mal seizures); or tonic, akinetic, atypical absence, myoclonic, complex partial, or generalized squires. Infantile spasms can occur as soon as the day of birth and are often difficult to recognize. Seizures can also be difficult to control by medication, and sometimes surgery or other measures are used.

About one-half to two-thirds of individuals with TSC have developmental delays ranging from mild learning disabilities to severe mental retardation. Behavior problems, including aggression, sudden rage, attention deficit hyperactivity disorder, acting out, obsessive-compulsive disorder, and repetitive, destructive, or self-harming behavior occur in children with TSC and can be difficult to manage. About one-third of children with TSC meet criteria for autism spectrum disorder.

Kidney involvement: Kidney problems such as cysts and angiomyolipomas occur in an estimated 70 to 80 percent of individuals with TSC, usually occurring between ages fifteen and thirty. Cysts are usually small, appear in limited numbers, and cause no serious problems. Approximately 2 percent of individuals with TSC develop large numbers of cysts in a pattern similar to polycystic kidney disease[2] during childhood. In these cases, kidney function is compromised and kidney failure occurs. In rare instances, the cysts may bleed, leading to blood loss and anemia.

Angiomyolipomas—benign growths consisting of fatty tissue and muscle cells—are the most common kidney lesions in TSC. These growths are seen in the majority of individuals with TSC, but are also found in about one of every three hundred people without TSC.

Angiomyolipomas caused by TSC are usually found in both kidneys and in most cases they produce no symptoms. However, they can sometimes grow so large that they cause pain or kidney failure. Bleeding from angiomyolipomas may also occur, causing both pain and weakness. If severe bleeding does not stop naturally, there may severe blood loss, resulting in profound anemia and a life-threatening drop in blood pressure, warranting urgent medical attention.

Other rare kidney problems include renal cell carcinoma, developing from an angiomyolipoma, and oncocytomas, benign tumors unique to individuals with TSC.

Tumors called cardiac rhabdomyomas are often found in the hearts of infants and young children with TSC, and they are often seen on prenatal fetus ultrasound exams. If the tumors are large or there are multiple tumors, they can block circulation and cause death. However, if they do not cause problems at birth—when in most cases they are at their largest size—they usually become smaller with time and do not affect the individual in later life.

Benign tumors called phakomas are sometimes found in the eyes of individuals with TSC, appearing as white patches on the retina. Generally they do not cause vision loss or other vision problems, but they can be used to help diagnose the disease.

Additional tumors and cysts may be found in other areas of the body, including the liver, lung, and pancreas. Bone cysts, rectal polyps, gum fibromas, and dental pits may also occur.

A wide variety of skin abnormalities may occur in individuals with TSC. Most cause no problems but are helpful in diagnosis. Some cases may cause disfigurement, necessitating treatment. The most common skin abnormalities include the following:

- Hypomelanotic macules ("ash leaf spots"), which are white or lighter patches of skin that may appear anywhere on the body and are caused by a lack of skin pigment or melanin—the substance that gives skin its color.

- Reddish spots or bumps called facial angiofibromas (also called adenoma sebaceum), which appear on the face (sometimes resembling acne) and consist of blood vessels and fibrous tissue.

- Raised, discolored areas on the forehead called forehead plaques, which are common and unique to TSC and may help doctors diagnose the disorder.

- Areas of thick, leathery, pebbly skin called shagreen patches, usually found on the lower back or nape of the neck.

- Small fleshy tumors called ungual or subungual fibromas that grow around and under the toenails or fingernails and may need to be surgically removed if they enlarge or cause bleeding. These usually appear later in life, ages twenty to fifty.

- Other skin features that are not unique to individuals with TSC, including molluscum fibrosum or skin tags, which typically occur across the back of the neck and shoulders, café au lait spots or flat brown marks, and poliosis, a tuft or patch of white hair that may appear on the scalp or eyelids.

Lung lesions are present in about one-third of adult women with TSC and are much less commonly seen in men. Lung lesions include lymphangioleiomyomatosis (LAM) and multinodular multifocal pneumocyte hyperplasia (MMPH). LAM is a tumor-like disorder in which cells proliferate in the lungs, and there is lung destruction with cyst formation. There is a range of symptoms with LAM, with many TSC individuals having no symptoms, while others suffer with breathlessness, which can progress and be severe. MMPH is a more benign tumor that occurs in men and women equally.

How is TSC diagnosed?

The diagnosis of TSC is based upon clinical criteria. In many cases the first clue to recognizing TSC is the presence of seizures or delayed development. In other cases, the first sign may be white patches on the skin (hypomelanotic macules) or the identification of cardiac tumor rhabdomyoma.

Diagnosis of the disorder is based on a careful clinical exam in combination with computed tomography (CT) or magnetic resonance imaging (MRI) of the brain, which may show tubers in the brain, and an ultrasound of the heart, liver, and kidneys, which may show tumors in those organs. Doctors should carefully examine the skin for the wide variety of skin features, the fingernails and toenails for ungual fibromas, the teeth and gums for dental pits and/or gum fibromas, and the eyes for retinal lesions. A Wood's lamp or ultraviolet light may be used to locate the hypomelanotic macules, which are sometimes hard to see on infants and individuals with pale or fair skin. Because of the wide variety of signs of TSC, it is best if a doctor experienced in the diagnosis of TSC evaluates a potential patient.

In infants TSC may be suspected if the child has cardiac rhabdomyomas or seizures (infantile spasms) at birth. With a careful examination of the skin and brain, it may be possible to diagnose TSC in a very young infant. However, many children are not diagnosed until later in life when their seizures begin and other symptoms such as facial angiofibromas appear.

How is TSC treated?

In October 2010 the U.S. Food and Drug Administration (FDA) approved the use of everolimus to treat benign tumors called subependymal giant cell astrocytomas in individuals with TSC who require treatment but are not candidates for surgery. There is no cure for TSC, although treatment is available for a number of the symptoms. Antiepileptic drugs may be used to control seizures. Vigabatrin is a particularly useful medication in TSC, and has been approved by the FDA for treatment of infantile spasms in TSC, although it has significant side effects. Specific medications may be prescribed for behavior problems. Intervention programs including special schooling and occupational therapy may benefit individuals with special needs and developmental issues. Surgery may be needed in case of complications connected to tubes, SEN, or SEGA, as well as in risk of hemorrhage from kidney tumors. Respiratory insufficiency due to LAM can be treated with supplemental oxygen therapy or lung transplantation if severe.

Because TSC is a lifelong condition, individuals need to be regularly monitored by a doctor to make sure they are receiving the best possible treatments. Due to the many varied symptoms of TSC, care by a clinician experienced with the disorder is recommended.

Basic laboratory studies have revealed insight into the function of the TSC genes and has led to recent use of rapamycin and related drugs for treating some manifestations of TSC. Rapamycin has been shown to be effective in treating SEGA, the brain tumor seen in TSC. However, its benefit for a variety of other aspects of and tumors seen in people with TSC is less certain, and clinical trials looking at the benefit carefully are continuing. Rapamycin and related drugs are not yet approved by the FDA for any purpose in individuals with TSC.

What is the prognosis?

The prognosis for individuals with TSC is highly variable and depends on the severity of symptoms. Those individuals with mild symptoms usually do well and have a normal life expectancy, while paying attention to TSC-specific issues. Individuals who are severely affected can suffer from severe mental retardation and persistent epilepsy.

All individuals with TSC are at risk for life-threatening conditions related to the brain tumors, kidney lesions, or LAM. Continued monitoring by a physician experienced with TSC is important. With appropriate medical care, most individuals with the disorder can look forward to normal life expectancy.

What research is being done?

Scientists who study TSC seek to increase our understanding of the disorder by learning more about the TSC1 and TSC2 genes that can cause the disorder and the function of the proteins—tuberin and hamartin—produced by these genes. Scientists hope knowledge gained from their current research will improve the genetic test for TSC and lead to new avenues of treatment, methods of prevention, and, ultimately, a cure for this disorder.

Research studies run the gamut from very basic scientific investigation to clinical translational research. For example, some investigators are trying to identify all the protein components that are in the same "signaling pathway" in which the TSC1 and TSC2 protein products and the mTOR protein are involved. Other studies are focused on understanding in detail how the disease develops, both in animal models and in patients, to better define new ways of controlling or preventing the development of the disease. Finally, clinical trials of rapamycin are underway to rigorously test the potential benefit of this compound for some of the tumors that are problematic in TSC patients.

Notes

1. Tuberous sclerosis is often referred to as tuberous sclerosis complex (TSC) in medical literature to help distinguish it from Tourette syndrome, an unrelated neurological disorder.

2. Polycystic kidney disease is a genetic disorder characterized by the growth of numerous fluid-filled cysts in the kidneys.

Chapter 35

Vision Disorders

Chapter Contents

Section 35.1

Color Vision Deficiency

Excerpted from "Color Vision Deficiency,"
Genetics Home Reference (http://ghr.nlm.nih.gov), March 2006.
Reviewed by David A. Cooke, M.D., FACP, May 2013.

What is color vision deficiency?

Color vision deficiencies are a group of conditions that affect the perception of color. They cause a range of changes in color vision, from mild difficulty with distinguishing shades to a total inability to detect color. These conditions are divided into three major categories: red-green color vision defects, blue-yellow color vision defects, and a complete absence of color vision.

Red-green color vision defects are the most common form of color vision deficiency. Affected individuals have trouble distinguishing between shades of red and green. They see these colors differently than most people and may have trouble naming different hues. Blue-yellow color vision defects, which are rarer, cause problems with differentiating shades of blue and green. These two forms of color vision deficiency disrupt color perception but do not affect the sharpness of vision (visual acuity).

An absence of color vision, called achromatopsia, is uncommon. People with complete achromatopsia cannot perceive any colors. They see only black, white, and shades of gray. A milder form of this condition, incomplete achromatopsia, may allow some color discrimination. People with achromatopsia almost always have additional problems with vision including reduced visual acuity, increased sensitivity to light (photophobia), and small involuntary eye movements called nystagmus.

How common is color vision deficiency?

Red-green color vision defects are the most common form of color vision deficiency. This condition affects males more often than females. Among populations with Northern European ancestry, it occurs in about 8 percent of males and 0.5 percent of females. Red-green color vision defects have a lower incidence in almost all other populations studied.

Blue-yellow color vision defects affect males and females equally. This condition occurs in fewer than one in ten thousand people worldwide.

Complete achromatopsia affects an estimated one in thirty thousand people. This condition is much more common among Pingelapese islanders, who live on one of the Eastern Caroline Islands of Micronesia. Five percent to 10 percent of this population have a total absence of color vision.

What genes are related to color vision deficiency?

Mutations in the CNGA3, CNGB3, GNAT2, OPN1LW, OPN1MW, and OPN1SW genes cause color vision deficiency.

The retina, a light-sensitive tissue at the back of the eye, contains two types of light receptor cells called rods and cones. These cells transmit visual signals from the eye to the brain. Rods are responsible for vision in low light. Cones provide vision in bright light, including color vision. Three types of cones each contain a special pigment (a photopigment) that is most sensitive to a particular wavelength of light. The brain combines input from all three types of cones to produce normal color vision.

Specific genes provide instructions for making the three photopigments. The OPN1LW gene makes a pigment that is more sensitive to light at the red end of the visible spectrum, and cones with this pigment are sometimes called long-wavelength-sensitive or L cones. The OPN1MW gene makes a pigment that is more sensitive to light in the middle of the visible spectrum (yellow/green light), and cones with this pigment are often called middle-wavelength-sensitive or M cones. The OPN1SW gene makes a pigment that is more sensitive to light at the blue/violet end of the visible spectrum, and cones with this pigment are usually called short-wavelength-sensitive or S cones.

Genetic changes involving the OPN1LW and OPN1MW genes cause red-green color vision defects. These changes lead to an absence of L or M cones or the production of cones with abnormal visual properties that affect red-green color vision. Blue-yellow color vision defects result from mutations in the OPN1SW gene. These mutations inactivate the short-wave-sensitive pigment, which probably leads to the premature destruction of S cones or the production of defective cones. A loss of S cones impairs perception of the color blue and makes it difficult or impossible to detect differences between shades of blue and green.

Changes in the CNGA3, CNGB3, and GNAT2 genes are responsible for achromatopsia. Each of these genes provides instructions for making a protein that is involved in the normal function of cones in the retina. Mutations in any of these genes prevent all three types of cones from reacting appropriately to light. As a result, most people with mutations in one of these genes must depend on rods alone for vision. They typically have no color vision and often have other visual problems as well. Some people with mutations in the CNGA3 gene have incomplete achromatopsia, which may allow some cone function and limited color vision.

A particular form of incomplete achromatopsia, called blue cone monochromacy, occurs when genetic changes prevent both L and M cones from functioning normally. People with this condition have only S cones. Because the brain must compare input from at least two types of cones to detect color, people who have only functional S cones have very poor color vision.

Some problems with color vision are not caused by gene mutations. These nonhereditary conditions, which are described as acquired color vision deficiencies, occur in people with other eye disorders. Specifically, acquired color vision deficiencies can result from diseases involving the retina, the nerve that carries visual information from the eye to the brain (the optic nerve), or areas of the brain involved in processing visual information.

How do people inherit color vision deficiency?

The types of color vision deficiency have different patterns of inheritance. Red-green color vision defects and blue cone monochromacy are inherited in an X-linked recessive pattern. A condition is considered X-linked if the mutated gene that causes the disorder is located on the X chromosome, one of the two sex chromosomes. In males (who have only one X chromosome), one altered copy of the gene in each cell is sufficient to cause the condition. In females (who have two X chromosomes), a mutation must be present in both copies of the gene to cause the disorder. Males are affected by X-linked recessive disorders much more frequently than females. A characteristic of X-linked inheritance is that fathers cannot pass X-linked traits to their sons.

Blue-yellow color vision defects are inherited in an autosomal dominant pattern, which means one copy of the altered OPN1SW gene in each cell is sufficient to cause the condition.

Complete achromatopsia is inherited in an autosomal recessive pattern, which means both copies of the CNGA3, CNGB3, or GNAT2 gene in each cell have mutations. Most often, the parents of an individual with an autosomal recessive condition each carry one copy of the mutated gene, but do not show signs and symptoms of the condition.

Section 35.2

Early-Onset Glaucoma

Excerpted from "Early-Onset Glaucoma," Genetics Home Reference
(http://ghr.nlm.nih.gov), February 2009.

What is early-onset glaucoma?

Glaucoma is a group of eye disorders in which the optic nerves connecting the eyes and the brain are progressively damaged. This damage can lead to reduction in side (peripheral) vision and eventual blindness. Other signs and symptoms may include bulging eyes, excessive tearing, and abnormal sensitivity to light (photophobia). The term "early-onset glaucoma" may be used when the disorder appears before the age of forty.

In most people with glaucoma, the damage to the optic nerves is caused by increased pressure within the eyes (intraocular pressure). Intraocular pressure depends on a balance between fluid entering and leaving the eyes.

Usually glaucoma develops in older adults, in whom the risk of developing the disorder may be affected by a variety of medical conditions including high blood pressure (hypertension) and diabetes mellitus, as well as family history. The risk of early-onset glaucoma depends mainly on heredity.

Structural abnormalities that impede fluid drainage in the eye may be present at birth and usually become apparent during the first year of life. Such abnormalities may be part of a genetic disorder that affects many body systems, called a syndrome. If glaucoma appears before the age of five without other associated abnormalities, it is called primary congenital glaucoma.

Other individuals experience early onset of primary open-angle glaucoma, the most common adult form of glaucoma. If primary open-angle glaucoma develops during childhood or early adulthood, it is called juvenile open-angle glaucoma.

How common is early-onset glaucoma?

Primary congenital glaucoma affects approximately one in ten thousand people. Its frequency is higher in the Middle East. Juvenile open-angle glaucoma affects about one in fifty thousand people. Primary open-angle glaucoma is much more common after the age of forty, affecting about 1 percent of the population worldwide.

What genes are related to early-onset glaucoma?

Approximately 10 percent to 33 percent of people with juvenile open-angle glaucoma have mutations in the MYOC gene. MYOC gene mutations have also been detected in some people with primary congenital glaucoma.

The MYOC gene provides instructions for producing a protein called myocilin. Myocilin is found in certain structures of the eye, called the trabecular meshwork and the ciliary body, that regulate the intraocular pressure.

Researchers believe that myocilin functions together with other proteins as part of a protein complex. Mutations may alter the protein in such a way that the complex cannot be formed. Defective myocilin that is not incorporated into functional complexes may accumulate in the trabecular meshwork and ciliary body. The excess protein may prevent sufficient flow of fluid from the eye, resulting in increased intraocular pressure and causing the signs and symptoms of early-onset glaucoma.

Between 20 percent and 40 percent of people with primary congenital glaucoma have mutations in the CYP1B1 gene. CYP1B1 gene mutations have also been detected in some people with juvenile open-angle glaucoma.

The CYP1B1 gene provides instructions for producing a form of the cytochrome P450 protein. Like myocilin, this protein is found in the trabecular meshwork, ciliary body, and other structures of the eye.

It is not well understood how defects in the CYP1B1 protein cause signs and symptoms of glaucoma. Recent studies suggest that the defects may interfere with the early development of the trabecular meshwork.

In the clear covering of the eye (the cornea), the CYP1B1 protein may also be involved in a process that regulates the secretion of fluid inside the eye. If this fluid is produced in excess, the high intraocular pressure characteristic of glaucoma may develop.

The CYP1B1 protein may interact with myocilin. Individuals with mutations in both the MYOC and CYP1B1 genes may develop glaucoma at an earlier age and have more severe symptoms than do those with mutations in only one of the genes. Mutations in other genes may also be involved in early-onset glaucoma.

How do people inherit early-onset glaucoma?

Early-onset glaucoma can have different inheritance patterns. Primary congenital glaucoma is usually inherited in an autosomal recessive pattern, which means both copies of the gene in each cell have mutations. Most often, the parents of an individual with an autosomal recessive condition each carry one copy of the mutated gene, but do not show signs and symptoms of the condition.

Juvenile open-angle glaucoma is inherited in an autosomal dominant pattern, which means one copy of the altered gene in each cell is sufficient to cause the disorder. In some families, primary congenital glaucoma may also be inherited in an autosomal dominant pattern.

Section 35.3

X-Linked Juvenile Retinoschisis

Excerpted from "X-linked Juvenile Retinoschisis,"
Genetics Home Reference (http://ghr.nlm.nih.gov), August 2008.
Reviewed by David A. Cooke, M.D., FACP, May 2013.

What is X-linked juvenile retinoschisis?

X-linked juvenile retinoschisis is a genetic eye disorder that impairs normal vision. This disorder affects the retina, which is a specialized light-sensitive tissue that lines the back of the eye. Damage to the retina impairs the sharpness of vision (visual acuity). Typically, X-linked juvenile retinoschisis affects cells in the central area of the retina called the macula. The macula is responsible for sharp central vision, which is needed for detailed tasks such as reading, driving, and recognizing faces. X-linked juvenile retinoschisis is one type of a broader disorder called macular degeneration, which involves disruption in the normal functioning of the macula. Occasionally, side (peripheral) vision is affected in people with X-linked juvenile retinoschisis.

X-linked juvenile retinoschisis occurs almost exclusively in males. It is usually diagnosed when affected boys start school and poor vision and difficulty with reading become apparent. In more severe cases, eye squinting and involuntary movement of the eyes (nystagmus) can be seen in infancy. Visual acuity remains unchanged in most people between their teenage years and their forties or fifties, when a significant decline in visual acuity typically occurs. Rarely, severe complications develop, such as separation of the retinal layers (retinal detachment) or leakage of blood vessels in the retina (vitreous hemorrhage). These eye abnormalities can cause impaired vision or blindness.

How common is X-linked juvenile retinoschisis?

The prevalence of X-linked juvenile retinoschisis is estimated to be one in five thousand to twenty-five thousand males worldwide.

What genes are related to X-linked juvenile retinoschisis?

Mutations in the RS1 gene cause most cases of X-linked juvenile retinoschisis. The RS1 gene provides instructions for producing a protein called retinoschisin, which is found in the retina. Studies suggest that retinoschisin plays a role in the development and maintenance of the retina and in specialized cells within the retina that detect light and color (photoreceptor cells).

RS1 gene mutations lead to a reduced amount of retinoschisin, which can cause tiny splits (schisis) or tears to form in the retina. This damage often forms a "spoke-wheel" pattern in the macula, which can be seen during an eye examination. These abnormalities are typically seen in the area of the macula, affecting visual acuity, but can also occur in the sides of the retina, resulting in impaired peripheral vision.

Some individuals with X-linked juvenile retinoschisis do not have a mutation in the RS1 gene. In these individuals, the cause of the disorder is unknown.

How do people inherit X-linked juvenile retinoschisis?

This condition is inherited in an X-linked recessive pattern. The gene associated with this condition is located on the X chromosome, which is one of the two sex chromosomes. In males (who have only one X chromosome), one altered copy of the gene in each cell is sufficient to cause the condition. In females (who have two X chromosomes), a mutation would have to occur in both copies of the gene to cause the disorder. Because it is unlikely that females will have two altered copies of this gene, males are affected by X-linked recessive disorders much more frequently than females. A characteristic of X-linked inheritance is that fathers cannot pass X-linked traits to their sons.

Chapter 36

Wilson Disease

What is Wilson disease?

Wilson disease is a genetic disorder that prevents the body from getting rid of extra copper. A small amount of copper obtained from food is needed to stay healthy, but too much copper is poisonous. In Wilson disease, copper builds up in the liver, brain, eyes, and other organs. Over time, high copper levels can cause life-threatening organ damage.

Who gets Wilson disease?

People who get Wilson disease inherit two abnormal copies of the ATP7B gene, one from each parent. Wilson disease carriers, who have only one copy of the abnormal gene, do not have symptoms. Most people with Wilson disease have no known family history of the disease. A person's chances of having Wilson disease increase if one or both parents have it.

About one in forty thousand people get Wilson disease.[1] It equally affects men and women. Symptoms usually appear between ages five and thirty-five, but new cases have been reported in people aged two to seventy-two years.

Excerpted from "Wilson Disease," National Institute of Diabetes and Digestive and Kidney Diseases, National Institutes of Health, April 30, 2012.

What causes Wilson disease?

Wilson disease is caused by a buildup of copper in the body. Normally, copper from the diet is filtered out by the liver and released into bile, which flows out of the body through the gastrointestinal tract. People who have Wilson disease cannot release copper from the liver at a normal rate, due to a mutation of the ATP7B gene. When the copper storage capacity of the liver is exceeded, copper is released into the bloodstream and travels to other organs—including the brain, kidneys, and eyes.

What are the symptoms of Wilson disease?

Wilson disease first attacks the liver, the central nervous system, or both.

A buildup of copper in the liver may cause ongoing liver disease. Rarely, acute liver failure occurs; most patients develop signs and symptoms that accompany chronic liver disease, including the following:

- Swelling of the liver or spleen

- Jaundice, or yellowing of the skin and whites of the eyes

- Fluid buildup in the legs or abdomen

- A tendency to bruise easily

- Fatigue

A buildup of copper in the central nervous system may result in neurologic symptoms, including the following:

- Problems with speech, swallowing, or physical coordination

- Tremors or uncontrolled movements

- Muscle stiffness

- Behavioral changes

Other signs and symptoms of Wilson disease include the following:
- Anemia

- Low platelet or white blood cell count

- Slower blood clotting, measured by a blood test

- High levels of amino acids, protein, uric acid, and carbohydrates in urine

- Premature osteoporosis and arthritis

Kayser-Fleischer rings result from a buildup of copper in the eyes and are the most unique sign of Wilson disease. They appear in each eye as a rusty-brown ring around the edge of the iris and in the rim of the cornea. The iris is the colored part of the eye surrounding the pupil. The cornea is the transparent outer membrane that covers the eye.

How is Wilson disease diagnosed?

Wilson disease is diagnosed through a physical examination and laboratory tests.

During the physical examination, a doctor will look for visible signs of Wilson disease. A special light called a slit lamp is used to look for Kayser-Fleischer rings in the eyes. Kayser-Fleischer rings are present in almost all people with Wilson disease who show signs of neurologic damage but are present in only 50 percent of those with signs of liver damage alone.

Laboratory tests measure the amount of copper in the blood, urine, and liver tissue. Most people with Wilson disease will have a lower than normal level of copper in the blood and a lower level of corresponding ceruloplasmin, a protein that carries copper in the bloodstream. In cases of acute liver failure caused by Wilson disease, the level of blood copper is often higher than normal. A twenty-four-hour urine collection will show increased copper in the urine in most patients who display symptoms. A liver biopsy—a procedure that removes a small piece of liver tissue—can show if the liver is retaining too much copper. The analysis of biopsied liver tissue with a microscope detects liver damage, which often shows a pattern unique to Wilson disease.

Genetic testing may help diagnose Wilson disease in some people, particularly those with a family history of the disease.

Wilson disease can be misdiagnosed because it is rare and its symptoms are similar to those of other conditions.

Who should be screened for Wilson disease?

Anyone with unexplained liver disease or neurologic symptoms with evidence of liver disease, such as abnormal liver tests and symptoms of liver disease, should be screened for Wilson disease. People with a family history of Wilson disease, especially those with an affected sibling or parent, should also be screened. A doctor can diagnose Wilson disease before the appearance of symptoms. Early treatment can reduce or even prevent illness.

How is Wilson disease treated?

Wilson disease requires lifelong treatment to reduce and control the amount of copper in the body.

Initial therapy includes the removal of excess copper, a reduction of copper intake, and the treatment of any liver or central nervous system damage.

The drugs d-penicillamine (Cuprimine) and trientine hydrochloride (Syprine) release copper from organs into the bloodstream. Most of the copper is then filtered out by the kidneys and excreted in urine. A potential major side effect of both drugs is that neurologic symptoms can become worse—a possible result of the newly released copper becoming reabsorbed by the central nervous system. About 20 to 30 percent of patients using d-penicillamine will also initially experience other reactions to the medication, including fever, rash, and other drug-related effects on the kidneys and bone marrow. The risk of drug reaction and neurologic worsening appears to be lower with trientine hydrochloride, which should be the first choice for the treatment of all symptomatic patients.

Pregnant women should take a lower dose of d-penicillamine or trientine hydrochloride during pregnancy to reduce the risk of birth defects. A lower dose will also help reduce the risk of slower wound healing if surgical procedures are performed during childbirth.

Zinc, administered as zinc salts such as zinc acetate (Galzin), blocks the digestive tract's absorption of copper from food. Zinc removes copper too slowly to be used alone as an initial therapy for people who already have symptoms, but it is often used in combination with d-penicillamine or trientine hydrochloride. Zinc is safe to use at full dosage during pregnancy.

Maintenance therapy begins when symptoms improve and tests show that copper has been reduced to a safe level. Maintenance therapy typically includes taking zinc and low doses of either d-penicillamine or trientine hydrochloride. Blood and urine should be monitored by a health care provider to ensure treatment is keeping copper at a safe level.

People with Wilson disease should reduce their dietary copper intake. They should not eat shellfish or liver, as these foods may contain high levels of copper. Other foods high in copper—including mushrooms, nuts, and chocolate—should be avoided during initial therapy but, in most cases, may be eaten in moderation during maintenance therapy. People with Wilson disease should have their drinking water checked for copper content and should not take multivitamins that contain copper.

If the disorder is detected early and treated effectively, people with Wilson disease can enjoy good health.

Hope through Research

The National Institute of Diabetes and Digestive and Kidney Diseases conducts and supports Wilson disease research.

The U.S. Food and Drug Administration is evaluating a new anticopper drug called tetrathiomolybdate (Coprexa). A National Institutes of Health–supported clinical trial found tetrathiomolybdate to be as effective as trientine hydrochloride in removing copper but with less risk of worsening neurologic symptoms.

References

1. Olivarez M, Caggana M, Pass KA, Ferguson P, Brewer GJ. Estimate of the frequency of Wilson's disease in the US Caucasian population: a mutation analysis approach. *Annals of Human Genetics*. 2001;65:459–63.

Part Three

Chromosome Abnormalities

Chapter 37

Angelman Syndrome

What is Angelman syndrome?

Angelman syndrome is a complex genetic disorder that primarily affects the nervous system. Characteristic features of this condition include delayed development, intellectual disability, severe speech impairment, and problems with movement and balance (ataxia). Most affected children also have recurrent seizures (epilepsy) and a small head size (microcephaly). Delayed development becomes noticeable by the age of six to twelve months, and other common signs and symptoms usually appear in early childhood.

Children with Angelman syndrome typically have a happy, excitable demeanor with frequent smiling, laughter, and hand-flapping movements. Hyperactivity, a short attention span, and a fascination with water are common. Most affected children also have difficulty sleeping and need less sleep than usual.

With age, people with Angelman syndrome become less excitable, and the sleeping problems tend to improve. However, affected individuals continue to have intellectual disability, severe speech impairment, and seizures throughout their lives. Adults with Angelman syndrome have distinctive facial features that may be described as "coarse." Other common features include unusually fair skin with light-colored hair and an abnormal side-to-side curvature of the spine (scoliosis). The life expectancy of people with this condition appears to be nearly normal.

Excerpted from "Angelman Syndrome," Genetics Home Reference (http://ghr.nlm.nih.gov), October 2011.

How common is Angelman syndrome?

Angelman syndrome affects an estimated one in twelve thousand to twenty thousand people.

What are the genetic changes related to Angelman syndrome?

Many of the characteristic features of Angelman syndrome result from the loss of function of a gene called UBE3A. People normally inherit one copy of the UBE3A gene from each parent. Both copies of this gene are turned on (active) in many of the body's tissues. In certain areas of the brain, however, only the copy inherited from a person's mother (the maternal copy) is active. This parent-specific gene activation is caused by a phenomenon called genomic imprinting. If the maternal copy of the UBE3A gene is lost because of a chromosomal change or a gene mutation, a person will have no active copies of the gene in some parts of the brain.

Several different genetic mechanisms can inactivate or delete the maternal copy of the UBE3A gene. Most cases of Angelman syndrome (about 70 percent) occur when a segment of the maternal chromosome 15 containing this gene is deleted. In other cases (about 11 percent), Angelman syndrome is caused by a mutation in the maternal copy of the UBE3A gene.

In a small percentage of cases, Angelman syndrome results when a person inherits two copies of chromosome 15 from his or her father (paternal copies) instead of one copy from each parent. This phenomenon is called paternal uniparental disomy. Rarely, Angelman syndrome can also be caused by a chromosomal rearrangement called a translocation, or by a mutation or other defect in the region of DNA that controls activation of the UBE3A gene. These genetic changes can abnormally turn off (inactivate) UBE3A or other genes on the maternal copy of chromosome 15.

The causes of Angelman syndrome are unknown in 10 to 15 percent of affected individuals. Changes involving other genes or chromosomes may be responsible for the disorder in these cases.

In some people who have Angelman syndrome, the loss of a gene called OCA2 is associated with light-colored hair and fair skin. The OCA2 gene is located on the segment of chromosome 15 that is often deleted in people with this disorder. However, loss of the OCA2 gene does not cause the other signs and symptoms of Angelman syndrome. The protein produced from this gene helps determine the coloring (pigmentation) of the skin, hair, and eyes.

Can Angelman syndrome be inherited?

Most cases of Angelman syndrome are not inherited, particularly those caused by a deletion in the maternal chromosome 15 or by paternal uniparental disomy. These genetic changes occur as random events during the formation of reproductive cells (eggs and sperm) or in early embryonic development. Affected people typically have no history of the disorder in their family.

Rarely, a genetic change responsible for Angelman syndrome can be inherited. For example, it is possible for a mutation in the UBE3A gene or in the nearby region of DNA that controls gene activation to be passed from one generation to the next.

Chapter 38

Cri du Chat Syndrome

What is cri du chat syndrome?

Cri du chat syndrome—also known as 5p- syndrome and cat cry syndrome—is a rare genetic condition that is caused by the deletion (a missing piece) of genetic material on the small arm (the p arm) of chromosome 5. The cause of this rare chromosomal deletion is unknown.

What are the symptoms of cri du chat syndrome?

The symptoms of cri du chat syndrome vary among individuals. The variability of the clinical symptoms and developmental delays may be related to the size of the deletion of the 5p arm.

The clinical symptoms of cri du chat syndrome usually include a high-pitched cat-like cry, mental retardation, delayed development, distinctive facial features, small head size (microcephaly), widely spaced eyes (hypertelorism), low birth weight, and weak muscle tone (hypotonia) in infancy. The cat-like cry typically becomes less apparent with time.

Most individuals who have cri du chat syndrome have difficulty with language. Half of children learn sufficient verbal skills to communicate. Some individuals learn to use short sentences, while others express themselves with a few basic words, gestures, or sign language.

Reprinted from "Learning about Cri du Chat Syndrome," National Human Genome Research Institute (www.genome.gov), April 18, 2013.

Other characteristics may include feeding difficulties, delays in walking, hyperactivity, scoliosis, and significant retardation. A small number of children are born with serious organ defects and other life-threatening medical conditions, although most individuals with cri du chat syndrome have a normal life expectancy.

Both children and adults with this syndrome are usually friendly and happy, and enjoy social interaction.

How is cri du chat syndrome diagnosed?

The diagnosis of cri du chat syndrome is generally made in the hospital at birth. A health care provider may note the clinical symptoms associated with the condition. The cat-like cry is the most prominent clinical feature in newborn children and is usually diagnostic for the cri du chat syndrome.

Additionally, analysis of the individual's chromosomes may be performed. The missing portion (deletion) of the short arm of chromosome 5 may be seen on a chromosome analysis. If not, a more detailed type of genetic test called fluorescence in situ hybridization (FISH) analysis may be needed to reveal the deletion.

What is the treatment for cri du chat syndrome?

No specific treatment is available for this syndrome. Children born with this genetic condition will most likely require ongoing support from a team made up of the parents, therapists, and medical and educational professionals to help the child achieve his or her maximum potential. With early and consistent educational intervention, as well as physical and language therapy, children with cri du chat syndrome are capable of reaching their fullest potential and can lead full and meaningful lives.

Is cri du chat syndrome inherited?

Most cases of cri du chat syndrome are not inherited. The chromosomal deletion usually occurs as a random event during the formation of reproductive cells (eggs or sperm) or in early fetal development. People with cri du chat typically have no history of the condition in their family.

About 10 percent of people with cri du chat syndrome inherit the chromosome with a deleted segment from an unaffected parent. In these cases, the parent carries a chromosomal rearrangement called a balanced translocation, in which no genetic material is gained or lost.

Balanced translocations usually do not cause any medical problems; however, they can become unbalanced as they are passed to the next generation. A deletion in the short arm of chromosome 5 is an example of an unbalanced translocation, which is a chromosomal rearrangement with extra or missing genetic material. Unbalanced translocations can cause birth defects and other health problems such as those seen in cri-du-chat syndrome.

Chapter 39

Down Syndrome and Other Trisomy Disorders

Chapter Contents

Section 39.1

Down Syndrome

Reprinted from "Learning about Down Syndrome," National Human Genome Research Institute (www.genome.gov), May 15, 2013.

What is Down syndrome?

Down syndrome is a chromosomal condition related to chromosome 21. It affects one in eight hundred to one in one thousand live born infants.

What are the symptoms of Down syndrome?

People who have Down syndrome have learning difficulties, mental retardation, a characteristic facial appearance, and poor muscle tone (hypotonia) in infancy.

Individuals with Down syndrome also have an increased risk for having heart defects, digestive problems such as gastroesophageal reflux or celiac disease, and hearing loss. Some people who have Down syndrome have low activity of the thyroid gland (hypothyroidism), an organ in the lower neck that produces hormones.

How is Down syndrome diagnosed?

Down syndrome can be diagnosed in infancy based on the characteristic clinical findings. When Down syndrome is suspected in a person, a genetic test called a chromosome analysis is performed on a blood or skin sample to look for an extra chromosome 21 (trisomy 21). Trisomy 21 means that each cell in the body has three copies of chromosome 21 instead of the usual two copies.

Having an extra number 21 chromosome interrupts the normal course of development, causing the characteristic clinical features of Down syndrome. Some people who have Down syndrome have an extra number 21 chromosome in only some of their body's cells. This type of Down syndrome is called mosaic Down syndrome.

A small number of individuals have Down syndrome because part of chromosome 21 becomes attached (translocated) to another chromosome before or at the time of conception. These individuals have two copies of chromosome 21, and additional material from chromosome 21 that is attached to another chromosome. The chromosomes of parents of a child with Down syndrome caused by a translocation are studied to see whether the translocation was inherited.

What is the treatment for Down syndrome?

Treatment for Down syndrome is based on the person's physical problems and intellectual challenges. Many babies who have Down syndrome do not have good muscle tone, which makes it harder for them to roll over and walk. Physical therapy can help with these problems.

About 40 to 60 percent of babies born with Down syndrome have a heart defect. Therefore, all newborns with Down syndrome have their heart checked with an electrocardiogram and an echocardiogram. When there is a heart defect present in an infant with Down syndrome, the infant is referred to a pediatric cardiologist for medical management or to a pediatric cardiac surgeon for early surgical repair.

Some infants with Down syndrome have difficulties with swallowing or they may have blockages in their bowels. Surgery can be performed to correct these problems. Once corrected, they usually cause no further health issues.

Children with Down syndrome may have frequent colds and sinus and ear infections. These are treated early and aggressively to prevent hearing loss and chronic infections.

Low thyroid levels are more common in infants who have Down syndrome. It is recommended that thyroid level testing be performed at least yearly.

Some infants with Down syndrome have eye problems such as cataracts (cloudy lenses) or crossed eyes (strabismus). Surgery can help with these problems.

Sucking problems related to low muscle tone or heart problems may make breast feeding difficult initially. Occupational therapists, speech therapists, breast feeding consultants, and support groups usually have specific resources for the mothers of infants with Down syndrome.

Intelligence in individuals with Down syndrome ranges from low normal to very slow to learn. At birth it is not possible to tell the level of intelligence a baby with Down syndrome will have. All areas of development, including motor skills, language, intellectual abilities, and social and adaptive skills, are followed closely in children with Down syndrome. Early referral, beginning at birth, to an early intervention program will help enhance development. Preschool programs for children with Down syndrome include physical, occupational, speech, and educational therapies.

Many adults with Down syndrome have jobs and live independently.

Is Down syndrome inherited?

Most cases of Down syndrome are not inherited, but occur as random events during the formation of reproductive cells (eggs and sperm). An error in cell division called nondisjunction results in reproductive cells with an abnormal number of chromosomes. For example, an egg or sperm cell may gain an extra copy of chromosome 21. If one of these atypical reproductive cells contributes to the genetic makeup of a child, the child will have an extra chromosome 21 in each of the body's cells.

Mosaic Down syndrome is also not inherited. It occurs as a random error during cell division early in fetal development. As a result, some of the body's cells have the usual two copies of chromosome 21, and other cells have three copies of the chromosome. Translocation Down syndrome can be inherited. An unaffected person can carry a rearrangement of genetic material between chromosome 21 and another chromosome. This rearrangement is called a balanced translocation because there is no extra material from chromosome 21. Although they do not have signs of Down syndrome, people who carry this type of balanced translocation are at an increased risk of having children with the condition.

Section 39.2

Edwards Syndrome (Trisomy 18)

Excerpted from "Trisomy 18," © 2013 A.D.A.M., Inc.
Reprinted with permission.

Trisomy 18 is a genetic disorder in which a person has a third copy of material from chromosome 18, instead of the usual two copies.

Causes

Trisomy 18 is a somewhat common syndrome. It is three times more common in girls than boys.

The syndrome occurs when there is extra material from chromosome 18. The extra material affects normal development.

Symptoms

- Clenched hands
- Crossed legs
- Feet with a rounded bottom (rocker-bottom feet)
- Low birth weight
- Low-set ears
- Mental delay
- Poorly developed fingernails
- Small head (microcephaly)
- Small jaw (micrognathia)
- Undescended testicle
- Unusual shaped chest (pectus carinatum)

Exams and Tests

An exam during pregnancy may show an unusually large uterus and extra amniotic fluid. There may be an unusually small placenta when the baby is born.

A physical exam of the infant may show unusual fingerprint patterns. X-rays may show a short breastbone. Chromosome studies will show trisomy 18, partial trisomy, or translocation.

Other signs include:

• hole, split, or cleft in the iris of the eye (coloboma);

• separation between the left and right side of the abdominal muscle (diastasis recti);

• umbilical hernia or inguinal hernia.

There are often signs of congenital heart disease, such as:

• atrial septal defect (ASD);

• patent ductus arteriosus (PDA);

• ventricular septal defect (VSD).

Tests may also show kidney problems, including:

• horseshoe kidney;

• hydronephrosis;

• polycystic kidney.

Treatment

Treatment of children with trisomy 18 is planned on a case-by-case basis. Which treatments are used depend on the patient's individual condition.

Outlook (Prognosis)

Half of infants with this condition do not survive beyond the first week of life. Some children have survived to the teenage years, but with serious medical and developmental problems.

Possible Complications

Complications depend on the specific defects and symptoms.

When to Contact a Medical Professional

Genetic counseling can help families understand the condition, the risks of inheriting it, and how to care for the patient.

Prevention

Tests can be done during pregnancy to find out if the child has this syndrome.

Genetic testing is recommended for parents who have a child with this syndrome and who want to have more children.

Alternative Names

Edwards syndrome

Section 39.3

Patau Syndrome (Trisomy 13)

Excerpted from "Trisomy 13," © 2013 A.D.A.M., Inc.
Reprinted with permission.

Trisomy 13 (also called Patau syndrome) is a genetic disorder in which a person has three copies of genetic material from chromosome 13, instead of the usual two copies. Rarely, the extra material may be attached to another chromosome (translocation).

Causes

Trisomy 13 occurs when extra DNA from chromosome 13 appears in some or all of the body's cells:

- **Trisomy 13:** The presence of an extra (third) chromosome 13 in all of the cells.

- **Trisomy 13 mosaicism:** the presence of an extra chromosome 13 in some of the cells.

- **Partial trisomy:** The presence of a part of an extra chromosome 13 in the cells.

The extra material interferes with normal development.

Trisomy 13 occurs in about one out of every ten thousand newborns. Most cases are not passed down through families (inherited). Instead, the events that lead to trisomy 13 occur in either the sperm or the egg that forms the fetus.

Symptoms

- Cleft lip or palate
- Clenched hands (with outer fingers on top of the inner fingers)
- Close-set eyes—eyes may actually fuse together into one
- Decreased muscle tone
- Extra fingers or toes (polydactyly)
- Hernias: umbilical hernia, inguinal hernia
- Hole, split, or cleft in the iris (coloboma)
- Low-set ears
- Intellectual disability, severe
- Scalp defects (missing skin)
- Seizures
- Single palmar crease
- Skeletal (limb) abnormalities
- Small eyes
- Small head (microcephaly)
- Small lower jaw (micrognathia)
- Undescended testicle (cryptorchidism)

Exams and Tests

The infant may have a single umbilical artery at birth. There are often signs of congenital heart disease, such as:

- abnormal placement of the heart toward the right side of the chest instead of the left;
- atrial septal defect;
- patent ductus arteriosus;
- ventricular septal defect.

Gastrointestinal x-rays or ultrasound may show rotation of the internal organs.

Magnetic resonance imaging (MRI) or computed tomography (CT) scans of the head may reveal a problem with the structure of the brain. The problem is called holoprosencephaly. It is the joining together of the two sides of the brain.

Chromosome studies show trisomy 13, trisomy 13 mosaicism, or partial trisomy.

Treatment

Treatment varies from child to child and depends on the specific symptoms.

Outlook (Prognosis)

More than 80 percent of children with trisomy 13 die in the first year.

Possible Complications

Complications begin almost immediately. Most infants with trisomy 13 have congenital heart disease.

Complications may include:

- breathing difficulty or lack of breathing (apnea);

- deafness;

- feeding problems;

- heart failure;

- seizures;

- vision problems.

When to Contact a Medical Professional

Call for an appointment with your health care provider if you have had a child with trisomy 13 and you plan to have another child. Genetic counseling can help families understand the condition, the risk of inheriting it, and how to care for the patient.

Prevention

Trisomy 13 can be diagnosed before birth by amniocentesis with chromosome studies of the amniotic cells.

Parents of infants with trisomy 13 that is caused by a translocation should have genetic testing and counseling, which may help them avoid having another child with the condition.

Alternative Names

Patau syndrome

Section 39.4

Triple X Syndrome

Excerpted from "XXX Syndrome (Trisomy X)," http://www.med.umich.edu/yourchild/topics/xxxsyn.htm, compiled by Kyla Boyse, RN, reviewed by Autumn Tansky, MS, updated July 2010. Content provided by the University of Michigan Health System, © 2010. All rights reserved. Reprinted with permission.

What is XXX or triple X syndrome?

XXX syndrome (also called trisomy X or triple X) is caused by the presence of an extra "X" chromosome in every cell. Typically, a female has two X chromosomes in every cell of their body, so the extra "X" is unusual. The extra "X" chromosome is typically inherited from the mother, but is a random event—not caused by anything she did or could prevent. Trisomy X is often not diagnosed until later in life, if ever. The risk of having a second child with an extra chromosome is approximately 1 percent, until mom is older than thirty-eight years of age, as it is thought that this random event becomes more common as a woman ages. Prenatal testing is available in future pregnancies.

How common is trisomy X?

The extra "X" chromosome occurs in about one in every one thousand newborn girls.

What are the features of triple X syndrome?

Many girls and women with triple X have no signs or symptoms. Signs and symptoms vary a lot between individuals, but can include:

- **Physical:** Tall stature (height);

- **Possible mild facial characteristics:** Increased width between eyes, skin fold at inner eyelid (epicanthal fold), proportionately smaller head size;

- **Developmental:** Learning disabilities (70 percent): Normal IQ, but may be 10 to 15 points below siblings;

- **Speech and language delays (50 percent);**

- **Delayed motor skills:** Poor coordination, awkwardness, clumsiness;

- **Behavioral:** Introverted, difficulty with interpersonal relationships.

How is Triple X diagnosed and treated?

XXX syndrome is diagnosed prenatally, through CVS or amniocentesis, or after the child is born by a blood test. These tests are all able to look at a person's chromosomes (karyotype.) There is no way to remove the extra X chromosome. Treatment depends on what needs the child has. Girls with XXX syndrome may need to be seen by physical, developmental, occupational, or speech therapists if they have developmental or speech problems. Additionally, a pediatric psychologist or group therapy may be helpful if they have social troubles. Girls with trisomy X are treated as any other child with a developmental or psychological concern would be treated.

What is 46,XX/47,XXX mosaicism?

This describes a chromosome study that shows a mixture of normal cells and cells with an extra X chromosome. A girl with mosaicism will usually have fewer effects of the extra chromosome, because not all of her cells have this extra genetic material. She will probably not be much different than she would be if her chromosome study showed all normal cells.

Chapter 40

Fragile X Syndrome

What is fragile X syndrome?

Fragile X syndrome is the most common form of inherited mental retardation in males and is also a significant cause of mental retardation in females. It affects about one in four thousand males and one in eight thousand females and occurs in all racial and ethnic groups.

Nearly all cases of fragile X syndrome are caused by an alteration (mutation) in the FMR1 gene where a deoxyribonucleic acid (DNA) segment, known as the CGG triplet repeat, is expanded. Normally, this DNA segment is repeated from five to about forty times. In people with fragile X syndrome, however, the CGG segment is repeated more than two hundred times. The abnormally expanded CGG segment inactivates (silences) the FMR1 gene, which prevents the gene from producing a protein called fragile X mental retardation protein. Loss of this protein leads to the signs and symptoms of fragile X syndrome. Both boys and girls can be affected, but because boys have only one X chromosome, a single fragile X is likely to affect them more severely.

What are the symptoms of fragile X syndrome?

A boy who has the full FMR1 mutation has fragile X syndrome and will have moderate mental retardation. They have a particular facial

---

"Learning about Fragile X Syndrome," National Human Genome Research Institute (www.genome.gov), September 16, 2010.

appearance, characterized by a large head size, a long face, prominent forehead and chin, and protruding ears. In addition, males who have fragile X syndrome have loose joints (joint laxity), and large testes (after puberty).

Affected boys may have behavioral problems such as hyperactivity, hand flapping, hand biting, temper tantrums, and autism. Other behaviors in boys after they have reached puberty include poor eye contact, perseverative speech, problems in impulse control, and distractibility. Physical problems that have been seen include eye, orthopedic, heart, and skin problems.

Girls who have the full FMR1 mutation have mild mental retardation.

Family members who have fewer repeats in the FMR1 gene may not have mental retardation, but may have other problems. Women with less severe changes may have premature menopause or difficulty becoming pregnant.

Both men and women may have problems with tremors and poor coordination.

What does it mean to have a fragile X premutation?

People with about fifty-five to two hundred repeats of the CGG segment are said to have an FMR1 premutation (an intermediate variation of the gene). In women, the premutation is liable to expand to more than two hundred repeats in cells that develop into eggs. This means that women with the FMR1 premutation have an increased risk of having a child with fragile X syndrome. By contrast, the premutation CGG repeat in men remains at the same size or shortens as it is passed to the next generation.

Males and females who have a fragile X premutation have normal intellect and appearance. A few individuals with a premutation have subtle intellectual or behavioral symptoms, such as learning difficulties or social anxiety. The difficulties are usually not socially debilitating, and these individuals may still marry and have children.

Males who have a premutation with fifty-nine to two hundred CGG trinucleotide repeats are usually unaffected and are at risk for fragile X–associated tremor/ataxia syndrome (FXTAS). The fragile X–associated tremor/ataxia syndrome (FXTAS) is characterized by late-onset, progressive cerebellar ataxia and intention tremor in males who have a premutation. Other neurologic findings include short-term memory loss, executive function deficits, cognitive decline, parkinsonism, peripheral neuropathy, lower-limb proximal muscle weakness, and autonomic dysfunction.

The degree to which clinical symptoms of fragile X are present (penetrance) is age related; symptoms are seen in 17 percent of males aged fifty to fifty-nine years, in 38 percent of males aged sixty to sixty-nine years, in 47 percent of males aged seventy to seventy-nine years, and in 75 percent or males aged eighty years or older. Some female premutation carriers may also develop tremor and ataxia.

Females who have a premutation usually are unaffected, but may be at risk for premature ovarian failure and FXTAS. Premature ovarian failure (POF) is defined as cessation of menses before age forty years and has been observed in carriers of premutation alleles. A review by Sherman (2005) concluded that the risk for POF was 21 percent in premutation carriers compared to 1 percent for the general population.

How is fragile X syndrome diagnosed?

There are very few outward signs of fragile X syndrome in babies, but one is a tendency to have a large head circumference. An experienced geneticist may note subtle differences in facial characteristics. Mental retardation is the hallmark of this condition and, in females, this may be the only sign of the problem.

A specific genetic test (polymerase chain reaction [PCR]) can now be performed to diagnose fragile X syndrome. This test looks for an expanded mutation (called a triplet repeat) in the FMR1 gene.

How is fragile X syndrome treated?

There is no specific treatment available for fragile X syndrome. Supportive therapy for children who have fragile X syndrome includes the following:

- Special education and anticipatory management including avoidance of excessive stimulation to decrease behavioral problems.

- Medication to manage behavioral issues, although no specific medication has been shown to be beneficial.

- Early intervention, special education, and vocational training.

- Vision, hearing, connective tissue, and heart problems, when present, are treated in the usual manner.

Is fragile X syndrome inherited?

This condition is inherited in an X-linked dominant pattern. A condition is considered X-linked if the mutated gene that causes the disorder is located on the X chromosome, one of the two sex chromosomes. The inheritance is dominant if one copy of the altered gene in each cell is sufficient to cause the condition. In most cases, males experience more severe symptoms of the disorder than females. A striking characteristic of X-linked inheritance is that fathers cannot pass X-linked traits to their sons.

Chapter 41

Klinefelter Syndrome

What Is Klinefelter Syndrome?

Klinefelter syndrome is a group of conditions that affects the health of males who are born with at least one extra X chromosome. Chromosomes, found in all body cells, contain genes. Genes provide specific instructions for body characteristics and functions. For example, some genes determine height and hair color. Other genes influence language skills and reproductive functions. Each person typically has 23 pairs of chromosomes. One of these pairs (sex chromosomes) determines a person's sex. A baby with two X chromosomes (XX) is female. A baby with one X chromosome and one Y chromosome (XY) is male.

Most males with Klinefelter syndrome, also called XXY males, have two X chromosomes instead of one. The extra X usually occurs in all body cells. Sometimes the extra X only occurs in some cells, resulting in a less severe form of the syndrome (called mosaic Klinefelter syndrome). Rarely, a more severe form occurs when there are two or more extra X chromosomes.

Did You Know?

Klinefelter syndrome is the most common sex-chromosome abnormality, affecting about one in every 500 to 700 men.

What Causes Klinefelter Syndrome?

The addition of extra chromosomes seems to occur by chance. The syndrome is not inherited from the parents. The addition occurs in the sperm, the egg, or after conception.

What Are the Signs and Symptoms of Klinefelter Syndrome?

Signs and symptoms can vary. Some males have no symptoms but a doctor will be able to see subtle physical signs of the syndrome. Many males are not diagnosed until puberty or adulthood. As many as two-thirds of men with the syndrome may never be diagnosed. Many men with mosaic Klinefelter syndrome have few obvious signs except very small testicles.

Signs and Symptoms by Age Group

Infants and young boys may have:

- problems at birth, such as testicles that haven't dropped into the scrotum or a hernia (when an internal organ bulges through a body cavity wall into the scrotum);
- a small penis;
- weak muscles;
- speech and language problems, such as delayed speech;
- problems with learning and reading;
- problems fitting in socially;
- mood and behavioral problems.

Adolescents may also have:

- very small, firm testicles;
- enlarged breasts, called gynecomastia;
- long legs but a short trunk;
- above-average height;
- reduced muscle bulk;
- sparse facial and body hair;
- delayed puberty;
- low energy levels.

Adults may also have:

- low testosterone (male hormone) levels;
- infertility from a lack of sperm;
- decreased sex drive;
- problems getting or keeping an erection;
- other difficulties, such as being unable to make plans or solve problems.

Health Problems Linked to Klinefelter Syndrome

Klinefelter syndrome can lead to weak bones (osteoporosis), varicose veins, and autoimmune diseases (when the immune system acts against the body), such as lupus or rheumatoid arthritis. XXY males have an increased risk for breast cancer and cancers that affect blood, bone marrow, or lymph nodes, such as leukemia. They also tend to have excess fat around the abdomen (which raises the risk of health problems), heart and blood vessel disease, and type 2 diabetes.

How Is Klinefelter Syndrome Diagnosed?

Diagnosis is based on a physical examination, hormone testing, and chromosome analysis. The syndrome can also be diagnosed before birth but testing is not routinely done at that time.

What Is the Treatment for Klinefelter Syndrome?

Treatment can help males overcome many of the physical, social, and learning problems that are part of the syndrome. Males with Klinefelter syndrome should be seen by a team of health care providers. The team may include endocrinologists, general practitioners, pediatricians, urologists, speech therapists, genetic counselors, and psychologists. Surgery may be needed to reduce breast size. With treatment, men can lead very normal lives.

Experts recommend testosterone replacement, starting during puberty, for proper development of muscles, bones, male sex characteristics such as facial hair, and sexual function. Continued treatment throughout life helps prevent long-term health problems. Testosterone replacement does not cure infertility, however. Infertility treatments require specialized—and costly—techniques, but some men with Klinefelter syndrome have been able to father children.

Questions to Ask Your Doctor

- Will diagnostic tests and treatment be covered by my insurance?

- What are my (or my child's) options for testosterone therapy? What are the benefits and risks?

- What can I do manage other health problems linked to Klinefelter syndrome?

- Will I (or my child) be able to have children?

- Will I (or my child) have normal sexual function?

- Should I see an endocrinologist for my (or my child's) care?

Chapter 42

Prader-Willi Syndrome

What is Prader-Willi syndrome (PWS)?

Prader-Willi syndrome (PWS) is a genetic syndrome that affects one in every twelve thousand to fifteen thousand people of both sexes and all races and ethnic groups. It is caused by a disorder of chromosome 15.

What are the features of children with PWS?

Any of these symptoms may show up in your child and can vary from mild to severe:

- Low muscle tone (hypotonia or floppy baby).

- Feeding problems and poor weight gain in infancy.

- Extreme hunger, overeating, obsession with food after infancy.

- Big weight gain between one and six years of age. This leads to serious obesity if no steps are taken to help.

- Distinctive facial features: narrow face, almond-shaped eyes, small mouth with thin upper lip and down-turned corners.

- Hypogonadism (less than normal sex hormones), leading to incomplete sexual development, undescended testicles, small penis, delayed puberty.

- Developmental delay, including mild to moderate intellectual disability and learning difficulties.

- Infants and children are typically happy and loving and exhibit few behavior problems.

- Older children and adults have problems with behavior regulation, such as difficulties with transitions and unanticipated changes.

- Other behavior problems may include: temper tantrums, violent outbursts, obsessive/compulsive behavior, stealing, lying, and being argumentative, rigid, manipulative, and possessive.

- Short stature, small hands and feet.

- Fair skin.

- Speech problems.

- Skin picking, which can cause sores.

What causes Prader-Willi syndrome? Is there a test for it?

The syndrome is caused by genetic deletions (missing genetic material) on chromosome 15. Genetic tests for PWS are available. People with the signs and symptoms of PWS should get tested.

What are the major health concerns for people with PWS?

- Severe obesity is the major medical problem.

- Obesity-related problems—including diabetes, high blood pressure, chronic venous insufficiency (leading to ulcers or sores on legs and feet), cellulitis, and hypoventilation.

- Strabismus (crossed eyes) may require surgical correction.

- Scoliosis.

- Osteoporosis can occur earlier than usual and can cause fractures.

- Sleep disturbances and sleep apnea.

- Bedwetting.

- Dental problems—including soft tooth enamel, thick saliva, poor oral hygiene, teeth grinding.

How is PWS treated?

There is no cure for PWS, but PWS comes with lots of health problems that need to be treated. With early diagnosis and a proactive approach, kids with PWS can thrive.

Weight management is a major task of parents of kids with PWS. These kids need a balanced, low-calorie diet with vitamin and calcium supplements, along with plenty of exercise. You will probably need to restrict access to food by locking your cabinets and refrigerator. No medication or surgical intervention has been found to eliminate the need for strict dieting.

Growth hormone is a common medication used in PWS. It increases muscle mass and function, may allow for a higher daily calorie intake, and helps kids grow taller.

Sleep apnea may need to be checked out with a sleep study, and may require treatment. Growth hormone treatment can worsen sleep apnea, according to recent research, so kids on growth hormone should be carefully followed and monitored for problems.

Sex hormone replacement can lead to more normal physical development in puberty.

Behavioral management—daily routines, structure, firm rules and limits, and positive rewards work best.

Psychotropic medications may help with obsessive-compulsive symptoms and mood swings if behavior management alone is not enough.

Physical and occupational therapy help promote motor development along with growth hormone.

Speech and language therapy may help with speech delays.

Early intervention and special education can help your child reach his or her full potential.

Reviewer's note: While all cases appear to involve the same genes, the genetic causes are quite complex, and may not to be the same in everyone with Prader-Willi syndrome. Interestingly, the same gene mutations can cause either Prader-Willi syndrome or Angelman syndrome, and it matters which parent provided the abnormal gene. People with Prader-Willi syndrome have usually inherited the abnormality from their mother, while those with Angelman syndrome have usually inherited it from their father.

Chapter 43

Smith-Magenis Syndrome

What is Smith-Magenis syndrome?

Smith-Magenis syndrome is a developmental disorder that affects many parts of the body. The major features of this condition include mild to moderate intellectual disability, delayed speech and language skills, distinctive facial features, sleep disturbances, and behavioral problems.

Most people with Smith-Magenis syndrome have a broad, square-shaped face with deep-set eyes, full cheeks, and a prominent lower jaw. The middle of the face and the bridge of the nose often appear flattened. The mouth tends to turn downward with a full, outward-curving upper lip. These facial differences can be subtle in early childhood, but they usually become more distinctive in later childhood and adulthood. Dental abnormalities are also common in affected individuals.

Disrupted sleep patterns are characteristic of Smith-Magenis syndrome, typically beginning early in life. Affected people may be very sleepy during the day, but have trouble falling asleep and awaken several times each night.

People with Smith-Magenis syndrome have affectionate, engaging personalities, but most also have behavioral problems. These include frequent temper tantrums and outbursts, aggression, anxiety, impulsiveness, and difficulty paying attention. Self-injury, including biting,

Excerpted from "Smith-Magenis Syndrome," Genetics Home Reference (http://ghr.nlm.nih.gov), February 2007. Reviewed by David A. Cooke, M.D., FACP, May 2013.

hitting, head banging, and skin picking, is very common. Repetitive self-hugging is a behavioral trait that may be unique to Smith-Magenis syndrome. People with this condition also compulsively lick their fingers and flip pages of books and magazines (a behavior known as "lick and flip").

Other signs and symptoms of Smith-Magenis syndrome include short stature, abnormal curvature of the spine (scoliosis), reduced sensitivity to pain and temperature, and a hoarse voice. Some people with this disorder have ear abnormalities that lead to hearing loss. Affected individuals may have eye abnormalities that cause nearsightedness (myopia) and other vision problems. Although less common, heart and kidney defects also have been reported in people with Smith-Magenis syndrome.

How common is Smith-Magenis syndrome?

Smith-Magenis syndrome affects at least one in twenty-five thousand individuals worldwide. Researchers believe that many people with this condition are not diagnosed, however, so the true prevalence may be closer to one in fifteen thousand individuals.

What are the genetic changes related to Smith-Magenis syndrome?

Most people with Smith-Magenis syndrome have a deletion of genetic material from a specific region of chromosome 17. Although this region contains multiple genes, researchers believe that the loss of one particular gene, RAI1, in each cell is responsible for most of the characteristic features of this condition. The loss of other genes in the deleted region may help explain why the features of Smith-Magenis syndrome vary among affected individuals.

A small percentage of people with Smith-Magenis syndrome have a mutation in the RAI1 gene instead of a chromosomal deletion. Although these individuals have many of the major features of the condition, they are less likely than people with a chromosomal deletion to have short stature, hearing loss, and heart or kidney abnormalities. The RAI1 gene provides instructions for making a protein whose function is unknown. Mutations in one copy of this gene lead to the production of a nonfunctional version of the RAI1 protein or reduce the amount of this protein that is produced in cells. Researchers are uncertain how changes in this protein result in the physical, mental, and behavioral problems associated with Smith-Magenis syndrome.

Can Smith-Magenis syndrome be inherited?

Smith-Magenis syndrome is typically not inherited. This condition usually results from a genetic change that occurs during the formation of reproductive cells (eggs or sperm) or in early fetal development. Most often, people with Smith-Magenis syndrome have no history of the condition in their family.

Chapter 44

Turner Syndrome

What is Turner syndrome?

Turner syndrome is a chromosomal condition that alters development in females. Women with this condition tend to be shorter than average and are usually unable to conceive a child (infertile) because of an absence of ovarian function. Other features of this condition that can vary among women who have Turner syndrome include: extra skin on the neck (webbed neck), puffiness or swelling (lymphedema) of the hands and feet, skeletal abnormalities, heart defects, and kidney problems.

This condition occurs in about 1 in 2,500 female births worldwide, but is much more common among pregnancies that do not survive to term (miscarriages and stillbirths).

Turner syndrome is a chromosomal condition related to the X chromosome.

Researchers have not yet determined which genes on the X chromosome are responsible for most signs and symptoms of Turner syndrome. They have, however, identified one gene called SHOX that is important for bone development and growth. Missing one copy of this gene likely causes short stature and skeletal abnormalities in women with Turner syndrome.

"Learning about Turner Syndrome," National Human Genome Research Institute (www.genome.gov), September 26, 2011.

What are the symptoms of Turner syndrome?

Girls who have Turner syndrome are shorter than average. They often have normal height for the first three years of life, but then have a slow growth rate. At puberty they do not have the usual growth spurt.

Nonfunctioning ovaries are another symptom of Turner syndrome. Normally a girl's ovaries begin to produce sex hormones (estrogen and progesterone) at puberty. This does not happen in most girls who have Turner syndrome. They do not start their periods or develop breasts without hormone treatment at the age of puberty.

Even though many women who have Turner have nonfunctioning ovaries and are infertile, their vagina and womb are totally normal.

In early childhood, girls who have Turner syndrome may have frequent middle ear infections. Recurrent infections can lead to hearing loss in some cases.

Girls with Turner syndrome are usually of normal intelligence with good verbal skills and reading skills. Some girls, however, have problems with math, memory skills, and fine-finger movements.

Additional symptoms of Turner syndrome include the following:

- An especially wide neck (webbed neck) and a low or indistinct hairline.

- A broad chest and widely spaced nipples.

- Arms that turn out slightly at the elbow.

- A heart murmur, sometimes associated with narrowing of the aorta (blood vessel exiting the heart).

- A tendency to develop high blood pressure (so this should be checked regularly).

- Minor eye problems that are corrected by glasses.

- Scoliosis (deformity of the spine) occurs in 10 percent of adolescent girls who have Turner syndrome.

- The thyroid gland becomes underactive in about 10 percent of women who have Turner syndrome. Regular blood tests are necessary to detect it early and if necessary treat with thyroid replacement.

- Older or overweight women with Turner syndrome are slightly more at risk of developing diabetes.

- Osteoporosis can develop because of a lack of estrogen, but this can largely be prevented by taking hormone replacement therapy.

How is Turner syndrome diagnosed?

A diagnosis of Turner syndrome may be suspected when there are a number of typical physical features observed such as webbed neck, a broad chest, and widely spaced nipples. Sometimes diagnosis is made at birth because of heart problems, an unusually wide neck, or swelling of the hands and feet.

The two main clinical features of Turner syndrome are short stature and the lack of the development of the ovaries.

Many girls are diagnosed in early childhood when a slow growth rate and other features are identified. Diagnosis sometimes takes place later when puberty does not occur.

Turner syndrome may be suspected in pregnancy during an ultrasound test. This can be confirmed by prenatal testing—chorionic villous sampling or amniocentesis—to obtain cells from the unborn baby for chromosomal analysis. If a diagnosis is confirmed prenatally, the baby may be under the care of a specialist pediatrician immediately after birth.

Diagnosis is confirmed by a blood test, called a karyotype. This is used to analyze the chromosomal composition of the female.

What is the treatment for Turner syndrome?

During childhood and adolescence, girls may be under the care of a pediatric endocrinologist, who is a specialist in childhood conditions of the hormones and metabolism.

Growth hormone injections are beneficial in some individuals with Turner syndrome. Injections often begin in early childhood and may increase final adult height by a few inches.

Estrogen replacement therapy is usually started at the time of normal puberty, around twelve years to start breast development. Estrogen and progesterone are given a little later to begin a monthly "period," which is necessary to keep the womb healthy. Estrogen is also given to prevent osteoporosis.

Babies born with a heart murmur or narrowing of the aorta may need surgery to correct the problem. A heart expert (cardiologist) will assess and follow up any treatment necessary.

Girls who have Turner syndrome are more likely to get middle ear infections. Repeated infections may lead to hearing loss and should be evaluated by the pediatrician. An ear, nose, and throat specialist (ENT) may be involved in caring for this health issue.

High blood pressure is quite common in women who have Turner syndrome. In some cases, the elevated blood pressure is due to narrowing of the aorta or a kidney abnormality. However, most of the time, no specific cause for the elevation is identified. Blood pressure should be checked routinely and, if necessary, treated with medication. Women who have Turner syndrome have a slightly higher risk of having an underactive thyroid or developing diabetes. This should also be monitored during routine health maintenance visits and treated if necessary.

Regular health checks are very important. Special clinics for the care of girls and women who have Turner syndrome are available in some areas, with access to a variety of specialists. Early preventive care and treatment is very important.

Almost all women are infertile, but pregnancy with donor embryos may be possible.

Having appropriate medical treatment and support allows a woman with Turner syndrome to lead a normal, healthy and happy life.

Is Turner syndrome inherited?

Turner syndrome is not usually inherited in families. Turner syndrome occurs when one of the two X chromosomes normally found in women is missing or incomplete. Although the exact cause of Turner syndrome is not known, it appears to occur as a result of a random error during the formation of either the eggs or sperm.

Humans have forty-six chromosomes, which contain all of a person's genes and deoxyribonucleic acid (DNA). Two of these chromosomes, the sex chromosomes, determine a person's gender. Both of the sex chromosomes in females are called X chromosomes. (This is written as XX.) Males have an X and a Y chromosome (written as XY). The two sex chromosomes help a person develop fertility and the sexual characteristics of their gender.

In Turner syndrome, the girl does not have the usual pair of two complete X chromosomes. The most common scenario is that the girl has only one X chromosome in her cells. Some girls with Turner syndrome do have two X chromosomes, but one of the X chromosomes is incomplete. In another scenario, the girl has some cells in her body with two X chromosomes, but other cells have only one. This is called mosaicism.

Chapter 45

Velocardiofacial Syndrome

What is velocardiofacial syndrome?

Velocardiofacial syndrome (VCFS) is a genetic condition that is sometimes hereditary. VCFS is characterized by a combination of medical problems that vary from child to child. These medical problems include: cleft palate, or an opening in the roof of the mouth, and other differences in the palate; heart defects; problems fighting infection; low calcium levels; differences in the way the kidneys are formed or work; a characteristic facial appearance; learning problems; and speech and feeding problems.

The name "velocardiofacial syndrome" comes from the Latin words "velum," meaning palate, "cardia," meaning heart, and "facies," having to do with the face. Not all of these identifying features are found in each child who is born with VCFS. The most common features are palatal differences (~75 percent), heart defects (75 percent), problems fighting infection (77 percent), low calcium levels (50 percent), differences in the kidney (35 percent), characteristic facial appearance (numbers vary depending on the individual's ethnic and racial background), learning problems (~90 percent), and speech (~75 percent) and feeding problems (35 percent).

Two genes—COMT and TBX1—are associated with VCFS. However, not all of the genes that cause VCFS have been identified. Most children who have been diagnosed with this syndrome are missing a

Reprinted from "Learning about Velocardiofacial Syndrome," National Human Genome Research Institute (www.genome.gov), October 13, 2011.

small part of chromosome 22. Chromosomes are threadlike structures found in every cell of the body. Each chromosome contains hundreds of genes. A human cell normally contains forty-six chromosomes (twenty-three from each parent). The specific location or address of the missing segment in individuals with VCFS is 22q11.2.

VCFS is also called the 22q11.2 deletion syndrome. It also has other clinical names such as DiGeorge syndrome, conotruncal anomaly face syndrome (CTAF), autosomal dominant Opitz G/BBB syndrome, or Cayler cardiofacial syndrome. As a result of this deletion, about thirty genes are generally absent from this chromosome.

VCFS affects about one in four thousand newborns. VCFS may affect more individuals, however, because some people who have the 22q11.2 deletion may not be diagnosed, as they have very few signs and symptoms.

What are the symptoms of VCFS?

Despite the involvement of a very specific portion of chromosome 22, there is great variation in the symptoms of this syndrome. At least thirty different symptoms have been associated with the 22q11 deletion. Most of these symptoms are not present in all individuals who have VCFS.

Symptoms include: cleft palate, usually of the soft palate (the roof of the mouth nearest the throat, which is behind the bony palate); heart problems; similar faces (elongated face, almond-shaped eyes, wide nose, small ears); eye problems; feeding problems that include food coming through the nose (nasal regurgitation) because of the palatal differences; middle-ear infections (otitis media); low calcium due to hypoparathyroidism (low levels of the parathyroid hormone that can result in seizures); immune system problems that make it difficult for the body to fight infections; differences in the way the kidneys are formed or how they work; weak muscles; differences in the spine, such as curvature of the spine (scoliosis) or bony abnormalities in the neck or upper back; and tapered fingers. Children are born with these features.

Children who have VCFS also often have learning difficulties and developmental delays. About 65 percent of individuals with the 22q11.2 deletion are found to have a nonverbal learning disability. When tested, their verbal IQ scores are greater than ten points higher than their performance IQ scores. This combination of test scores brings down the full-scale IQ scores but they won't represent the abilities of the individual accurately. As a result of this type of learning disability, students will have relative strengths in reading and rote memorization but will struggle with math and abstract reasoning. These individuals may also have communication and social interaction problems such as autism. As adults, these individuals have an increased risk for developing mental illness such as depression, anxiety, and schizophrenia.

How is VCFS diagnosed?

VCFS is suspected as a diagnosis based on clinical examination and the presence of the signs and symptoms of the syndrome.

A special blood test called FISH (fluorescence in situ hybridization) is then done to look for the deletion in chromosome 22q11.2. More than 95 percent of individuals who have VCFS have a deletion in chromosome 22q11.2.

Those individuals who do not have the 22q11.2 deletion by standard FISH testing may have a smaller deletion that may only be found using more sophisticated lab studies such as comparative genomic hybridization, multiplex ligation-dependent probe amplification (MLPA), additional FISH studies performed in a research laboratory, or using specific gene studies to look for mutations in the genes known to be in this region. Again, these studies may be available only through a research lab.

What is the treatment for VCFS?

Treatment is based on the type of symptoms that are present. For example, heart defects are treated as they would normally be via surgical interventions in the newborn period. Individuals who have low calcium levels are given calcium supplements and frequently vitamin D to help them absorb the calcium. Palate problems are treated by a team of specialists called a cleft palate or craniofacial team and again often require surgical interventions and intensive speech therapy. Infections are generally treated aggressively with antibiotics in infants and children with immune problems.

Early intervention and speech therapies are started when possible at one year of age to assess and treat developmental delays.

Is VCFS inherited?

VCFS is due to a 22q11.2 deletion. Most often neither parent has the deletion and so it is new in the child (93 percent) and the chance for the couple to have another child with VCFS is quite low (close to zero). However, once the deletion is present in a person, he or she has a 50 percent chance for having children who also have the deletion. The 22q11 deletion happens as an accident when either the egg or sperm are being formed or early in fetal development.

In less than 10 percent of cases, a person with VCFS inherits the deletion in chromosome 22 from a parent. When VCFS is inherited in families, this means that other family members may be affected as well.

Since some people with the 22q11.2 deletion are very mildly affected, it is suggested that all parents of children with the deletion have testing. Furthermore, some people with the deletion have no symptoms but they have the deletion in some of their cells but not all. This is called mosaicism. Even other people have the deletion only in their egg cells or sperm cells but not in their blood cells. It is recommended that all parents of a child with a 22q11.2 deletion seek genetic counseling before or during a subsequent pregnancy to learn more about their chances of having another child with VCFS.

Chapter 46

Williams Syndrome

Williams syndrome is a rare genetic disorder that can lead to problems with development.

Causes

Williams syndrome is a rare condition caused by missing genes. Parents may not have any family history of the condition. However, a person with Williams syndrome has a 50 percent chance of passing the disorder on to each of his or her children. The cause usually occurs randomly.

Williams syndrome occurs in about one in eight thousand births.

One of the twenty-five missing genes is the gene that produces elastin, a protein that allows blood vessels and other tissues in the body to stretch. It is likely that having only one copy of this gene results in the narrowing of blood vessels seen in this condition.

Symptoms

- Delayed speech that may later turn into strong speaking ability and strong learning by hearing

- Developmental delay

- Easily distracted, attention deficit disorder (ADD)
- Feeding problems including colic, reflux, and vomiting
- Inward bend of the small finger (clinodactyly)
- Learning disorders
- Mild-to-moderate intellectual disability
- Personality traits including being very friendly, trusting strangers, fearing loud sounds or physical contact, and being interested in music
- Short compared to the rest of the person's family
- Sunken chest (pectus excavatum)
- Unusual appearance of the face:
  - Flattened nasal bridge with small upturned nose
  - Long ridges in the skin that run from the nose to the upper lip (philtrum)
  - Prominent lips with an open mouth
  - Skin that covers the inner corner of the eye (epicanthal folds)
  - Partially missing teeth, defective tooth enamel, or small, widely spaced teeth

Exams and Tests

Signs include:

- blood vessel narrowing including supravalvular aortic stenosis, pulmonary stenosis, and pulmonary artery stenosis;
- farsightedness;
- high blood calcium level (hypercalcemia) that may cause seizures and rigid muscles;
- high blood pressure;
- slack joints that may change to stiffness as patient gets older;
- unusual pattern ("stellate" or star-like) in iris of the eye.

Tests for Williams syndrome:

- blood pressure check;
- blood test for missing chromosome (fluorescence in situ hybridization [FISH] test);
- echocardiography combined with Doppler ultrasound;
- kidney ultrasound.

Treatment

There is no cure for Williams syndrome. Avoid taking extra calcium and vitamin D. Treat high levels of blood calcium, if present. Blood vessel narrowing can be a significant health problem and is treated based on its severity.

Physical therapy is helpful to patients with joint stiffness. Developmental and speech therapy can also help these children (for example, verbal strengths can help make up for other weaknesses). Other treatments are based on a patient's symptoms.

It can help to have treatment coordinated by a geneticist who is experienced with Williams syndrome.

Outlook (Prognosis)

About 75 percent of those with Williams syndrome have some intellectual disability.

Most patients will not live as long as normal, due to complications.

Most patients require full-time caregivers and often live in supervised group homes.

Possible Complications

- Calcium deposits in the kidney and other kidney problems
- Death (in rare cases from anesthesia)
- Heart failure due to narrowed blood vessels
- Pain in the abdomen

When to Contact a Medical Professional

Many of the symptoms and signs of Williams syndrome may not be obvious at birth. Call your health care provider if your child has features similar to those of Williams syndrome. Seek genetic counseling if you have a family history of Williams syndrome.

Prevention

There is no known way to prevent the genetic problem that causes Williams syndrome. Prenatal testing is available for couples with a family history of Williams syndrome who wish to conceive.

Alternative Names

Williams-Beuren syndrome

Part Four

Complex Disorders with Genetic and Environmental Components

Chapter 47

Genes, Behavior, the Environment, and Health

Yesterday

People observed for thousands of years that diseases run in families, but it was only with twentieth-century genetic discoveries that we began to understand how specific genes affect health.

Research showed that some diseases, including cystic fibrosis, Duchenne muscular dystrophy, and sickle cell disease, are caused by changes in a single gene. However, it became apparent that multiple genes, acting in concert, confer risk for other complex diseases, including diabetes and hypertension, psychiatric disorders like schizophrenia and depression, and alcohol and drug dependence.

Genes alone were not the whole story. Identical twins who had exactly the same genetic makeup but who were raised in different families sometimes developed different diseases or health outcomes. These types of findings suggested that our living conditions or environments were also very important contributors to health and disease.

Today

The now completed mapping of the entire human genome gives researchers powerful tools to identify genetic contributions to health and disease.

Reprinted from "Genes, Behavior, the Environment, and Health," Research Portfolio Online Reporting Tools (RePORT), a service of the National Institutes of Health, March 29, 2013.

We know that genes alone do not cause many common diseases like heart disease, diabetes, cancer, and depression, as well as alcohol, tobacco, and other drug addictions. Rather, many genes influence our risk of developing diseases, and whether or not that risk actually leads to disease depends on a lifetime of complex interactions between our genes and our environments. Similarly, certain environments or experiences that are known to increase our chances of physical or mental health problems are especially risky for people who also have a particularly vulnerable genetic makeup.

Major stressful events, such as job loss, divorce, abuse, or caring for a seriously ill family member, may lead to depression. Research on gene-environment interactions show that children experiencing highly stressful environments are more likely to become depressed as adults if they also have a particular version of a gene that influences the level of the brain chemical serotonin. Individuals experiencing high levels of stress as children but devoid of this genetic variation aren't as likely to become depressed.

This same serotonin-related gene may be involved in alcohol consumption. National Institutes of Health (NIH) researchers revealed that female monkeys with a particular version of the gene prefer to drink alcohol more than monkeys with a different version of the gene. If the monkeys with the version of the gene that prefer alcohol are reared in groups of other young monkeys rather than by their mothers, they show an even greater preference for alcohol and drink more of it when they are young adults. This is an example of how a genetic risk is made worse by specific conditions during early stages of development. These monkey studies, in which researchers can better control the environment, allow us to pinpoint more specifically how gene-environment interactions lead to disorders and diseases in an animal model that closely resembles humans.

Scientists doing research on rats discovered that the behavior of rat moms toward their newborn pups—how they nurse, lick, and groom the pups—changes the lifelong responses of those offspring to stress. The mothers' behaviors change the activity of genes in their offspring's brains—specifically, genes that are involved in the response to stress hormones.

Toxic environments also contribute to influencing our behavior. Studies with children have shown that cumulative exposure to lead contributes to risk for delinquent behavior. Exposures to certain pesticides and industrial chemicals increase the risk of developing attention deficit hyperactivity disorder in children. Animals similarly exposed also show abnormal patterns in the developing brain. Moreover, different strains of rodents show different outcomes from similar chemical exposures, indicating that genetic differences can influence the response to an environmental exposure.

More and more studies are showing that gene-environment interactions during early development may have long-lasting effects on health that do not show up until adulthood.

In order to develop successful treatments for the many disorders caused by gene/environment interactions, the NIH launched the Genes and Environment Initiative and the Genetic Association Information Network to explore and catalogue how genes and environment interact to influence the occurrence of common diseases.

Tomorrow

The identification of subsets of individuals with high disease risks due to particular combinations of genetic variations and environmental exposures or stressors will allow development of more targeted screening, interventions, and preventative strategies, as well as more effective maintenance of health.

Prevention of neurological disease and behavioral dysfunction caused by chemical exposures can be implemented by identifying and eliminating exposures to chemicals that cause risk, especially for those with known genetic susceptibility.

We can develop more personalized, and therefore more effective, behavioral treatments like changing social support, improving diet and exercise habits, or helping to cope with stress, to counteract higher risks for disease among those with certain genetic vulnerabilities or to enhance the effects of other genetic factors that offer protection against health problems.

Knowledge gained from research on gene-environment interactions can also be used by policymakers to design more "user-friendly" living conditions that delay or prevent the genetic risks of disease from being realized.

Chapter 48

Addiction and Genetics

Chapter Contents

Section 48.1

Genetics of Alcohol Use Disorders

Reprinted from the National Institute on Alcohol Abuse and
Alcoholism, National Institutes of Health, 2010.

How do genes influence alcoholism?

Alcoholism often seems to run in families, and we may hear about
scientific studies of an "alcoholism gene." Genetics certainly influence
our likelihood of developing alcoholism, but the story isn't so simple.

Research shows that genes are responsible for about half of the risk
for alcoholism. Therefore, genes alone do not determine whether someone will become an alcoholic. Environmental factors, as well as gene
and environment interactions, account for the remainder of the risk.[1]

Multiple genes play a role in a person's risk for developing alcoholism. There are genes that increase a person's risk, as well as those that
may decrease that risk, directly or indirectly. For instance, some people
of Asian descent carry a gene variant that alters their rate of alcohol
metabolism, causing them to have symptoms like flushing, nausea, and
rapid heartbeat when they drink. Many people who experience these effects avoid alcohol, which helps protect them from developing alcoholism.[2]

As we have learned more about the role genes play in our health,
researchers have discovered that different factors can alter the expression of our genes. This field is called epigenetics. Scientists are
learning more and more about how epigenetics can affect our risk for
developing alcoholism.

Can our genes affect alcohol treatment?

Scientists are also exploring how genes may influence the effectiveness of treatments for alcoholism. For instance, the drug naltrexone
has been shown to help some, but not all, alcohol-dependent patients
to reduce their drinking. Research has shown that alcoholic patients
with variations in a specific gene respond positively to treatment with
the drug, while those without the specific gene do not. A fuller understanding of how genes influence treatment outcomes will help doctors
prescribe the treatment that is most likely to help each patient.[3]

References

1. A Family History of Alcoholism—Are You at Risk?

2. Spectrum 1: 1.

3. AR&H Volume 31, Number 4, 2008

Section 48.2

Genetic Variation May Contribute to Risk of Alcoholism

Researchers at the University of Michigan Health System have uncovered a new link between genetic variations associated with alcoholism, impulsive behavior, and a region of the brain involved in craving and anxiety.

The results, published online on April 12, 2011, in *Molecular Psychiatry*, suggest that variations in the GABRA2 gene contribute to the risk of alcoholism by influencing impulsive behaviors, at least in part through a portion of the cerebral cortex known as the insula, says study senior author Margit Burmeister, Ph.D., research professor at U-M's Molecular and Behavioral Neuroscience Institute.

"Scientists often find a statistical association between behaviors and various genes, but the mechanism that's at work frequently remains unclear," Burmeister says. "Here we took some steps toward explaining how specific genetic risk factors are influencing behavior and the brain."

Individuals under distress who also have the risky genetic variant tend to act impulsively, a behavior that may lead to the development of alcohol problems, says lead author Sandra Villafuerte, Ph.D., a research investigator at U-M's Molecular and Behavioral Neuroscience Institute and Department of Psychiatry.

"Developing deeper understandings of the various genetic and environmental factors involved in risky behaviors may guide prevention and treatment efforts in the future," Villafuerte says.

The study included 449 people, who came from 173 families—129 of whom had at least one member diagnosed with alcohol dependence or abuse. Those with certain variations in the GABRA2 gene were more likely to have alcohol dependence symptoms and higher measures of impulsiveness in response to distress, the study found. Stronger associations were found in women than in men.

"This wouldn't be a surprise to an alcohol researcher," Burmeister says. "Men and women tend to have different pathways to alcoholism. Drinking to relieve anxiety and distress is seen more in women."

Researchers also used functional magnetic resonance imaging (fMRI) to observe changes of blood flow in the brains of forty-four young adults from these families as they performed a task in which they anticipated winning or losing money.

"The neuroimaging allowed us to see for the first time how these genetic variants create differences in how the brain responds in certain situations," says Mary M. Heitzeg, Ph.D., a research assistant professor in U-M's Department of Psychiatry and U-M's Addiction Research Center.

They found that individuals with one form of the GABRA2 gene associated with alcoholism showed significantly higher activation in the insula when anticipating rewards and losses than those with other combinations. This higher activation was also related to a greater level of impulsiveness in response to distress.

The insula's association with addictive behavior is well known: smokers who had insula damage due to stroke found it much easier to give up cigarettes, *Science* reported in 2007.

"We believe these results suggest GABRA2 exerts an influence on an underlying neural system that impacts early risk factors and, later, alcohol dependency," says Burmeister, also a professor of psychiatry and human genetics at the U-M Medical School. "In the future, we hope to further examine the effects of family environment and other behavioral and environmental factors."

The authors stress that genetic risk factors don't act alone, and simply having them does not mean that someone will become an alcoholic.

Section 48.3

Genes Influence Amount of Alcohol Consumption

Scientists have found that the genes which influence the amount of alcohol people drink may be distinct from those that affect the risk of alcoholism.

A large number of studies have focused on a genetic predisposition to alcoholism. They presume that the genes involved in this disorder, combined with environmental factors, influence susceptibility to alcohol dependence.

The various genetic pathways affecting alcohol drinking behavior have been investigated by Dr. Boris Tabakoff and his team at the University of Colorado–Denver using both rats and humans.

They compared genes involved in alcohol pathways in rats with human genes, using male study participants from Montreal, Canada, and Sydney, Australia, to identify common genetic factors across species. Alcohol consumption among the participants ranged from abstinence to heavy intake, and drinking patterns were recorded.

The researchers discovered that drinking behavior is linked to the "pleasure and reward" pathways in the brain, and also to some of the systems that control food intake. In the journal *BMC Biology*, they write that the results emphasize the importance of looking at signaling pathways rather than single genes, and show cross-species similarities in predisposition to alcohol consumption.

"Our results also suggest that different genetic factors predispose to alcohol dependence versus alcohol consumption," they add.

Dr. Tabakoff said, "We know that high levels of alcohol consumption can increase the risk of becoming alcohol dependent in those who have a genetic makeup that predisposes to dependence. This is a case of interaction between genes and environment.

"Indeed, in our study we found that higher alcohol consumption in humans was positively correlated with alcohol dependence. However, because different sets of genes seem to influence the level of alcohol consumption, as opposed to propensity for alcohol dependence, we are confronted with great variation in humans."

He explains that people with genes that predispose them to drink only moderate amounts of alcohol may still have the genetic predisposition to lose control over their drinking behavior, and perhaps become alcohol dependent. On the other hand, those with a tendency to drink larger amounts of alcohol may not have the genes that predispose them to become dependent.

The reasons for differences in alcohol intake between people are the subject of an immense amount of research. Both environmental and genetic factors are thought to contribute, but there is often a lack of discrimination between alcohol consumption in dependent and nondependent individuals. There is no clear reason to assume that the same genetic factors are responsible. In fact, say the team, "one can interpret some of the data collected with mice to show a dissociation between a propensity for high alcohol consumption and propensity for physical dependence."

They conclude, "The genetic factors that contribute to the full range of alcohol consumption versus alcohol dependence in humans are distinct."

In 2008, experts from the National Institute on Alcohol Abuse and Alcoholism in Maryland carried out a review of the work done so far on genes and alcohol. Dr. Francesca Ducci and colleagues write, "Alcoholism is a chronic relapsing disorder with an enormous societal impact. Understanding the genetic basis of alcoholism is crucial to characterize individuals' risk and to develop efficacious prevention and treatment strategies."

They found that genetic factors account for 40 to 60 percent of the variance between people in risk of alcoholism. The genes involved in susceptibility to alcoholism include both alcohol-specific genes and those that affect neuronal pathways to do with reward, behavioral control, and resilience to stress.

Major progress in gene identification has occurred in recent years, they write, but "the genetic determinants of alcoholism remain to be discovered." Nevertheless, a technological revolution has occurred, allowing genome-wide searches. Genomes can now be assessed at a level of detail that was previously inconceivable, they explain, and new technologies and different approaches "promise to increase our understanding of the mechanisms by which genetic variation alters molecular function and predisposes individuals to alcoholism and other diseases."

The experts conclude that, "Although the genetic bases of alcoholism remain largely unknown, there are reasons to think that more genes will be discovered in the future. Multiple and complementary approaches will be required to piece together the mosaic of causation."

This work demonstrates the value of linking animal studies with genome-wide screening in humans to produce valuable findings on alcoholism and other drinking patterns.

References

Tabakoff, B. et al. Genetical genomic determinants of alcohol consumption in rats and humans. *BMC Biology*, published online October 27, 2009.

Tabakoff, B. et al. The genomic determinants of alcohol preference in mice. *Mammalian Genome*, Vol. 19, May 2008, pp, 352–65.

Ducci, F. and Goldman, D. Genetic approaches to addiction: genes and alcohol. *Addiction*, Vol. 103, September 2008, pp. 1414–28.

Section 48.4

Genetic Research Leads to Advance in Treatment of Alcoholism

"The Future of Alcohol Addiction Treatment?" (http://www.medicine
.virginia.edu/clinical/departments/psychiatry/news/ondansetron) © 2011
by the Rector and the Board of Visitors of the University of Virginia.
Reprinted with permission. All rights reserved.

For the first time in alcohol addiction research—and a first in the entire field of addiction treatment—University of Virginia (UVA) investigators have successfully treated alcohol-dependent individuals with medication that is tailored specifically to match their genetic profile.

"Our findings suggest a new paradigm for the treatment of alcoholism, as well as a major breakthrough in individualized medicine for predetermined genotypes," says Bankole Johnson, MD, PhD, study leader and professor and chair of the UVA Department of Psychiatry and Neurobehavioral Sciences.

The study, published in the March 2011 issue of the *American Journal of Psychiatry* and available online, tested 283 genetically profiled alcoholics for the efficacy of ondansetron, a serotonin antagonist drug.

Previous research by UVA scientists has found that specified variations in the serotonin transporter gene, SLC6A4, play a significant role in influencing drinking intensity. Furthermore, past UVA research has identified ondansetron as a likely pharmaceutical target for serotonin-related genes.

Serotonin is a brain chemical that is involved in the regulation of pain perception, sleep, mood, and other psychological processes. Studies have shown that serotonin mediates the rewarding effects of alcohol.

In this latest study, UVA researchers randomized alcoholics by genotype (LL vs. Sx and TT vs. Gx) in a controlled, double-blind clinical trial. Subjects received either ondansetron or placebo for eleven weeks, and all received standard cognitive behavioral therapy. A majority of subjects were white males, and more than 65 percent of subjects completed the study in its entirety.

The study was funded by the National Institute on Alcohol Abuse and Alcoholism (NIAAA) of the National Institutes of Health (NIH).

Study findings show that ondansetron is indeed a promising therapeutic agent for the treatment of severe alcohol consumption among alcohol-dependent individuals with the predicted genetic marker—a marker that's responsible for the amount of pleasure certain people may perceive while drinking or may perceive as a craving when they stop drinking, Johnson explains.

"The treatment response among those who received ondansetron was remarkable," says Johnson. "What this tells us is that we have measurable evidence that personalized medicine is indeed a viable treatment for alcohol dependence."

The primary outcome tested by researchers involved ondansetron's effects on the severity of alcohol consumption in selected alcohol-dependent individuals. The study was confined to one secondary variable—the percentage of days abstinent, in order to provide clinicians additional efficacy information. Study findings demonstrated a predicted therapeutic response to ondansetron, which increased the percentage of days abstinent relative to placebo for predetermined genotypes.

For men, who comprised 73 percent of all subjects, high-risk drinking of alcohol is defined as consuming five or more drinks per drinking day. This high risk has been associated with such severe health consequences as accidental injuries, deaths from external sources, aggression (both victim and perpetrator of), as well as numerous medical, legal, and occupational problems.

For subjects with the LL/TT genotype, those treated with ondansetron, on average, fell below the high-risk drinking category, while those who received placebo remained in the high-risk category. In addition, these same genotype categories responded more positively to ondansetron, versus placebo, in increasing the days of abstinence.

The benefits of this type of personalized treatment approach are remarkably promising. Personalized medicine, or genome-based medicine, has the potential to give patients and their physicians the ability to make more informed treatment decisions.

"By being able to do genetic screening beforehand, clinicians can eliminate a great deal of the trial and error approach to prescribing medicine," Johnson says. "Personalized medicine allows them to better predict a successful treatment option, as well as reducing both premature medication changes and simultaneous multiple medication regimens."

Not all alcohol-dependent individuals are treated successfully with ondansetron.

"Although this treatment approach accounts for nearly one-third of patients with alcohol dependence, more research is needed to identify alcoholics with other genetic variations who will respond significantly to alternative medications," says Johnson. "Our findings, however, are a major step into the forefront of modern medicine."

Section 48.5

Genes Influence How Much People Smoke and Risk of Lung Cancer

Your deoxyribonucleic acid (DNA) influences how much you smoke and whether you will develop lung cancer or chronic obstructive pulmonary disease (COPD), according to an international team of researchers led by Washington University School of Medicine in St. Louis.

The study is the first large-scale effort to match genetics with smoking, lung cancer, and COPD combined. The investigators studied thirty-eight thousand smokers and found that two groups of gene variants on chromosome 15 influence risk for all three problems. Their findings appear in the journal *Public Library of Science (PLoS) Genetics*.

"We put together a consortium from around the world and analyzed DNA variants that we know cause biological changes in smokers," says the study's senior investigator Laura Jean Bierut, MD. "We were able to demonstrate that both of the variants affect the amount a person smokes. Then we showed that the same pattern of variants contributes to lung cancer and COPD."

Nicotine, the main, addictive ingredient in cigarettes, binds to nicotinic receptors in cells. Past genetic studies had implicated a section of chromosome 15 that includes important nicotinic receptor genes, and in this study, the investigators looked specifically at those genes (CHRNA5, CHRNA3, and CHRNB4). Various forms of the nicotinic receptor genes were associated with how much a person smoked, and not surprisingly, heavy smokers turned out to be at greatest risk for lung cancer and COPD.

430

Bierut, a professor of psychiatry and principal investigator of the Collaborative Genetic Study of Nicotine Dependence, and Nancy L. Saccone, PhD, assistant professor of genetics and lead author of the study, joined forces with geneticists who study addiction, lung cancer, and COPD as the Consortium for the Genetic Analysis of Smoking Phenotypes (CGASP). It is one of four consortia organized to study genetic data in smokers. All four groups have identified nicotinic receptor genes on chromosome 15 as important to smoking or lung disease.

"Previous studies have shown associations between gene variants and smoking," Saccone says. "The important finding from our analysis is that a new group of variants also is associated with smoking behavior, further highlighting this area as an important target for follow-up studies to better understand the mechanisms underlying those associations we observed."

The CGASP group took a different approach than the other groups. Scientists in the other groups simply surveyed the genome and looked for DNA regions that looked different in smokers. The CGASP study started with the hypothesis that cigarette smoking, lung cancer, and COPD are linked at the genetic level and concentrated in particular on nicotinic receptor genes. But the two different approaches yielded similar results, finding that DNA differences on chromosome 15, particularly in the CHRNA5 nicotine receptor gene, made significant contributions to nicotine addiction, lung cancer, and COPD.

Another difference between the various studies was that the CGASP group also looked at all three problems—nicotine addiction, lung cancer, and COPD—rather than just one.

"Demonstrating that all three diseases are related to smoking behavior does not prove that there is a direct, biological effect linking nicotine addiction to cancer and COPD, but you certainly can't rule it out," Bierut says. "It's really striking that this one gene is strongly driving addictive behavior and that it's also related to lung cancer and COPD."

The CHRNA5 gene functions both in the lung and in the brain. It is active in regions of the brain involved in addictive behavior.

"There's a reward center in the brain," Bierut says. "The center becomes activated with addiction, and the gene is clearly active in that brain region. But the gene also functions in the lung, meaning we need to ask the question of whether this gene is both driving the pathology of addiction in the brain while also working in the lung to contribute to COPD and cancer."

She says the gene variants identified by the CGASP consortium don't determine whether a person will smoke, but rather how much they will smoke, from light-smoking people who smoke fewer than ten cigarettes per day to heavy smokers who light up more than twenty times daily. And how much an individual smokes is one of the strongest contributors to lung cancer and COPD.

Depending on which gene variants a person has, that individual will tend to smoke different amounts. Bierut says people respond to nicotine differently, based in part on their genetic makeup, and then they adjust the amount they smoke according to nicotine's addictive effects.

And Saccone says as the researchers continue to study the connections between genes, smoking, lung cancer, and COPD, it will be important to pay close attention to the combined effects of small genetic variations.

"What we've identified in this study was detectable only after we accounted for the effects of other genetic variants in the same region of chromosome 15," she says. "I think this study illustrates that important effects can be obscured unless we move beyond separate analyses of single gene variants to joint analyses of multiple variants."

Section 48.6

Odds of Quitting Smoking Are Affected by Genetics

Excerpted from "Odds of Quitting Smoking Affected by Genetics," an NIH News Release, National Institutes of Health (www.nih.gov), May 30, 2012.

Genetics can help determine whether a person is likely to quit smoking on his or her own or need medication to improve the chances of success, according to research published in the May 30, 2012, issue of the *American Journal of Psychiatry*. Researchers say the study moves health care providers a step closer to one day providing more individualized treatment plans to help patients quit smoking.

The study was supported by multiple components of the National Institutes of Health, including the National Institute on Drug Abuse (NIDA), the National Human Genome Research Institute, the National Cancer Institute, and the Clinical and Translational Science Awards program, administered by the National Center for Advancing Translational Sciences.

"This study builds on our knowledge of genetic vulnerability to nicotine dependence, and will help us tailor smoking cessation strategies accordingly," said NIDA Director Nora D. Volkow, M.D. "It also highlights the potential value of genetic screening in helping to identify individuals early on and reduce their risk for tobacco addiction and its related negative health consequences."

Researchers focused on specific variations in a cluster of nicotinic receptor genes, CHRNA5-CHRNA3-CHRNB4, which prior studies have shown contribute to nicotine dependence and heavy smoking. Using data obtained from a previous study supported by the National Heart Lung and Blood Institute, researchers showed that individuals carrying the high-risk form of this gene cluster reported a two-year delay in the median quit age compared to those with the low-risk genes. This delay was attributable to a pattern of heavier smoking among those with the high-risk gene cluster. The researchers then conducted a clinical trial, which confirmed that persons with the high-risk genes were more likely to fail in their quit attempts compared to those with the low-risk genes when treated with placebo. However, medications approved for nicotine cessation (such as nicotine replacement therapies or bupropion) increased the likelihood of abstinence in the high-risk groups. Those with the highest risk had a threefold increase in their odds of being abstinent at the end of active treatment compared to placebo, indicating that these medications may be particularly beneficial for this population.

"We found that the effects of smoking cessation medications depend on a person's genes," said first author Li-Shiun Chen, M.D., of the Washington University School of Medicine, St. Louis. "If smokers have the risk genes, they don't quit easily on their own and will benefit greatly from the medications. If smokers don't have the risk genes, they are likely to quit successfully without the help of medications such as nicotine replacement or bupropion."

According to the Centers for Disease Control and Prevention External Web Site Policy, tobacco use is the single most preventable cause of disease, disability, and death in the United States. Smoking or exposure to secondhand smoke results in more than 440,000 preventable deaths each year—about one in five U.S. deaths overall. Another 8.6 million live with a serious illness caused by smoking. Despite these well-documented health costs, over 46 million U.S. adults continue to smoke cigarettes.

Chapter 49

Alzheimer Disease and Genetics

Chapter Contents

Section 49.1

Genes Related to Alzheimer Disease

Excerpted from "Alzheimer Disease," Genetics Home Reference
(http://ghr.nlm.nih.gov), December 2008. Revised by David A.
Cooke, M.D., FACP, May 2013.

What is Alzheimer disease?

Alzheimer disease is a degenerative disease of the brain that causes dementia, which is a gradual loss of memory, judgment, and ability to function. This disorder usually appears in people older than age sixty-five, but less common forms of the disease appear earlier in adulthood.

Memory loss is the most common sign of Alzheimer disease. Forgetfulness may be subtle at first, but the loss of memory worsens over time until it interferes with most aspects of daily living. Even in familiar settings, a person with Alzheimer disease may get lost or become confused. Routine tasks such as preparing meals, doing laundry, and performing other household chores can be challenging. Additionally, it may become difficult to recognize people and name objects. Affected people increasingly require help with dressing, eating, and personal care.

As the disorder progresses, some people with Alzheimer disease experience personality and behavioral changes and have trouble interacting in a socially appropriate manner. Other common symptoms include agitation, restlessness, withdrawal, and loss of language skills. People with this disease usually require total care during the advanced stages of the disease. Affected individuals usually survive eight to ten years after the appearance of symptoms, but the course of the disease can range from one to twenty-five years. Death usually results from pneumonia, malnutrition, or general body wasting (inanition).

Alzheimer disease can be classified as early-onset or late-onset. The signs and symptoms of the early-onset form appear before age sixty-five, while the late-onset form appears after age sixty-five. The early-onset form is much less common than the late-onset form, accounting for less than 5 percent of all cases of Alzheimer disease.

How common is Alzheimer disease?

Alzheimer disease currently affects an estimated 2.4 million to 4.5 million Americans. Because the risk of developing Alzheimer disease increases with age and more people are living longer, the number of people with this disease is expected to increase significantly in coming decades.

What genes are related to Alzheimer disease?

Most cases of early-onset Alzheimer disease are caused by gene mutations that can be passed from parent to child. Researchers have found that this form of the disorder can result from mutations in one of three genes: APP, PSEN1, or PSEN2. When any of these genes is altered, large amounts of a toxic protein fragment called amyloid beta peptide are produced in the brain. This peptide can build up in the brain to form clumps called amyloid plaques, which are characteristic of Alzheimer disease. A buildup of toxic amyloid beta peptide and amyloid plaques may lead to the death of nerve cells and the progressive signs and symptoms of this disorder.

Some evidence indicates that people with Down syndrome have an increased risk of developing Alzheimer disease. Down syndrome, a condition characterized by intellectual disability and other health problems, occurs when a person is born with an extra copy of chromosome 21 in each cell. As a result, people with Down syndrome have three copies of many genes in each cell, including the APP gene, instead of the usual two copies. Although the connection between Down syndrome and Alzheimer disease is unclear, the production of excess amyloid beta peptide in cells may account for the increased risk. People with Down syndrome account for less than 1 percent of all cases of Alzheimer disease.

The causes of late-onset Alzheimer disease are less clear, and most cases are probably not caused by a single gene abnormality. The late-onset form does not clearly run in families, although clusters of cases have been reported in some families. This disorder is probably related to variations in one or more genes in combination with lifestyle and environmental factors. A gene called APOE has been studied extensively as a risk factor for the disease. In particular, a variant of this gene called the e4 allele seems to increase an individual's risk for developing late-onset Alzheimer disease. Researchers are investigating many additional genes that may play a role in Alzheimer disease risk.

How do people inherit Alzheimer disease?

The early-onset form of Alzheimer disease is inherited in an autosomal dominant pattern, which means one copy of the altered gene in each cell is sufficient to cause the disorder. In most cases, an affected person inherits the altered gene from one affected parent.

The inheritance pattern of late-onset Alzheimer disease is uncertain. People who inherit one copy of the APOE e4 allele have an increased chance of developing the disease; those who inherit two copies of the allele are at even greater risk. It is important to note that people with the APOE e4 allele inherit an increased risk of developing Alzheimer disease, not the disease itself. Not all people with Alzheimer disease have the e4 allele, and most people who have the e4 allele will not develop the disease.

Section 49.2

Gene Mutation May Triple Alzheimer Risk

A rare mutation in a gene called TREM2 appears to nearly triple the risk for Alzheimer disease in adults, a new study finds.

This gene is involved in immune and inflammatory responses, and may be yet another piece of the mystery of the causes of Alzheimer disease and a target for treatment, the researchers added.

"We found a mutation that confers a large risk for Alzheimer's disease," said lead researcher Dr. Kari Stefansson, the CEO of deCODE Genetics based in Reykjavik, Iceland.

Although only 1.2 percent of the population has the TREM2 mutation, when comparing adults aged eighty-five and older with and without it, those who do have it are almost seven times more likely to have Alzheimer disease, he said.

Of course, having this mutation doesn't mean that one is destined to develop Alzheimer disease. Alzheimer is a complex disease and a person probably needs to have several risk factors that combine to produce the condition, Stefansson said.

"This has implications for treatment," he said. The mutation might be a target for new drugs that blunt the mutation's action, he said.

The report was published in the November 14, 2012, online edition of the *New England Journal of Medicine.*

An Alzheimer expert praised the new study.

"This shows the value of basic research," said William Thies, chief medical and scientific officer at the Alzheimer's Association. "This kind of science is very important, and can accelerate our finding better therapies for Alzheimer disease."

Thies noted this finding doesn't mean people should run out and be tested for this mutation. The mutation might, in the future, be important for treatments, but that's a long way off, he said.

The need to develop treatments for Alzheimer disease is a pressing issue, he added.

"The imperative for finding new therapies is obvious," Thies said. "When we get to fifteen or sixteen million people with the disease by the middle of the century, which is what the demographics would suggest, we can't take care of that many people and the dislocation in society is just going to be a mess."

For the study, Stefansson's group obtained gene sequences from more than 2,200 Icelanders. The researchers looked for gene variants in those with and without Alzheimer disease.

To check their results, the researchers looked at other populations in the United States, Norway, the Netherlands and Germany, where they confirmed their findings.

Another expert noted that the inflammation finding is important.

"Inflammation is certainly part of the conventional wisdom in the pathogenesis of Alzheimer's," said Dr. Sam Gandy, associate director of the Mount Sinai Alzheimer's Disease Research Center in New York City.

What this study says is that inflammation is so important that imbalance in the inflammatory component can affect the risk for disease, he said.

"We don't have a new drug today, but TREM2 highlights potentially druggable steps in the pathogenesis of Alzheimer's that we might have never ever even studied were it not for this genetic information," Gandy said.

Another expert, Greg Cole, a neuroscientist at the Greater Los Angeles VA Healthcare System and associate director of the Alzheimer's

Disease Research Center at the UCLA David Geffen School of Medicine, weighed in on the findings.

Cole said that "together with other discoveries of genetic variants in genes expressed in the same population of immune cells, this study adds to the now compelling data for a causal role for the brain's innate immune cells in the development of Alzheimer's disease, the most common dementia."

Understanding the role of genetic mutations "should help researchers devise drugs that achieve the opposite effect and modulate innate immune system function to reduce the risk," he said.

Another study in the same journal issue came to the same conclusion.

A team lead by John Hardy, at the University College London Institute of Neurology, and Andrew Singleton, at the U.S. National Institute on Aging (NIA), also found that the TREM2 mutation increased the risk for Alzheimer's disease.

"We have hypothesized for many years that a rare genetic variant can confer moderate risk for disease," Singleton said in an NIA statement. "These are the first studies to identify such a variant related to Alzheimer's disease."

Section 49.3

Additional Genes Linked to Alzheimer Risk

"Studies Find Possible New Genetic Risk Factors for Alzheimer's Disease," an NIH News Release, National Institutes of Health (www.nih.gov), April 4, 2011.

Scientists have confirmed one gene variant and have identified several others that may be risk factors for late-onset Alzheimer disease, the most common form of the disorder. In the largest genome-wide association study, or GWAS, ever conducted in Alzheimer research, investigators studied deoxyribonucleic acid (DNA) samples from more than fifty-six thousand study participants and analyzed shared data sets to detect gene variations that may have subtle effects on the risk for developing Alzheimer. The National Institutes of Health funded the study, which appeared April 3, 2011, in the online issue of *Nature Genetics*.

"New technologies are allowing us to look at subtle genetic differences among large groups of study participants. By comparing people diagnosed with Alzheimer with people free of disease symptoms, researchers are now able to discern elusive genetic factors that may contribute to risk of developing this very devastating disease," said Richard J. Hodes, M.D., director of the National Institute on Aging (NIA). "We are entering an exciting period of discoveries in genetics that may provide new insights about novel disease pathways that can be explored for development of therapies."

The Alzheimer's Disease Genetics Consortium (ADGC), a collaborative body established and funded by the NIA, part of the National Institutes of Health (NIH), coordinated the study. The research reported involved investigators at universities and research centers across the country. Datasets were funded in part by the NIA, the National Institute of Mental Health, the National Institute of Neurological Disorders and Stroke, and the National Center for Research Resources, all part of the NIH. The Alzheimer's Association, U.S. Department of Veterans Affairs, Wellcome Trust, Howard Hughes Medical Institute, and the Canadian

441

Institute of Health Research also lent support. Gerard Schellenberg, Ph.D., University of Pennsylvania School of Medicine, Philadelphia, directs the ADGC, which also received Recovery Act funds in 2009.

Until recently, only one gene variant, Apolipoprotein E-e4 (APOE-e4), had been confirmed as a significant risk factor gene for the common form of late-onset Alzheimer disease, which typically occurs after age sixty. In 2009 and 2010, however, researchers confirmed additional gene variants of CR1, CLU and PICALM as possible risk factors for late-onset Alzheimer. This newest GWAS confirms that a fifth gene variant, BIN 1, affects development of late-onset Alzheimer. It also identified genetic variants significant for Alzheimer at EPHA 1, MS4A, CD2AP, and CD33. The genes identified by this study may implicate pathways involved in inflammation, movement of proteins within cells, and lipid transport as being important in the disease process.

In addition, a second paper appearing online in the journal presented GWAS findings for Alzheimer by another scientific team. The United Kingdom–based group, led by Julie Williams, Ph.D., Cardiff University School of Medicine, Wales, found the same genes as risk factors and identified a gene variant ABCA7 as an additional gene of interest. Components of the NIH involved in or supporting the study included the NIA, the National Heart, Lung and Blood Institute, and the National Institute of Diabetes and Digestive and Kidney Diseases. Some private support came through the independent Foundation for the National Institutes of Health.

"Researchers conducting GWAS are looking for genetic variations that may have a smaller effect but still play a role in the disease," said Schellenberg. "Our findings bring us one step closer to a fuller understanding of the genetic basis of this complex disease, although more study is needed to determine the role these genetic factors may play in the onset and progression of Alzheimer's."

Schellenberg said the study was made possible by the research infrastructures established and funded by the NIA, including twenty-nine Alzheimer's Disease Centers, the National Alzheimer's Coordinating Center, the Genetics of Alzheimer's Disease Data Storage Site, the Late-onset Alzheimer's Disease Family Study, and the National Cell Repository for Alzheimer's Disease. They collect, store, and make available to qualified researchers DNA samples, datasets containing biomedical and demographic information about participants, and genetic analysis data.

Chapter 50

Asthma and Genetics

Chapter Contents

Section 50.1

Basic Facts about Genes and Asthma

Excerpted from "Asthma and Genetics,"
© 2009 Utah Department of Health Asthma Program
(www.health.utah.gov/asthma). Reprinted with permission.

Health problems that run in your family can increase your chances of developing the problem too. This is because families share their genetics, environment, and behaviors. These can be passed down in families and affect your health. But by knowing your past, you can make choices to protect your future.

Asthma is a complex disease. We don't know for certain what causes asthma, but studies have shown that both genetics and the environment can affect your risk of getting asthma.

Is there a genetic component to asthma?

Yes. Asthma can run in families. Since the 1920s studies done have shown that family history is a significant risk factor for asthma. There are many genes that may increase your risk of getting asthma.

Is there an environmental component to asthma?

Yes. The environment in which you live, work, and play can affect your risk of developing asthma.

Genomics—the study of how your genes interact with the environment—may hold the key to understanding why some people get asthma while others don't.

If I have a family history of asthma, does that mean I will get asthma, too?

Having a family history of asthma may increase your risk or your family members' risk of also getting asthma.

If you have a parent, sibling, or child with asthma you have an increased risk of getting asthma.

If both your parents have asthma, you have a greater risk of getting asthma than if only one parent had asthma.

Your family health history can help you and your doctor understand what your risk may be for asthma. It can also help you learn what your triggers may be and medications that may help you control your asthma.

Remember though, that just because asthma runs in your family, it doesn't mean you are destined to get it too.

If I don't have a family history of asthma, does that mean I won't get it?

No. You can still get asthma even if no one else in your family has it. Although a person with a family history of asthma has an increased risk of getting asthma, not everyone who is diagnosed with asthma has a family history of asthma.

Your genetics and environment can affect your risk of getting asthma. Many environmental factors have been thought to be risk factors in the development and exacerbation of asthma.

What should I do if asthma runs in my family?

Talk to your doctor about your family history and any allergy or breathing problems you have. This may help your doctor diagnose your asthma earlier, identify your triggers, and help you control your asthma.

Protect your lungs. Don't use tobacco and limit your exposure to secondhand smoke.

Be aware of common asthma triggers, like chemicals, pests, pollen, smoke, mold, air quality, pets, and exercise.

Learn what the signs and symptoms of asthma are. They include wheezing, coughing, chest tightness, and stuffy nose.

Section 50.2

New Research on the Genetics of Asthma

Gene Variant Increases Risk of Asthma

A tiny variation in a gene known as CHI3L1 increases susceptibility to asthma, bronchial hyperresponsiveness, and decline in lung function, researchers reported online in the *New England Journal of Medicine*. (The printed version appeared in the April 17 issue). The gene variant causes increased blood levels of YKL-40, a biomarker for asthma. A slightly different version of the genetic variation lowers YKL-40 levels and protects against asthma.

Although the original discovery came from a study of a genetically isolated population, the Hutterites of South Dakota, the researchers were able to confirm the same connections between the CHI3L1 variations, YKL-40 levels, and asthma susceptibility in three genetically diverse Caucasian populations from Chicago; Madison, Wisconsin; and Freiberg, Germany.

This gene, "may have important implications in the early identification of, susceptibility to, and prevention and treatment of asthma," said Elizabeth G. Nabel, MD, director, the National Heart, Lung, and Blood Institute.

"This is exciting because it connects asthma susceptibility to a whole new pathway at the protein and the genetic levels," said study author Carole Ober, professor of human genetics at the University of Chicago Medical Center. "There is a good deal more we need to find out about this connection, but now we know where to look."

"This is also the most significant genetic discovery based on our years of gathering data on asthma in the Hutterites," Ober added. "This is a group with enormous potential to advance our understanding of the genetic underpinnings of disease. We now have a remarkable collection of data, which we expect will lead us to many more insights."

Ober and colleagues at the University of Chicago had long been searching for genetic factors that could influence the risk of common diseases, such as asthma. To simplify this quest, they have focused since 1994 on the Hutterites, a genetically isolated U.S. religious community descended from about 90 people. The Hutterites came to the United States in 1874 and settled in small communal farming colonies in what is now South Dakota. Today Hutterite communities are present in the Dakotas, Minnesota, Montana, Washington, and Canada.

They provide an ideal community for genetic studies because they are all members of a large pedigree that is known back to the 1700s and they live communally, sharing resources and maintaining a traditional lifestyle. "They eat the same food, live off the same allowance and have the same education," said Ober, who has been working with them since 1979. They have similar, but not identical genomes. "So the genes that make a difference are easier to detect."

In 1996 and 1997, Ober's team gathered clinical data about asthma from more than seven hundred members of the Hutterite communities, and stored blood samples that were recently used to measure YKL-40 levels. About 11 percent of Hutterites had asthma and another 12 percent had bronchial hyperresponsiveness.

The genetic studies took on a sharper focus in 2007, when a team led by Geoffrey Chupp of Yale University showed that, on average, patients with asthma had higher levels of the protein YKL-40 in their blood than people without asthma, and that those with more severe asthma had even higher levels.

YKL-40, a natural suspect as a cause of asthma, belongs to a family of enzymes called chitinases. These enzymes are part of the innate immune system's response to chitin, a common biologic polymer found especially in insects—including dust mites and cockroaches, which have been associated with asthma—as well as in certain disease-causing organisms, including fungi and parasitic worms. The chitinases help break down chitin. They also trigger inflammation, which is a central component of asthma.

Working with Chupp's laboratory, Ober found that mean YKL-40 levels were also increased among Hutterites with asthma or hyperresponsive airways. Ober's group also showed that these elevated YKL-40 levels were handed down from generation to generation, indicating that differences between individuals were due nearly entirely to genetic differences.

So they began looking for variations in the CHI3L1 gene on chromosome 1 that codes for YKL-40. They found one very slight genetic difference between those with asthma and those without. Hutterites with asthma were more likely to have a small but consistent variation in one part of the gene, called a promoter, which regulates when the gene is expressed.

That variation changes one DNA base pair, out of the three billion in the human genome, at a location in the CHI3L1gene known as -131C/G. Those with asthma were more likely to have a cytosine (C), rather than guanine (G) at this location.

Those inheriting two copies of a C at -131 had higher YKL-40 levels and an asthma prevalence of 0.20. Those with CG had intermediate YKL-40 levels and an asthma prevalence of 0.12. Those with GG had the lowest YKL-40 levels and a prevalence of only 0.08, less than half that of the CC allele.

To see if these results could be generalized from the genetically isolated Hutterite population to a more diverse group, the researchers tested the same variations in the CHI3L1 gene in 178 Caucasian children enrolled in prospective birth cohort, known as COAST, a collaboration led by Robert Lemanske of the University of Wisconsin at Madison.

They also looked for correlations between asthma and SNP -131C/G in two clinical samples, one from the Children's University Hospital in Freiberg, Germany (344 children with asthma and 294 without), and one from the asthma clinics at the University of Chicago Medical Center (99 children and adults with asthma and 197 without).

In the two clinical samples, those with the CC configuration at position 131 were more likely to have asthma, with CG intermediate and GG the lowest risk of the disease. In the COAST cohort, many subject were still too young to have developed asthma, but the genetic pattern was closely associated with YKL-40 levels, and this association was already present at birth.

The authors suspect that the change from C to G at this site reduces expression of the gene, resulting in lower levels of YKL-40 and protection from asthma.

Although variation in CHI3L1 appears to be one of the most significant genetic triggers yet discovered for susceptibility to asthma, it is far from the sole cause of the disease, the researchers caution. In the Hutterites, it explains 9.4 percent of the variance in YKL-40 levels, suggesting that additional genetic variants also influence these levels. Finding those variations "could identify additional genes," they add, "with significant impact on asthma risk and lung function."

"This evolutionarily ancient pathway involving the innate immune system plays a surprisingly important role in asthma pathogenesis," said Ober, "and a single genetic variant in the CHI3L1 gene may account for most of this risk."

This could have a significant impact on drug development, she added. "For some people, if you block YKL-40 you might dramatically reduce the severity of the disease. Knowing the genotype at SNP -131C might identify those who most likely to benefit from such a treatment."

Asthma is a chronic, treatable disease that causes narrowing of the airways, making breathing difficult at times. More than 22 million people in the United States have asthma, including 6.5 million children under age eighteen, according to the Centers for Disease Control and Prevention (CDC). The disease generates annual health care costs estimated at $14 billion.

National Asthma Genetics Consortium Releases First Results

A new national collaboration of asthma genetics researchers has revealed a novel gene associated with the disease in African Americans, according to a new scientific report.

By pooling data from nine independent research groups looking for genes associated with asthma, the newly created EVE Consortium identified a novel gene association specific to populations of African descent. In addition, the new study confirmed the significance of four gene associations recently reported by a European asthma genetics study.

The findings, published in *Nature Genetics*, are a promising first step for a new national scientific effort to hunt for the genetic roots of asthma.

"We now have a really good handle on at least five genes that anyone would be comfortable saying are asthma risk loci," said Carole Ober, PhD, co-chair of the EVE Consortium, senior author of the study, and Blum-Riese Professor of human genetics and obstetrics/gynecology at the University of Chicago. "I think it's an exciting time in asthma genetics."

"Asthma rates have been on the rise in recent years, with the greatest rise among African Americans," said Susan B. Shurin, M.D., acting director of the National Heart, Lung, and Blood Institute (NHLBI) of the National Institutes of Health, which co-funded the study. "Understanding these genetic links is an important first step towards our goal of relieving the increased burden of asthma in this population."

Genome-wide association studies, or GWAS, are a popular method used by geneticists to find genetic variants associated with elevated risk for a particular disease. Genetic data from a group of patients with the target disease are compared to data from a control group without the disease, and researchers look for variants that appear significantly more often in the disease group.

But the ability, or power, of GWAS to find disease-associated variants is dependent on the number of participants enrolled in a study. To find variants involved in complex diseases, thousands of participants may be necessary—a logistical and financial demand often beyond the capacity of an individual research team.

"It has become clear to geneticists studying nearly every common disease that GWAS are often under-powered, and unless you pull together many researchers doing the same thing you're just not going to have the power to find genes," said Dan Nicolae, PhD, associate professor of medicine, statistics, and human genetics at University of Chicago, co-chair of the consortium and another senior author of the study. "That was the motivation for nine groups of investigators coming together to form EVE."

Spurred by support from the NHLBI and the National Institutes of Health, research groups from the nine institutions discussed pooling their GWAS data to create a larger, shared dataset. But it wasn't until they received a $5.6 million grant from the American Recovery and Reinvestment Act of 2009 that the EVE Consortium could officially form and hire the necessary personnel to execute the collaboration.

"It would never have been possible without the grant, this was a huge amount of work," said Nicolae, "The key was the ARRA funding that allowed us to move it faster."

In addition to increased power to find variants associated with asthma risk, the EVE dataset comprised a more ethnically diverse population than similar efforts in other countries by including European Americans, African Americans/African Caribbeans, and Latinos.

"We believe that this heterogeneity is important," Ober said. "There are differences in asthma prevalence in these three groups, so it's important to understand whether these are caused by environmental exposures or by differences in genetic risk factors."

The diverse sample enabled the researchers to discover a novel genetic association with asthma observed exclusively in African Americans and African Caribbeans. The polymorphism, located in a gene called PYHIN1, was not present in European Americans and may be the first asthma susceptibility gene variant specific to populations of African descent.

Four more gene variants were found significant for asthma risk by the meta-analysis: the 17q21 locus, and IL1RL1, TSLP, and IL33 genes. All four of these sites were concurrently identified in a separate dataset by the GABRIEL Study of more than forty thousand European asthma cases published last year in the *New England Journal of Medicine*. Confirming these associations in the more diverse EVE population offers additional evidence that the gene variants are significant across ethnicities, the researchers reported.

"We were able to show that almost all of the genes other than PYHIN1 are trans-ethnic and important in all of the groups," Ober said.

The Nature Genetics study is only the first fruit of the EVE Consortium mission to understand the genetics of asthma. A deeper meta-analysis looking at a longer list of gene variants is currently underway, and individual groups within the consortium are using the pooled dataset to answer additional questions. Topics of interest include gene-environment interactions, genetic associations with asthma-associated phenotypes such as allergies and lung function, and the role of tissue-specific gene expression.

"What you see here in this paper is only the beginning," Nicolae said. "The foundation was to make people work together, share the data, and share research ideas, and that will generate a lot of research down the road."

The paper, "Meta-analysis of genome-wide association studies of asthma in ethnically diverse North American populations" by Dara Torgerson et al., was published online July 31, 2011, by *Nature Genetics*.

In addition to Ober and Nicolae, lead investigators of groups participating in the consortium include W. James Gauderman and Frank D. Gilliand of University of Southern California; Eugene R. Bleecker and Deborah A. Meyers of Wake Forest University; Benjamin A. Raby and Scott T. Weiss of Harvard Medical School; Stephanie J. London of the National Institute of Environmental Health Sciences; Esteban G. Burchard of University of California, San Francisco; Fernando D. Martinez of University of Arizona; L. Keoki Williams of Henry Ford Health System; and Kathleen C. Barnes of Johns Hopkins University. For a complete list of authors and funding agencies, see *Nature Genetics* (DOI: 10.1038/ng.888).

Chapter 51

Cancer and Genetics

Chapter Contents

Section 51.1

Breast Cancer and Heredity

Excerpted from "Learning about Breast Cancer,"
National Human Genome Research Institute (www.genome.gov),
February 27, 2012.

What do we know about heredity and breast cancer?

Breast cancer is a common disease. Each year, approximately two hundred thousand women in the United States are diagnosed with breast cancer, and one in nine American women will develop breast cancer in her lifetime. But hereditary breast cancer—caused by a mutant gene passed from parents to their children—is rare. Estimates of the incidence of hereditary breast cancer range from between 5 to 10 percent to as many as 27 percent of all breast cancers.

In 1994, the first gene associated with breast cancer—BRCA1 (for BReast CAncer1)—was identified on chromosome 17. A year later, a second gene associated with breast cancer—BRCA2—was discovered on chromosome 13. When individuals carry a mutated form of either BRCA1 or BRCA2, they have an increased risk of developing breast or ovarian cancer at some point in their lives. Children of parents with a BRCA1 or BRCA2 mutation have a 50 percent chance of inheriting the gene mutation.

What do we know about hereditary breast cancer in Ashkenazi Jews?

In 1995 and 1996, studies of deoxyribonucleic acid (DNA) samples revealed that Ashkenazi (Eastern European) Jews are ten times more likely to have mutations in BRCA1 and BRCA 2 genes than the general population. Approximately 2.65 percent of the Ashkenazi Jewish population has a mutation in these genes, while only 0.2 percent of the general population carries these mutations.

Further research showed that three specific mutations in these genes accounted for 90 percent of the BRCA1 and BRCA2 variants within this ethnic group. This contrasts with hundreds of unique mutations of these two genes within the general population. However, despite the relatively high prevalence of these genetic mutations in Ashkenazi Jews, only 7 percent of breast cancers in Ashkenazi women are caused by alterations in BRCA1 and BRCA2.

What other genes may cause hereditary breast cancer?

Not all hereditary breast cancers are caused by BRCA1 and BRCA2. In fact, researchers now believe that at least half of hereditary breast cancers are not linked to these genes. Scientists also now think that these remaining cases of hereditary breast cancer are not caused by another single, unidentified gene, but rather by many genes, each accounting for a small fraction of breast cancers.

Is there a test for hereditary breast cancer?

Hereditary breast cancer is suspected when there is a strong family history of breast cancer: occurrences of the disease in at least three first- or second-degree relatives (sisters, mothers, aunts). Currently the only tests available are DNA tests to determine whether an individual in such a high-risk family has a genetic mutation in the BRCA1 or BRCA2 genes.

When someone with a family history of breast cancer has been tested and found to have an altered BRCA1 or BRCA2 gene, the family is said to have a "known mutation." Positive test results only provide information about the risk of developing breast cancer. The test cannot tell a person whether or when cancer might develop. Many, but not all, women and some men who inherit an altered gene will develop breast cancer. Both men and women who inherit an altered gene, whether or not they develop cancer themselves, can pass the alteration on to their sons and daughters.

But even if the test is negative, the individual may still have a predisposition to hereditary breast cancer. Currently available technique can't identify all cancer-predisposing mutations in the BRCA1 and BRCA2 genes. Or, an individual may have inherited a mutation caused by other genes. And, because most cases of breast cancer are not hereditary, individuals may develop breast cancer whether or not a genetic mutation is present.

How do I decide whether to be tested?

Given the limitations of testing for hereditary breast cancer, should an individual at high risk get tested? Genetic counselors can help individuals and families make decisions regarding testing.

For those who do test positive for the BRCA1 or BRCA2 gene, surveillance (mammography and clinical breast exams) can help detect the disease at an early stage. A woman who tests positive can also consider taking the drug tamoxifen, which has been found to reduce the risk of developing breast cancer by almost 50 percent in women at high risk. Clinical trials are now under way to determine whether another drug, raloxifene, is also effective in preventing breast cancer.

Section 51.2

Colon Cancer and Heredity

Excerpted from "Learning about Colon Cancer," March 22, 2012, and "Study Shows Colon and Rectal Tumors Constitute a Single Type of Cancer," July 18, 2012, National Human Genome Research Institute (www.genome.gov).

Learning about Colon Cancer

What do we know about heredity and colon cancer?

Colon cancer, a malignant tumor of the large intestine, affects both men and women. In the United States, approximately 160,000 new cases of colorectal cancer are diagnosed each year.

The majority of colon cancer cases are sporadic, which means a genetic mutation may happen in that individual person. However, approximately 5 percent of individuals with colon cancer have a hereditary form, which means that they have inherited a mutation from one of their parents that causes the disease. In those families, the chance of developing colon cancer is significantly higher than in the average person. These hereditary cancers typically occur at an earlier age than sporadic (noninherited) cases of colon cancer. The risk of inheriting these mutated genes from an affected parent is 50 percent for both males and females.

Scientists have discovered several genes contributing to a susceptibility to two types of colon cancer:

- **FAP (familial adenomatous polyposis):** So far, only one gene has been discovered that leads to FAP: the APC gene, located on human chromosome 5. However, over three hundred different mutations have been identified in this APC gene. Individuals with this syndrome develop many polyps in their colon. People who inherit mutations in this gene have a nearly 100 percent chance of developing colon cancer by age forty.

- **HNPCC (hereditary nonpolyposis colon cancer) also called Lynch Syndrome:** Individuals with an HNPCC gene mutation have an estimated 80 percent lifetime risk of developing colon or rectal cancer. However, these cancers account for only 3 to 5 percent of all colorectal cancers. So far, five HNPCC genes have been discovered:
  - MSH2 on chromosome 2
  - MLH1 on chromosome 3
  - PMS2 on chromosome 7
  - MSH6 on chromosome 2
  - PMS1 on chromosome 2

Mutations in MSH2 and MLH1 are the most common mutations that cause HNPCC. A mutation in PMS1 was originally reported in a single family with HNPCC, however, this mutation was not found in all members of the family who had developed the disease. For this reason, the role of PMS1 in HNPCC is currently being questioned.

The genes that cause HNPCC and FAP were relatively easy to discover because they exert strong effects. Other genes that cause susceptibility to colon cancer are harder to discover because the cancers are caused by a number of genes, each of which individually exerts a weak effect.

Is there a test for hereditary colon cancer?

Gene testing can identify individuals who carry the more common gene mutations associated with FAP or HPNCC, such as those listed above. However, these tests may not identify all gene mutations that cause FAP or HNPCC. In some families, additional mutations may be present that cause the FAP or HNPCC, which cannot be detected by the commonly used gene tests.

The test for FAP syndrome involves examining deoxyribonucleic acid (DNA) in blood cells called lymphocytes (white blood cells), looking for mutations in the APC gene. No treatment to reduce cancer risk is currently available for people with APC mutations that are associated with FAP. But for those who test positive, frequent surveillance can detect the cancer at an early, more treatable stage. Because of the early age at which this syndrome appears, the test may be offered to children under the age of eighteen if they have a parent known to carry the mutated APC gene.

Researchers hope that an easier test, which is currently experimental, will become available for common use in three to five years. This new test looks for cancer cells with the APC mutation in a stool sample.

Genetic testing for HNPCC involves looking for mutations in four of the five genes identified that are associated with HNPCC—MLH1, MSH2, MSH6, and PMS2.

Individuals in families at high risk of genetic predisposition may consider testing. Genetic counselors can help individuals make decisions regarding testing.

New Study Shows Colon and Rectal Tumors Constitute a Single Type of Cancer

The pattern of genomic alterations in colon and rectal tissues is the same regardless of anatomic location or origin within the colon or the rectum, leading researchers to conclude that these two cancer types can be grouped as one, according to The Cancer Genome Atlas (TCGA) project's large-scale study of colon and rectal cancer tissue specimens.

In multiple types of genomic analyses, colon and rectal cancer results were nearly indistinguishable. Initially, the TCGA Research Network studied colon tumors as distinct from rectal tumors.

"This finding of the true genetic nature of colon and rectal cancers is an important achievement in our quest to understand the foundations of this disease," said National Institutes of Health (NIH) director Francis S. Collins, M.D., Ph.D. "The data and knowledge gained here have the potential to change the way we diagnose and treat certain cancers."

The study also found several of the recurrent genetic errors that contribute to colorectal cancer. The study, funded by the National Cancer Institute (NCI) and the National Human Genome Research Institute (NHGRI), both parts of the National Institutes of Health, was published online in the July 19, 2012, issue of the journal *Nature*.

There is a known negative association between aggressiveness of colorectal tumors and the phenomenon of hypermutation, in which the rate of genetic mutation is abnormally high because normal deoxyribonucleic acid (DNA) repair mechanisms are disrupted. In this study, 16 percent of the specimens were found to be hypermutated. Three-fourths of these cases exhibited microsatellite instability (MSI), which often is an indicator for better prognosis. Microsatellites are repetitive sections of DNA in the genome. If mutations occur in the genes responsible for maintaining those regions of the genome, the microsatellites may become longer or shorter; this is called MSI.

NCI estimates that more than 143,000 people in the United States will be diagnosed with colorectal cancer and that 51,500 are likely to die from the disease in 2012. Colorectal cancer is the fourth most common cancer in men, after non-melanoma skin, prostate, and lung cancer. It is also the fourth most common cancer in women, after non-melanoma skin, breast, and lung cancer.

The researchers observed that in the 224 colorectal cancer specimens examined, twenty-four genes were mutated in a significant number of cases. In addition to genes found through prior research efforts (e.g., APC, ARID1A, FAM123B/WTX, TP53, SMAD4, PIK3CA, and KRAS), the scientists identified other genes (ARID1A, SOX9, and FAM123B/WTX) as potential drivers of this cancer when mutated. It is only through a study of this scale that these three genes could be implicated in this disease.

"While it may take years to translate this foundational genetic data on colorectal cancers into new therapeutic strategies and surveillance methods, this genetic information unquestionably will be the springboard for determining what will be useful clinically against colorectal cancers," said Harold E. Varmus, M.D., NCI director.

The research network also identified the genes ERBB2 and IGF2 as mutated or overexpressed in colorectal cancer and as potential drug targets. These genes are involved in regulating cell proliferation and were observed to be frequently overexpressed in colorectal tumors. This finding points to a potential drug therapy strategy in which inhibition of the products of these genes would slow progression of the cancer.

A key part of this study was the analysis of signaling pathways. Signaling pathways control gene activity during cell development and regulate the interactions between cells as they form organs or tissues. Among other findings, the TCGA Research Network identified new mutations in a particular signaling cascade called the WNT pathway. According to the researchers, this finding will improve development of WNT signaling inhibitors, which show initial promise as a class of drugs that could benefit colorectal cancer patients.

In addition to examining the WNT pathway, the investigators also identified RTK/RAS and AKT-PI3K as pathways that are altered in a substantial set of colorectal tumors, which may show promise for targeting therapies for colorectal cancer. Because of these findings, drug developers may now be able to narrow their scope of investigation with an expectation of producing more focused therapeutic approaches, noted the researchers.

"It takes a critical group of researchers to conduct research at this scale and of this quality," said Eric. D. Green, M.D., Ph.D., NHGRI director. "This study is among the most comprehensive of its kind to date and vividly illustrates how TCGA data sets can shed new light on fundamental properties of human cancers."

Section 51.3

New Lung Cancer Gene Found

"New Lung Cancer Gene Found: Cancer Biologists Identify a Driving Force Behind the Spread of an Aggressive Type of Lung Cancer," by Anne Trafton, *MIT News*, July 19, 2011. Reprinted with permission of *MIT News* (http://web.mit.edu/newsoffice/).

A major challenge for cancer biologists is figuring out which among the hundreds of genetic mutations found in a cancer cell are most important for driving the cancer's spread.

Using a new technique called whole-genome profiling, Massachusetts Institute of Technology (MIT) scientists have now pinpointed a gene that appears to drive progression of small cell lung cancer, an aggressive form of lung cancer accounting for about 15 percent of lung cancer cases.

The gene, which the researchers found overexpressed in both mouse and human lung tumors, could lead to new drug targets, says Alison Dooley, a recent PhD recipient in the lab of Tyler Jacks, director of MIT's David H. Koch Institute for Integrative Cancer Research. Dooley is the lead author of a paper describing the finding in the July 15, 2011, issue of *Genes and Development*.

Small cell lung cancer kills about 95 percent of patients within five years of diagnosis; scientists do not yet have a good understanding of which genes control it. Dooley and her colleagues studied the disease's progression using a strain of mice, developed in the laboratory of Anton Berns at the Netherlands Cancer Institute, that deletes two key tumor-suppressor genes, p53 and Rb.

"The mouse model recapitulates what is seen in human disease. It develops very aggressive lung tumors, which metastasize to sites where metastases are often seen in humans," such as the liver and adrenal glands, Dooley says.

This kind of model allows scientists to follow the disease progression from beginning to end, which can't normally be done with humans because the fast-spreading disease is often diagnosed very late. Using whole-genome profiling, the researchers were able to identify sections of chromosomes that had been duplicated or deleted in mice with cancer.

They found extra copies of a few short stretches of deoxyribonucleic acid (DNA), including a segment of chromosome 4 that turned out to include a single gene called Nuclear Factor I/B (NFIB). This is the first time NFIB has been implicated in small cell lung cancer, though it has been seen in a mouse study of prostate cancer. The gene's exact function is not known, but it is involved in the development of lung cells.

Researchers in Jacks's lab collaborated with scientists in Matthew Meyerson's lab at the Dana-Farber Cancer Institute and the Broad Institute to analyze human cancer cells, and found that NFIB is also amplified in human small cell lung tumors.

That makes a convincing case that the gene truly is playing an important role in human small cell lung cancer, says Barry Nelkin, a professor of oncology at Johns Hopkins University School of Medicine, who was not involved in this research.

"The question, always, with mouse models is whether they can tell you anything about a human disease," Nelkin says. "Some tell you something, but in others, there may be only a similarity in behavior, and the genetic changes are nothing like what is seen in humans."

The NFIB gene codes for a transcription factor, meaning it controls the expression of other genes, so researchers in Jacks's lab are now looking for the genes controlled by NFIB. "If we find what genes NFIB is regulating, that could provide new targets for small cell lung cancer therapy," Dooley says.

Section 51.4

Lung Cancer and Other Implicated Genes

"Familial Lung Cancer Gene Located" is reprinted from the National Human Genome Research Institute (NHGRI; www.genome.gov), December 27, 2012. "Genetic Variant Greatly Increases Lung Cancer Risk" is reprinted from "Genetic Variant Greatly Increases Lung Cancer Risk for Light, Non-Smokers," NHGRI, November 15, 2012. "Genetic Study Sheds New Light on Lung Cancer" is reprinted from "Large-Scale Genetic Study Sheds New Light on Lung Cancer, Opens Door to Individualized Treatment Strategies," NHGRI, July 24, 2012. "Potential Therapeutic Targets for Lung Squamous Cell Carcinoma Discovered" is reprinted from "TCGA Discovers Potential Therapeutic Targets for Lung Squamous Cell Carcinoma," National Human Genome Research Institute, September 10, 2012.

Familial Lung Cancer Gene Located

A consortium that includes scientists from the National Human Genome Research Institute (NHGRI) has identified a gene associated with an increased susceptibility to lung cancer in family members with a history of the disease. The new finding is reported in the April 15, 2009, issue of the journal *Clinical Cancer Research*.

Lung cancer, while often preventable, exacts a high toll. Each year, more than one million people worldwide die of the disease, including more than 150,000 in the United States. Smoking is by far the greatest risk factor for lung cancer, and is associated with more than 75 percent of lung cancer deaths. But some families bear more of the brunt of lung cancer than others.

The authors of the new report are part of a nationwide study of lung cancer called the Genetic Epidemiology of Lung Cancer Consortium (GELCC), which consists of twelve research institutions and universities, including NHGRI and the National Cancer Institute. GELCC is now in its tenth year of lung cancer research.

In a 2004 study conducted by GELCC, the researchers identified a large region on human chromosome 6 that conferred greater lung cancer risk in families with many affected individuals. Subsequent painstaking analysis to pinpoint the source of the elevated risk now has paid off with the identification of the precise culprit, a gene called RGS17.

"We sequenced many genes in our families. We found evidence for increased risk of lung cancer due to variation in RGS17 within our high-risk families and in two independent sets of lung cancer patients with a strong family history of the disease," said co-author Joan Bailey-Wilson, Ph.D., a statistical geneticist and co-chief of NHGRI's Inherited Disease Research Branch. "We don't see a strong influence of this gene in patients with no family history of lung cancer. Since we originally identified this genomic region in families with a strong family history of lung cancer, this is not unexpected. Our earlier results and current findings all hang together, making a lot of statistical and biological sense."

In their current study, researchers conducted fine-mapping of the suspect region of chromosome 6 in members of families in which five or more individuals over multiple generations were diagnosed with lung cancer. The region contains approximately one hundred genes. Precise computational analysis uncovered similar variants in the DNA sequence for members of the families with lung cancer. These variants, called single nucleotide polymorphisms (or SNPS) directed the researchers to the RGS17 gene.

Researchers validated this finding through laboratory experiments involving tumor samples from patients with lung cancer, as well as by growing human tumor cells in mice. Lung cancer samples were more likely to have a version of the RGS17 gene that produces high levels of the encoded protein than were normal tissue samples from individuals with no cancer. The tumor cells also multiplied more slowly when researchers took steps to suppress production of the encoded RGS17 protein. In addition, human lung cancer tumor cells with a suppressed version of the RGS17 gene had significantly decreased growth when injected into mice.

The conclusions of this analysis are that RGS17 plays a major role in lung cancer susceptibility, and individuals who carry the higher-risk version of this gene have an increased susceptibility to lung cancer when exposed to environmental risk factors, such as smoking.

While the research showed that RGS17 is an important gene for lung cancer susceptibility in families with a high incidence of lung cancer, the researchers did not see any correlation between this gene and lung cancer susceptibility in people without a strong family history of the disease.

Not content to rest upon its laurels, GELCC is already forging ahead into new areas of research. According to Dr. Bailey-Wilson, the group now plans to explore the mechanism by which RGS17 acts to increase lung cancer risk, as well as to continue its search for additional genes that influence susceptibility to familial lung cancer.

Genetic Variant Greatly Increases Lung Cancer Risk

National Institutes of Health (NIH) researchers and collaborators on a major, genetic epidemiology study of lung cancer have identified a genetic variant that greatly increases the risk of disease for individuals who inherit it, even if they have never smoked or are light smokers. The finding suggests that any level of tobacco exposure increases susceptibility for lung cancer in this group, underscoring the dangers from any type of cigarette smoke exposure. The study is published in the March 9, 2010, early online issue of the journal Cancer Research.

"Smoking is a poison for everybody," said co-author Joan Bailey-Wilson, Ph.D., a National Human Genome Research Institute (NHGRI) statistical geneticist and co-chief of NHGRI's Inherited Disease Research Branch. "For these folks, just a small amount of smoking puts them at high risk for lung cancer."

Each year, more than one million people worldwide die from lung cancer, including more than 150,000 in the United States. Smoking is by far the greatest risk factor for lung cancer and is associated with more than 75 percent of lung cancer deaths. The authors of the study point out the added importance of smoking prevention and early cancer detection procedures for individuals with a family history of lung cancer.

The analysis is part of a larger research initiative known as the Genetic Epidemiology of Lung Cancer Consortium (GELCC), a family study of lung cancer that has been ongoing for more than ten years. The NHGRI and the National Cancer Institute (NCI) are among twelve participating research institutions and universities across the country engaged in the research.

The researchers followed up on clues from the study of ninety-three families who have had at least two incidences of lung cancer among relatives. Among those 1,500 individuals, nearly 500 were affected with lung cancer. In a 2004 study conducted by GELCC, the researchers identified a large region on human chromosome 6 that conferred a greater lung cancer risk in a subset of families with many affected individuals. In April 2009, the group identified a gene, RGS17, that is located in this region on chromosome 6, and that is associated with an increased susceptibility to lung cancer in family members with a history of the disease. Work is ongoing to determine if variants in the RGS17 gene account for increased lung cancer risk in the GELCC families that are linked to chromosome 6q.

The goal of the present study was to further characterize this previously noted signature of genetic susceptibility on chromosome 6q. This signature for lung cancer susceptibility was within a longer stretch of deoxyribonucleic acid (DNA) than the RGS17 gene itself—a portion of chromosome 6q called a haplotype, containing multiple genes that tend to be inherited together.

To organize their data, the researchers divided smoking exposures into four categories: those whose smoking habit could be characterized as never, light, moderate, or heavy.

For family members without the genetic lung cancer risk haplotype, the risk of developing the disease tracked closely with the level of smoking. As would be expected, heavy smokers take on a significantly greater risk of developing lung cancer than moderate smokers, who are at a significantly greater risk than light smokers.

But in family members with the genetic risk haplotype, even light smoking resulted in a greatly increased risk for developing lung cancer, "about threefold higher than in light smokers with unknown carrier status or noncarrier status," said Dr. Bailey-Wilson. This result stands out further because the risk of developing lung cancer in light smokers who carried the risk haplotype was very similar to the risk in moderate and heavy smokers who carry the susceptibility variant. However, in smokers, the risk of lung cancer was higher in carriers of the risk haplotype than in noncarriers for all levels of exposure. This suggests that any degree of smoking exposure confers high risk of lung cancer in family members with the risk haplotype.

"The findings are really intriguing and are consistent with everything else we have seen in past studies looking for major risk alleles for lung cancer," said Dr. Bailey-Wilson, explaining that the work is an ongoing effort. "More studies will need to be done to further define the risks and to explain the linkage signal in this region. If we determine exactly which gene is involved and how it works to increase cancer risk, it may help us target people who have extremely high risk from secondhand smoke and it may help us understand how lung carcinogenesis occurs. This might allow for better treatments and for targeted smoking cessation efforts."

Currently, there is no publicly available genetic screening for the genetic variant on 6q responsible for this lung cancer susceptibility effect. Regarding advice to the public, Dr. Bailey-Wilson notes, "Anyone who smokes has a high risk of lung cancer, as well as increased risk for other diseases. Our best advice is to not smoke and to avoid exposure to passive tobacco smoke."

Genetic Study Sheds New Light on Lung Cancer

A multi-institution team, funded by the National Human Genome Research Institute (NHGRI) of the National Institutes of Health (NIH), today reported results of the largest effort to date to chart the genetic changes involved in the most common form of lung cancer, lung adenocarcinoma. The findings should help pave the way for more individualized approaches for detecting and treating the nation's leading cause of cancer deaths.

In a paper published in the October 23, 2008, issue of the journal *Nature*, the Tumor Sequencing Project (TSP) consortium identified twenty-six genes that are frequently mutated in lung adenocarcinoma—an achievement that more than doubles the number of genes known to be associated with the deadly disease. But the pioneering effort involved far more than just tallying up genes. Using a systematic, multidisciplinary approach, the TSP team also detailed key pathways involved in the disease, and described patterns of genetic mutations among different subgroups of lung cancer patients, including smokers and never-smokers.

More than one million people worldwide die of lung cancer each year, including more than 150,000 in the United States. Lung adenocarcinoma is the most frequently diagnosed form of lung cancer. The average five-year survival rate currently is about 15 percent, with survival being longest among people whose cancer has been detected early.

"By harnessing the power of genomic research, this pioneering work has painted the clearest and most complete portrait yet of lung cancer's molecular complexities. This big picture perspective will help to focus our research vision and speed our efforts to develop new strategies for disarming this common and devastating disease," said NHGRI Acting Director Alan E. Guttmacher, M.D.

Like most cancers, lung adenocarcinoma arises from changes that accumulate in people's deoxyribonucleic acid (DNA) over the course of their lives. However, little is known about the precise nature of these DNA changes, how they occur, and how they disrupt biological pathways to cause cancer's uncontrolled cell growth. To gain a more complete picture, researchers have joined together to form TSP and other large, collaborative projects that are using new tools and technologies to examine the complete set of DNA, or genome, found in various types of cancer.

"We found lung adenocarcinoma to be very diverse from a genetic standpoint. Our work uncovered many new targets for therapy of this deadly disease—oncogenes that drive particular forms of lung adenocarcinoma and tumor suppressor genes that would ordinarily prevent cancer cell growth," said Matthew Meyerson, M.D., Ph.D., a senior author of the paper. Dr. Meyerson is a senior associate member of the Broad Institute of MIT and Harvard and an associate professor at the Dana-Farber Cancer Institute and Harvard Medical School.

In the new study, the TSP team purified DNA from tumor samples and matching noncancerous tissue donated by 188 patients with lung adenocarcinoma. Next, they sequenced the DNA to look for mutations in 623 genes with known or potential relationships to cancer. Prior to the study, fewer than a dozen genes had been implicated in lung adenocarcinoma. The latest research identified twenty-six new genes that are mutated in a significant number of samples. Most of these genes had not previously been associated with lung adenocarcinoma.

Among the genes newly implicated in lung adenocarcinoma are the following:

- **Neurofibromatosis 1 (NF1):** Mutations in this gene have previously been shown to cause neurofibromatosis 1, a rare inherited disorder characterized by unchecked growth of tissue of the nervous system.

- **Ataxia telangiectasia mutated (ATM):** ATM mutations have previously been shown to play a role in ataxia telangiectasia, which is a rare inherited neurological disorder of childhood, and in various types of leukemia and lymphoma.

- **Retinoblastoma 1 (RB1):** Past research has tied RB1 mutations to retinoblastoma, a relatively uncommon type of childhood cancer that originates in the eye's retina.

- **Adenomatous polyposis coli (APC):** Mutations of this gene are common in colon cancer.

- **Ephrin receptors A3 and A5 (EPHA3 and EPHA5), neurotrophin receptors (NTRK1 and NTRK3) and other receptor-coupled tyrosine kinases (ERBB4, KDR and FGFR4):** These genes code for cell receptors coupled to members of the tyrosine kinase family of enzymes, which are considered prime targets for new cancer therapies.

After identifying the genetic mutations, the team went on to examine their impacts on biological pathways and determine which of those pathways were most crucial in lung adenocarcinoma. Such research is essential to efforts to develop new and better treatments for cancer.

For example, TSP researchers found more than two-thirds of the 188 tumors studied had at least one gene mutation affecting the mitogen-activated protein kinase (MAPK) pathway, indicating it plays a pivotal role in lung cancer. Based on those findings, the researchers suggested new treatment strategies for some subtypes of lung adenocarcinoma might include compounds that affect the MAPK pathway. One such group of compounds, called MEK inhibitors, has produced promising results in mouse models of colon cancer.

Likewise, the TSP's finding that more than 30 percent of tumors had mutations affecting the mammalian target of rapamycin (mTOR) pathway raises the possibility that the drug rapamycin might be tested in lung adenocarcinoma. Rapamycin is an mTOR-inhibiting compound approved for use in organ transplants and renal cancer.

In addition, the genetic findings suggest that certain lung cancer patients might benefit from chemotherapy drugs currently used to treat other types of cancer. For example, chemotherapy drugs known to inhibit the kinase insert domain receptor (KDR), such as sorafenib and sunitinib, might be tested in the relatively small percentage of lung adenocarcinoma patients whose tumors have mutations that activate the KDR gene.

In their *Nature* paper, TSP researchers also analyzed the patterns of genetic changes seen among different subgroups of lung adenocarcinoma patients, including smokers.

About 90 percent of lung cancer patients have significant histories of cigarette smoking, but 10 percent report no use of tobacco. In the TSP study, the number of genetic mutations detected in tumor samples from smokers was significantly higher than in tumors from never-smokers. Smokers' tumors contained as many as forty-nine mutations, while none of the never-smokers' tumors had more than five mutations. More work is needed to determine what these differences may mean for the management of lung cancer. However, doctors do know that in some other types of cancer, high mutation levels may cause a tumor to spread rapidly and/or be resistant to treatment.

"Our findings underscore the value of systematic, large-scale studies for exploring cancer. We now must move forward to apply this approach to even larger groups of samples and a wider range of cancers," said Richard K. Wilson, Ph.D., a senior author of the paper and director of the Genome Sequencing Center at Washington University School of Medicine, St. Louis.

The TSP team also included researchers from Baylor College of Medicine, Houston; Brigham and Women's Hospital, Boston; Memorial Sloan-Kettering Cancer Center, New York; the University of Cologne, Germany; the University of Michigan, Ann Arbor; and the University of Texas M.D. Anderson Cancer Center, Houston.

"Clearly, much still remains to be discovered. We have just begun to realize the tremendous potential of large-scale, genomic studies to unravel the many mysteries of cancer," said Richard Gibbs, Ph.D., a co-author of the lung adenocarcinoma paper and director of the Human Genome Sequencing Center at Baylor College of Medicine.

The TSP data are complementary to those from other large-scale cancer genome studies, such as The Cancer Genome Atlas (TCGA) project funded by NHGRI and the National Cancer Institute (NCI). In its pilot phase, TCGA is focusing on the most common form of brain tumor, called glioblastoma; a type of lung cancer called squamous cell lung cancer; and ovarian cancer. The first results from TCGA's glioblastoma study were published in the advance online edition of *Nature* on September 4, 2008, and published in *Nature*'s print edition on October 23, 2008.

The co-publication of these comprehensive cancer genome studies should provide hope to millions of people and families living with cancer. By applying advanced genomic tools to the complexities of cancer, these studies have helped to untangle the biological roots of these diseases, which will accelerate efforts by the worldwide scientific community to improve outcomes for cancer patients.

Potential Therapeutic Targets for Lung Squamous Cell Carcinoma Discovered

Researchers have identified potential therapeutic targets in lung squamous cell carcinoma, the second most common form of lung cancer. The Cancer Genome Atlas (TCGA) Research Network study that appeared online September 9, 2012, and in print September 27, 2012, in the journal *Nature*, comprehensively characterized the lung squamous cell carcinoma genome. The study found a large number and variety of DNA alterations, many of which seem to be driving forces behind pathways that are important to the initiation and progression of lung cancer. TCGA is jointly funded and managed by the National Human Genome Research Institute (NHGRI) and the National Cancer Institute (NCI), both part of the National Institutes of Health (NIH).

"With these findings, TCGA researchers have set the stage for the development, testing, and implementation of advanced diagnostics and therapeutics for lung squamous cell carcinoma," said NIH Director Francis S. Collins, M.D., Ph.D. "These findings also underscore the power and value of our nation's investment in The Cancer Genome Atlas."

Researchers have made important strides in understanding and developing precision medicine treatments for adenocarcinomas, which are the most common type of lung cancer. But these treatments have been largely ineffective in treating lung squamous cell carcinoma. Lung squamous cell carcinoma frequently develops in the large airways in the center of the lungs, while adenocarcinomas often arise at the edges of the lungs. Lung adenocarcinomas sometimes affect nonsmokers, while lung squamous cell carcinomas arise almost exclusively in smokers.

"This report provides an unprecedented view of the spectrum and high rate of genomic mutations that are found in lung squamous cell carcinoma," said Eric D. Green, M.D., Ph.D., NHGRI director. "We hope this report will spur basic research to better understand the genesis of the disease, and in clinical research as these new findings are factored into potential treatment approaches."

In this study, researchers identified promising therapeutic targets, including three families of tyrosine kinases, which are enzymes that function as on or off switches in many cellular functions and are frequently mutated in cancer. These enzymes were found to be mutated or amplified in many of the tumors analyzed by TCGA investigators. Importantly, enzymes in these families have been established as potential therapeutic targets in pre-clinical studies and investigated clinically as therapeutic targets in other cancer types. In an ancillary finding, in 69 percent of the tumors studied, investigators detected gene alterations in important signaling pathways that could also serve as therapeutic targets.

"Genomic analysis of lung adenocarcinomas has led to many important therapeutic advances, and this new research helps to explain why squamous lung cancers have not been responsive to drugs that work for adenocarcinomas," said Harold Varmus, M.D., director, NCI. "Because the spectrum of mutations is very different in each type, the identification of these new mutations by TCGA researchers has the potential to lead to therapeutic advances for squamous lung cancers."

For this study, researchers examined tissue samples from 178 patients with untreated lung squamous cell carcinomas. Notably, 96 percent of the patients in this study had a history of tobacco use. Researchers compared the tumor genome to the genome in normal tissue to make sure that a change in the tumor genome was the result of a mutation. The carcinomas exhibited a large number and variety of alterations, many of which appeared to deleteriously affect pathways that are important to the initiation and progression of cancer. Genes that help detoxify cells and repair damage, or are involved in cell specialization, were frequently altered.

Researchers also sequenced the whole genomes of nineteen tumor and normal tissue pairs to gather comprehensive information about genomic rearrangements. This is the first TCGA report to describe whole genome sequencing, which allows researchers to map the variety of changes that can occur in a tumor's genome, including the breaking and rejoining of chromosomes and other large structural alterations that might be involved in the genesis of the disease. These whole genome data will be freely available for future in-depth analysis that could help locate mutations in intergenic regions, which are stretches of DNA sequences located between clusters of genes that may not encode proteins but sometimes control nearby genes.

Researchers found alterations of the TP53 gene in 90 percent of the tumors and inactivation of the CDKN2A gene in 72 percent of tumors. In their nonmutated or unaltered state, both genes function as tumor suppressors to prevent cancer. When they are altered, however, cancer is able to grow unconstrained. Researchers also identified previously unreported mutations that reduce the function of the HLA-A gene in the tumors. HLA controls how the immune system distinguishes the body's own cells from foreign invaders.

Researchers speculate that mutations in the HLA gene may help the tumor escape the body's regular surveillance of mutated cells. Involvement of the HLA-A gene suggests that treatment strategies for some patients using customized immunotherapies could be effective. Recent clinical trials suggest that new biological agents, which work by decreasing the immune response and allow the immune system to react against cancer cells, may be effective treatments for some lung cancer patients.

"These TCGA findings should stimulate a wide variety of new clinical trials for patients with squamous cell lung cancer and specific genotypic alterations," said Matthew Meyerson, M.D., Ph.D., of the Dana-Farber Cancer Institute, the Broad Institute and Harvard Medical School, who co-led the project within TCGA. "These will include clinical trials of PI3 kinase inhibitors and other tyrosine kinase inhibitors, as well as ways to use genomics to select patients for trials of lung cancer treatments that dial down the immune response."

Section 51.5

Skin Cancer and Heredity

Reprinted from the following documents from the National Human Genome Research Institute (www.genome.gov): "Learning about Skin Cancer," October 30, 2012, and "NIH Researchers Achieve Better Understanding of Skin Cancer," July 31, 2012.

Learning about Skin Cancer

Skin cancer is the most common type of cancer in the United States. An estimated 40 to 50 percent of Americans who live to age sixty-five will have skin cancer at least once. The most common skin cancer is basal cell carcinoma, which accounts for more than 90 percent of all skin cancers in the United States.

The most virulent form of skin cancer is melanoma. In some parts of the world, especially in Western countries, the number of people who develop melanoma is increasing faster than any other cancer. In the United States, for example, the number of new cases of melanoma has more than doubled in the past twenty years.

What are the most common forms of skin cancer?

Three types of skin cancer are the most common:

- Basal cell carcinoma is a slow-growing cancer that seldom spreads to other parts of the body. Basal cells, which are round, form the layer just underneath the epidermis, or outer layer of the skin.

- Squamous cell carcinoma spreads more often than basal cell carcinoma, but still is considered rare. Squamous cells, which are flat, make up most of the epidermis.

- Melanoma is the most serious type of skin cancer. It occurs when melanocytes, the pigment cells in the lower part of the epidermis, become malignant, meaning that they start dividing uncontrollably. If melanoma spreads to the lymph nodes it may also reach other parts of the body, such as the liver, lungs, or brain. In such cases, the disease is called metastatic melanoma.

What are the symptoms of skin cancer?

The most commonly noticed symptom of skin cancer is a change on the skin, especially a new growth or a sore that doesn't heal. Both basal and squamous cell cancers are found mainly on areas of the skin that are exposed to the sun—the head, face, neck, hands and arms. However, skin cancer can occur anywhere.

For melanoma, the first sign often is a change in the size, shape, color, or feel of an existing mole. Melanomas can vary greatly in the way they look, but generally show one or more of the "ABCD" features:

- Their shape may be Asymmetrical.
- Their Borders may be ragged or otherwise irregular.
- Their Color may be uneven, with shades of black and brown.
- Their Diameter may change in size.

What do we know about the causes and heredity of skin cancer?

Ultraviolet (UV) radiation from the sun is the main cause of skin cancer, although artificial sources of UV radiation, such as sunlamps and tanning booths, also play a role. UV radiation can damage the deoxyribonucleic acid (DNA), or genetic information, in skin cells, creating "misspellings" in their genetic code and, as a result, alter the function of those cells.

Cancers generally are caused by a combination of environmental and genetic factors. With skin cancer, the environment plays a greater role, but individuals can be born with a genetic disposition toward or vulnerability to getting cancer. The risk is greatest for people who have light-colored skin that freckles easily—often those who also have red or blond hair and blue or light-colored eyes—although anyone can get skin cancer.

Skin cancer is related to lifetime exposure to UV radiation, and therefore most skin cancers appear after age fifty. However, the sun's damaging effects begin at an early age. People who live in areas that get high levels of UV radiation from the sun are more likely to get skin cancer. For example, the highest rates of skin cancer are found in South Africa and Australia, areas that receive high amounts of UV radiation.

About 10 percent of all patients with melanoma have family members who also have had the disease. Research suggests that a mutation in the CDKN2 gene on chromosome 9 plays a role in this form of melanoma. Studies have also implicated genes on chromosomes 1 and 12 in cases of familial melanoma.

Can I do anything to prevent or test for skin cancer?

When it comes to skin cancer, prevention is your best line of defense. Protection should start early in childhood and continue throughout life. Suggested protections include the following:

- Whenever possible, avoid exposure to the midday sun.
- Wear protective clothing—for example, long sleeves and broad-rimmed hats.
- Use sunscreen lotions with an SPF factor of at least 15.
- If a family member has had melanoma, have your doctor check for early warning signs regularly.

How is skin cancer treated?

Melanoma can be cured if it is diagnosed and treated when the tumor has not deeply invaded the skin. However, if a melanoma is not removed in its early stages, cancer cells may grow downward from the skin surface. When a melanoma becomes thick and deep, the disease often spreads to other parts of the body and is difficult to control.

Surgery is the standard treatment for melanoma, as well as other skin cancers. However, if the cancer has spread to other parts of the body, doctors may use other treatments, such as chemotherapy, immunotherapy, radiation therapy, or a combination of these methods.

Researchers Achieve Better Understanding of Skin Cancer

Melanocytes—the skin's pigments cells—are sensitive to the sun's ultraviolet radiation, which, along with chemical and other exposures, can trigger deoxyribonucleic acid (DNA) damage. The genetic material that fabricates, organizes, and invigorates the skin cells can undergo abnormal changes, or mutations.

Because mutations can cause faulty genetic instructions—some that control cell division and survival—affected melanocytes may start to grow and divide out of control. Such cells may spread to surrounding layers of the skin and to other parts of the body, resulting in a life-threatening cancer known as metastatic melanoma.

"Melanoma is very highly mutated and is in some cases mutated approximately on an order of magnitude higher than other cancer types," said Yardena Samuels, Ph.D., an investigator in the Cancer Genetics Branch of the National Human Genome Research Institute's (NHGRI)

Division of Intramural Research. Dr. Samuels is part of a National Institutes of Health (NIH)-led team studying the genetics of melanoma and is the senior author of an article in the September 25, 2011, early online issue of *Nature Genetics* that found that mutations in the metabotropic glutamate receptor-3 (GRM3) gene cause some cases of melanoma.

This newest melanoma-causing mutation joins a growing list of culprits. In April 2011, *Nature Genetics* published the team's first systematic genomic probe of melanoma. Using whole-exome sequencing, a technique that deciphers just the portions of the genome that code for proteins, the researchers identified fifteen new mutations that drive cancer development and one that had previously been detected. The researchers found that one of the mutated genes, GRIN2A, is mutated in 25 percent of melanoma cases. It is located in the signaling pathway for the nerve cell messenger glutamate—the same pathway as GRM3.

In the current study, the researchers focused on mutations in the largest human gene family, G protein–coupled receptors (GPCRs). The significance of the receptors coded by GPCR genes is underscored by the fact that they are the targets of more than half of the drugs approved by the U.S. Food and Drug Administration (FDA). Additionally, genes in the GPCR family regulate signal pathways for cell growth, the hallmark cellular activity in cancer.

NHGRI researchers and a colleague from the Johns Hopkins Sidney Kimmel Comprehensive Cancer Center in Baltimore designed and analyzed the new study, while National Cancer Institute (NCI) researchers, including Steven Rosenberg, M.D., Ph.D., chief of surgery at the NCI, and colleagues from the University of Texas MD Anderson Cancer Center in Houston and the University of Colorado Denver School of Medicine collected melanoma tumor samples.

The researchers obtained DNA from eleven melanoma tumor samples and sequenced the exon region—or protein-coding portion of the DNA sequence—that spanned the 734 GPCR genes. Mutational analysis narrowed the interest of the researchers to a group of 11 genes in the GPCR family that contained two or more mutations. The team accessed an additional eighty melanoma samples and detected that one particular gene, GRM3, had a high mutation rate in the tumor samples. Furthermore, multiple tumor samples contained the precise mutation in the very same location within the gene, an occurrence characterized as a mutational "hot spot." This prevalent recurrence indicates that the mutation has a selective advantage, elevating its importance as a mutation that drives the development of cancer.

To explore the function of this gene, the researchers studied melanoma cells that harbor the mutations. In an experiment that heightened the function of mutated GRM3, the researchers detected increased activity of a signal pathway called the MAP kinase pathway, already known to be involved in melanoma. A kinase is a type of protein enzyme that modifies other proteins to cause some particular cell function. The pathway includes a kinase known as MEK targeted by current melanoma drugs. While some targeted treatments have been effective, tumors become drug resistant within months of treatment. The pathway also is associated with the most highly mutated gene in melanoma, called BRAF.

The researchers performed a test to detect whether the cells with the newly identified mutation in GRM3 respond to the drug that inhibits the MEK pathway. They detected that mutated cells treated with an MEK inhibitor responded positively, dying off as they should rather than persistently replicating as cancer cells.

Further analysis showed that when the cells carry both a BRAF mutation and a GRM3 mutation, the inhibitor compound selectively killed the cells that had the GRM3 mutation. Dr. Samuels suggested that in some cases, failure of melanoma cells to respond to an MEK inhibitor might be due to those cells having a BRAF mutation but no GRM3 mutation. Dr. Samuels predicts that prospective genetic analysis will enable differentiation of melanoma into subclasses.

"Melanoma has been subdivided by pathological characteristics," she said. "With the advent of in-depth genetic analyses, it may become possible to classify melanoma by its genetic alterations. Based on our two recent studies, I predict several melanoma subclasses will be identified in the near future."

Section 51.6

Genetic Risks for Prostate, Breast, and Ovarian Cancers

New research has identified more than eighty genetic variations that can increase a person's risk of prostate, breast, and ovarian cancers.

Three Queensland University of Technology (QUT) scientists were part of the largest-ever study of its type, which could lead to improved early screening and new treatments.

The international team studied the deoxyribonucleic acid (DNA) of two hundred thousand people to identify genetic variations, called single nucleotide polymorphisms (SNPs), that are associated with the risk of developing prostate, breast, and ovarian cancer.

The research appeared in the March 28, 2013, edition of *Nature Genetics*.

Genetics scientist with QUT's Institute of Health and Biomedical Innovation (IHBI) Dr. Jyotsna Batra said each variation increased the risk of developing cancer by a small amount.

However, the cancer risk multiplied significantly with the number of variations within a person's DNA.

"Take prostate cancer, for instance, which was the focus of Queensland's contribution to the research," Dr. Batra said, also of QUT's Faculty of Health.

"If you're unlucky enough to be in the 1 percent of people with lots of these prostate-cancer related variations in your DNA, your risk of developing this disease could rise by nearly 50 percent compared to the population average."

The new SNP research means scientists now know of seventy-eight genetic variations linked to prostate cancer.

"We found twenty-three additional genetic variations linked to prostate cancer and sixteen of those relate to life-threatening forms of the disease," Dr. Batra said.

"We can now explain 35 percent of the hereditary risk of prostate cancer by combining the effects of these seventy-eight variations—but that means we have 65 percent to go."

Dr. Batra worked closely with fellow IHBI scientists Professor Judith Clements and Srilakshmi Srinivasan, as well as scientists from the Queensland Institute of Medical Research, to help design the SNP chip that analyzed the DNA for prostate cancer-released genetic variations.

The analysis involved Queensland prostate cancer patients, whose DNA were compared to that of healthy individuals.

The QUT scientists are currently designing a second chip to isolate the remaining variations.

The SNP research would be used to design genetic tests for prostate cancer, which would complement existing screening technologies.

"These genetic variations are inherited and don't change with age," Professor Clements said.

"That means it's possible to test for the cancer risks well before they actually develop in a person.

"About one in nine men will develop prostate cancer by eighty years of age but not all prostate cancer is life threatening.

"So knowing the genetic composition of a man's DNA becomes an important step in dealing with his disease.

"Doctors would likely opt for regular screening and early surgical removal for patients likely to develop aggressive prostate cancer, but opt for watchful waiting in patients with variations linked to nonaggressive forms."

The generic variation study was led by the UK's University of Cambridge and the Institute of Cancer Research.

It marked the first attempt to identify genetic variations associated with the risk of prostate, breast, and ovarian cancer in a very large number of people.

Section 51.7

Genetic Link to Prostate Cancer Risk in African Americans

"Genetic Link to Prostate Cancer Risk in African Americans Found," by Jeanne Galatzer-Levy, September 6, 2012. © Board of Trustees of the University of Illinois (www.uic.edu), 2012. Reprinted with permission.

Prostate cancer in African American men is associated with specific changes in the IL-16 gene, according to researchers at the University of Illinois at Chicago College of Medicine.

The study, published online in the journal *Cancer Epidemiology, Biomarkers & Prevention*, establishes the association of IL-16 with prostate cancer in men of both African and European descent.

"This provides us with a new potential biomarker for prostate cancer," says principal investigator Rick Kittles, University of Illinois at Chicago (UIC) associate professor of medicine in hematology/oncology.

Previously identified changes in the gene for IL-16, an immune system protein, were associated with prostate cancer in men of European descent. But the same changes in the gene's coded sequence—called "polymorphisms"—did not confer the same risk in African Americans.

Doubt was cast on IL-16's role in prostate cancer when researchers were unable to confirm that the IL-16 polymorphisms identified in whites were also important risk factors in African Americans, Kittles said.

Kittles and his colleagues used a technique called imputation—a type of statistical extrapolation—that allowed them to see new patterns of association and identify new places in the gene to look for polymorphisms. They found changes elsewhere in the IL-16 gene that were associated with prostate cancer and that were unique to African Americans.

Polymorphisms result from deoxyribonucleic acid (DNA) mutations and emerge in the ancestral history of different populations. People of African descent are much more genetically diverse than whites, Kittles said, making the search for polymorphisms associated with disease more difficult.

Although the effect of the particular changes to the gene appear to be different in men of African versus European descent, it is likely

479

that several of the polymorphisms in the gene alter the function of the IL-16 protein.

"This confirms the importance of IL-16 in prostate cancer and leads us in a new direction," Kittles said. "Very little research has been done on IL-16, so not much is known about it."

"We now need to explore the functional role of IL-16 to understand the role it is playing in prostate cancer," he said.

Chapter 52

Crohn Disease and Genetics

What is Crohn disease?

Crohn disease is a complex, chronic disorder that primarily affects the digestive system. This condition typically involves abnormal inflammation of the intestinal walls, particularly in the lower part of the small intestine (the ileum) and portions of the large intestine (the colon). Inflammation can occur in any part of the digestive system, however. The inflamed tissues become thick and swollen, and the inner surface of the intestine may develop open sores (ulcers).

Crohn disease most commonly appears in a person's late teens or twenties, although the disease can appear at any age. Signs and symptoms tend to flare up multiple times throughout life. The most common features of this condition are persistent diarrhea, abdominal pain and cramping, loss of appetite, weight loss, and fever. Some people with Crohn disease have chronic bleeding from inflamed tissues in the intestine; over time, this bleeding can lead to a low number of red blood cells (anemia). In some cases, Crohn disease can also cause medical problems affecting the joints, eyes, or skin.

Intestinal blockage is a common complication of Crohn disease. Blockages are caused by swelling or a buildup of scar tissue in the intestinal walls. Some affected individuals also develop fistulae, which are abnormal connections between the intestine and other tissues.

Excerpted from "Crohn Disease," Genetics Home Reference (http://ghr.nlm .nih.gov), August 2007. Reviewed by David A. Cooke, M.D., FACP, May 2013.

Fistulae occur when ulcers break through the intestinal wall to form passages between loops of the intestine or between the intestine and nearby structures (such as the bladder, vagina, or skin).

Crohn disease is one common form of inflammatory bowel disease (IBD). Another type of IBD, ulcerative colitis, also causes chronic inflammation of the intestinal lining. Unlike Crohn disease, which can affect any part of the digestive system, ulcerative colitis typically causes inflammation only in the colon. In addition, the two disorders involve different patterns of inflammation.

How common is Crohn disease?

Crohn disease is most common in western Europe and North America, where it affects 100 to 150 in 100,000 people. About one million Americans are currently affected by this disorder. Crohn disease occurs more often in Caucasians (whites) and people of eastern and central European (Ashkenazi) Jewish descent than among people of other ethnic backgrounds.

What are the genetic changes related to Crohn disease?

Crohn disease is related to chromosomes 5 and 10.

Variations of the ATG16L1, IRGM, and NOD2 genes increase the risk of developing Crohn disease.

The IL23R gene is associated with Crohn disease.

A variety of genetic and environmental factors likely play a role in causing Crohn disease. Although researchers are studying risk factors that may contribute to this complex disorder, many of these factors remain unknown. Cigarette smoking is thought to increase the risk of developing this disease, and it may also play a role in periodic flare-ups of signs and symptoms.

Studies suggest that Crohn disease may result from a combination of certain genetic variations, changes in the immune system, and the presence of bacteria in the digestive tract. Recent studies have identified variations in specific genes, including ATG16L1, IL23R, IRGM, and NOD2, that influence the risk of developing Crohn disease. These genes provide instructions for making proteins that are involved in immune system function. Variations in any of these genes may disrupt the ability of cells in the intestine to respond normally to bacteria. An abnormal immune response to bacteria in the intestinal walls may lead to chronic inflammation and the digestive problems characteristic of Crohn disease.

Researchers have also discovered genetic variations in certain regions of chromosome 5 and chromosome 10 that appear to contribute to Crohn disease risk. One area of chromosome 5, known as the IBD5 locus, contains several genetic changes that may increase the risk of developing this condition. Other regions of chromosome 5 and chromosome 10 identified in studies of Crohn disease risk are known as "gene deserts" because they include no known genes. Instead, these regions may contain stretches of DNA that regulate nearby genes. Additional research is needed to determine how genetic variations in these chromosomal regions are related to a person's chance of developing Crohn disease.

Can Crohn disease be inherited?

The inheritance pattern of Crohn disease is unclear because many genetic and environmental factors are likely to be involved. This condition tends to cluster in families, however, and having an affected family member is a significant risk factor for the disease.

Chapter 53

Mental Illness and Genetics

Chapter Contents

Section 53.1

Familial Recurrence of Mental Illness

"Family History of Mental Illness," © 2008 Emory University School of Medicine
Department of Human Genetics. Reprinted with permission. For additional
information, visit the Department of Genetics website at http://www.genetics
.emory.edu. Reviewed by David A. Cooke, M.D., FACP, May 2013.

Mental illness is a category of diseases/disorders known to cause
mild to severe disturbances in thought and/or behavior, which can
result in an inability to cope with the ordinary demands and routines
of life. There are more than two hundred classified forms of mental
illness. Common disorders are depression, bipolar disorder, dementia,
schizophrenia, and anxiety disorders. Symptoms may include changes
in mood, personality, personal habits, and/or social withdrawal. With
treatment, many individuals learn to cope or recover from a mental
illness or emotional disorder.

Mental disorders are common in the United States and around the
world. An estimated 57.5 million Americans eighteen years of age and
older—approximately one in four adults—are diagnosed with a mental
disorder in a given year. In addition, mental disorders are the leading
cause of disability in the United States and Canada for ages fifteen
to forty-four years. Many people suffer from more than one mental
disorder. Approximately 45 percent of those with a mental disorder
meet the criteria for two or more disorders.

Mental illnesses are multifactorial illnesses (caused by the interaction of various genetic and environmental factors). Causes may include a reaction to environmental stresses, genetic factors, biochemical
imbalances, or a combination of these. Because genetic factors are
involved, when one family member is affected, other close relatives
may be at increased risk. At this time, no genetic tests are available
for mental illness, and therefore prenatal diagnosis is not possible.

Mood Disorders

Mood disorders include major depressive disorder, dysthymia (a
milder, but longer-lasting form of depression), and bipolar disorder.

Approximately 20.9 million American adults (9.5 percent of the U.S. adult population) have a mood disorder. The median age of onset for mood disorders is thirty years:

- **Depression:** Major depressive disorder is the leading cause of disability in the United States for ages fifteen to forty-four. While major depressive disorder can occur at any age, the median age of onset is thirty-two years. Major depressive disorder is more prevalent in women than in men. Recurrence risks for first-degree relatives (children, parents, siblings) are approximately 10 percent for individuals with depression (two to four times the general population risk); however, this risk could be higher depending on the family history, number of affected family members, and age of onset. Relatives of individuals diagnosed with depression earlier in life are at a greater risk to develop depression than relatives of individuals diagnosed later in life.

- **Bipolar disorder:** More than two million American adults, or about 1 percent of the population age eighteen and older in any given year, have bipolar disorder. Bipolar disorder is also known as manic depression. The illness causes a person's mood to swing from excessively "high" (mania) to irritable, sad, and/or hopeless (depression), with periods of a normal mood in between. The median age of onset for bipolar disorder is twenty-five years. For information regarding recurrence risks, please refer to Table 53.1.

Schizophrenia

Schizophrenia is a disorder in which a person may have difficulty distinguishing between what is real and what is imaginary; may be unresponsive or withdrawn; and may have difficulty expressing normal emotions in social situations. Schizophrenia is not split personality or multiple personality. Most people with schizophrenia are not violent and do not pose a danger to others. Schizophrenia is not caused by childhood experiences, poor parenting, or lack of willpower, nor are the symptoms identical for each person. Schizophrenia often appears in men in their late teens or early twenties, while women are generally affected in their twenties or early thirties. Schizophrenia affects men and women with equal frequency. There is a slight increase in the risk of schizophrenia in the siblings of patients with other types of psychosis. For information regarding recurrence risks, please refer to Table 53.1.

Anxiety Disorders

Anxiety disorders include panic disorder, obsessive-compulsive disorder, post-traumatic stress disorder, generalized anxiety disorder, and phobias (social phobia, agoraphobia, and specific phobias). Approximately forty million Americans have an anxiety disorder. Most people with an anxiety disorder also have another mood disorder. Nearly three-quarters of those with an anxiety disorder will have their first episode by 21.5 years of age.

Table 53.1. Recurrence Risks

Affected Relative	Bipolar Disorder	Schizophrenia
General population risk	2–3%	1%
Sibling	13%	9%
Parent	15%	13%
Sibling and one parent	20%	15%
Both parents	50%	45%
Second-degree relative (aunt, uncle, grandparent)	5%	3%
Monozygotic twin	70%	40%
Dizygotic twin	20%	10%
First cousin	2–3%	1–2%

Source: Table from *Harper's Practical Genetic Counseling, 6th ed.*, 2004.

Section 53.2

Family History as Predictor of Severity of Mental Illness

We've all been asked at routine visits to the doctor to record our family's history with medical problems like cancer, diabetes, or heart disease. But when it comes to mental disorders, usually mum's the word.

New findings by researchers at the Duke Institute for Genome Sciences and Policy (IGSP) make a strong case for changing that status quo. They have found that thirty minutes or less of question-and-answer about the family history of depression, anxiety, or substance abuse is enough to predict a patient's approximate risks for developing each disorder and how severe their future illness is likely to be.

"There are lots of kids with behavior problems who may outgrow them on their own without medication, versus the minority with mental illnesses that need treatment," said Terrie Moffitt, a professor of psychology and neuroscience in the IGSP. "Family history is the quickest and cheapest way to sort that out."

Researchers who are on the hunt for genes responsible for mental disorders might also take advantage of the discovery, added Avshalom Caspi, an IGSP investigator and professor of psychology and neuroscience. "It suggests they may be better off selecting people with more serious illness or, better still, collecting family history information directly," he said.

That mental illnesses tend to run in families is certainly no surprise. In fact, psychiatric conditions are some of the most heritable of all disorders. But the link between family history and the seriousness of psychiatric disease has been less certain.

Moffitt, Caspi, and their colleagues looked to 981 New Zealanders born at a single hospital in 1972 or 1973, who are participants in what is known as the Dunedin Study. Researchers have been tracking the physical and mental health and lifestyles of those enrolled in the longitudinal study since they were three years old.

In this case, Caspi and Moffitt's team tested each individual's personal experience with depression, anxiety, alcohol dependence, and drug dependence in relation to their family history "scores"—the proportion of their grandparents, parents, and siblings over age ten who were affected. The analysis shows that family history can predict a more recurrent course of each of the four disorders. It is also indicative of those more likely to suffer a worse impairment and to make greater use of mental health services. Contrary to earlier reports, those with a stronger family history did not necessarily develop their disorders at an earlier age.

Family history could be used to identify those in need of early intervention or more aggressive treatment, the researchers said. But if a few, simple questions could have that much value, why has family history been ignored for so long?

Moffitt said that health professionals have shied away from questioning people about their family history of mental illnesses because of the stigma attached to them. "There's a sense that families are not as open about mental disorders—that people may not know or may make incorrect assumptions," she said.

The new findings suggest those concerns may be overblown. One key, they say, is in how you go about asking the questions.

For example, instead of asking each person if any of their relatives had a history of anxiety disorder outright, the researchers asked, "Has anyone on the list of family members ever had a sudden spell or attack in which they felt panicked?" If the interviewee came up with a name, they were then asked, "Did this person have several attacks of extreme fear or panic, even though there was nothing to be afraid of?"

There is another very practical reason that those in the mental health profession don't ask about family history. The "bible of psychiatry," officially known as the *Diagnostic and Statistical Manual of Mental Disorders (DSM)*, makes no mention of it. The DSM is the primary tool for making mental health diagnoses and delivering mental healthcare in the United States and, to some extent, in other countries around the world.

"There's nothing about family history in the *DSM* even though it may be the most important," Moffitt said. There will soon be an opening to fix that. Experts including Moffitt are now in the process of revising the *DSM*, which is currently in its fourth edition. The next edition, *DSM-V*, is due for publication in 2012.

Coauthors on the study include HonaLee Harrington of Duke; Barry Milne of the University of Auckland; Michael Rutter of King's College London; and Richie Poulton of the University of Otago. The original report appeared in the July 2009 issue of *Archives of General Psychiatry*.

Section 53.3

Genetic Links in Obsessive-Compulsive Disorder

Obsessive-compulsive disorder (OCD) tends to run in families, causing members of several generations to experience severe anxiety and disturbing thoughts that they ease by repeating certain behaviors. In fact, close relatives of people with OCD are up to nine times more likely to develop OCD themselves.

Now, new research is shedding new light on one of the genetic factors that may contribute to that pattern. And while no one gene "causes" OCD, the research is helping scientists confirm the importance of a particular gene that has been suspected to play a major role in OCD's development.

In two papers published simultaneously in the *Archives of General Psychiatry*, researchers from the University of Michigan, the University of Illinois at Chicago (UIC), the University of Chicago, and the University of Toronto report finding an association between OCD patients and a glutamate transporter gene called SLC1A1.

The gene encodes a protein called EAAC1 that regulates the flow of a substance called glutamate in and out of brain cells. So, variations in the gene might lead to alterations in that flow, perhaps putting a person at increased risk of developing OCD.

The new findings are especially important not only because of the simultaneous discoveries reported in the papers, but also because of previous studies that show a functional link between glutamate and OCD. Brain imaging and spinal fluid studies have shown differences in the glutamate system between OCD patients and healthy volunteers, including in areas of the brain where the EAAC1 protein is most common.

"Taken together, these findings suggest that SLC1A1 is a strong candidate gene for OCD, which if confirmed could lead to improvements in understanding and treating this condition, and screening those with an elevated risk," says Gregory Hanna, M.D., senior author on one of the papers and an associate professor of psychiatry at the U-M Medical School. "It's possible that altered glutamate activity in some brain regions may contribute to the obsessions and compulsions that are the hallmark of OCD."

Hanna and colleague Edwin Cook, Jr., M.D., of UIC together lead a major study of OCD genetics involving patients and their families who are willing to donate DNA samples and be interviewed by researchers. The study is still seeking OCD patients and their parents to participate in further research on the genetics of OCD.

While the new findings are exciting because they strengthen the evidence for glutamate's role in OCD vulnerability, the researchers caution that more work needs to be done before their discovery has any impact on OCD treatment.

Four years ago, the U-M and UIC team published a genome scan from young OCD patients and their parents that found signs of OCD-related genetic variations on chromosome 9, in the area of SLC1A1.

Since that time, they have been zeroing in on the gene and its nearby stretches of deoxyribonucleic acid (DNA), using analyses of single nucleotide polymorphisms that look at specific differences between individuals within the gene. At the same time, the Toronto group has been focusing on that same area in studies involving adults and children with OCD and their close relatives.

The new U-M, UC, and UIC paper is based on genetic samples from 71 OCD patients (children and adults) and their parents. It finds a significant association between early-onset OCD and genetic variations at several sites on the SLC1A1 gene. A strong association at two of those sites was only seen in male early-onset OCD patients, which surprised the researchers but may make sense in light of the fact that early-onset OCD is more common in boys than in girls. As many as half of all OCD patients experience their first symptoms in childhood or adolescence.

The new U-T paper is based on data from 157 OCD patients and 319 of their first-degree relatives. It finds linkages between OCD and three locations on the SLC1A1 gene.

In a commentary published in the same issue of the journal, two Yale University researchers call the new findings promising, and call for additional research. "These data add to a growing body of work that suggest that SLC1A1 is perhaps a primary candidate gene for OCD," they write.

Hanna notes that the finding of genetic vulnerabilities for OCD are important, but so is the understanding of how environmental factors—

including hormones and infections—may play a role in the onset of the disorder.

He directs the U-M Child & Adolescent Psychiatry Division's Pediatric Anxiety and Tic Disorders Program, which treats young patients whose OCD may be related to an infection. That disorder, called PANDAS for pediatric autoimmune neuropsychiatric disorders associated with streptococcal infections, causes both OCD and tics in patients.

As their research continues, Hanna and his colleagues hope to eventually conduct clinical trials of glutamate-targeting medications in OCD patients, and to collect more DNA and blood samples from patients and their families. They're also looking at other regions of the genome that might contain gene variations that are more common in people with OCD.

Editor's note: Follow up studies have strengthened the evidence for a link between OCD and the SLCIA1 gene. Other studies have also pointed to a connection between OCD and the SLC6A4 serotonin transporter gene. This suggests that there may be multiple genes that can cause OCD. It is also possible that more than one abnormal gene may be required to cause the disease.

Section 53.4

Genetic Links in Schizophrenia and Bipolar Disorder

A team of over 250 researchers from more than twenty countries have discovered that common genetic variations contribute to a person's risk of schizophrenia and bipolar disorder.

The study of more than fifty thousand adults ages eighteen and older provides new molecular evidence that eleven deoxyribonucleic acid (DNA) regions in the human genome have strong association with these diseases, including six regions not previously observed. The researchers also found that many of these DNA variants contribute to both diseases.

The findings, reported by the Psychiatric Genome-Wide Association Study Consortium and published online September 18, 2011 in two papers in the journal *Nature Genetics*, represent significant advances in the understanding the causes of these chronic, severe, and debilitating disorders.

Also known as a whole genome association study, a genome-wide association study examines all or most of the genes of different individuals to see how much the genes vary from individual to individual.

"This is the largest study of its kind by far," said Patrick F. Sullivan, M.D., Ray M. Hayworth and Family Distinguished Professor of Psychiatry and professor of genetics at the University of North Carolina (UNC) at Chapel Hill. Sullivan, a PGC coordinator and principal investigator in the study, is also a member of the UNC Lineberger Comprehensive Cancer Center and the Carolina Center for Genome Sciences.

The study that focused on schizophrenia identified "strong evidence for seven different places in the human genome, five of which were new and two previously implicated, that contain DNA changes that are significantly associated with schizophrenia," Sullivan said.

And in a joint analysis of a schizophrenia and bipolar disorder sample, the Consortium found three different DNA regions, or loci, in which both disorders reached genome-wide statistical significance. "This tells us that these disorders, which many of us have considered to be separate things, actually share fundamental similarity," Sullivan said.

Schizophrenia and bipolar disorder are common and often devastating brain disorders. Some of the most prominent symptoms in schizophrenia are persistent delusions, hallucinations, and cognitive problems. Bipolar disorder (or manic-depressive illness) is characterized by episodes of severe mood problems including mania and depression. Both affect about 1 percent of the world's population and usually strike in late adolescence or early adulthood. Despite the availability of treatments, these illnesses are usually chronic, and response to treatment is often incomplete, leading to prolonged disability and personal suffering. Family history, which reflects genetic inheritance, is a strong risk factor for both schizophrenia and bipolar disorder, and it has generally been assumed that dozens of genes, along with environmental factors, contribute to disease risk.

"The consortium is the largest research consortium ever in psychiatry and is certainly the largest biological experiment we've ever done in the field," Sullivan said. "We are studying on the order of ninety thousand individuals across multiple disorders, while trying to do something for the greater good, which is effectively to go as far and as deep as we can in understanding the genomics of mental illness."

The research was funded by numerous European, U.S., and Australian funding bodies. Funds for coordination of the consortium were provided by the National Institute of Mental Health in Bethesda, Maryland.

Chapter 54

Diabetes and Genetics

Major Collaboration Uncovers Surprising New Genetic Clues to Diabetes

An international team that included scientists from the National Human Genome Research Institute (NHGRI), part of the National Institutes of Health (NIH), reported on March 31, 2008, that it has identified six more genetic variants involved in type 2 diabetes, boosting to sixteen the total number of genetic risk factors associated with increased risk of the disease. None of the genetic variants uncovered by the new study had previously been suspected of playing a role in type 2 diabetes. Intriguingly, the new variant most strongly associated with type 2 diabetes also was recently implicated in a very different condition: prostate cancer.

The unprecedented analysis, published on March 31, 2008, in the advance online edition of *Nature Genetics*, combined genetic data from more than seventy thousand people. The work was carried out through the collaborative efforts of more than ninety researchers at more than forty centers in Europe and North America.

"Major Collaboration Uncovers Surprising New Genetic Clues to Diabetes," is excerpted from the National Human Genome Research Institute (NHGRI; www .genome.gov), March 31, 2008. Editor's note added by David A. Cooke, M.D., FACP, May 2013. "Researchers Identify Genetic Elements Influencing the Risk of Type 2 Diabetes" is excerpted from "NIH Researchers Identify Genetic Elements Influencing the Risk of Type 2 Diabetes," NHGRI, March 12, 2012.

"None of the genes we have found was previously on the radar screen of diabetes researchers," said one of the paper's senior authors, Mark McCarthy, M.D., of the University of Oxford in England. "Each of these genes, therefore, provides new clues to the processes that go wrong when diabetes develops, and each provides an opportunity for the generation of new approaches for treating or preventing this condition."

When considered individually, the genetic variants discovered to date account for only small differences in the risk of developing type 2 diabetes. But researchers say when all of the variants are analyzed together, some significant differences in risk are likely to emerge. "By combining information from the large number of genes now implicated in diabetes risk, it may be possible to use genetic tools to identify people at unusually high or low risk of diabetes. However, until we know how to use this information to prompt beneficial changes in people's treatment or lifestyle, widespread genetic testing would be premature," said another senior author, David Altshuler, M.D., Ph.D., of Massachusetts General Hospital in Boston and the Broad Institute of Massachusetts Institute of Technology and Harvard in Cambridge, Massachusetts.

Type 2 diabetes affects more than two hundred million people worldwide, including nearly twenty-one million people in the United States. Previously known as adult-onset, or non-insulin-dependent diabetes mellitus (NIDDM), type 2 diabetes usually appears after age forty, often in overweight, sedentary people. However, a growing number of younger people—and even children—are developing the disease.

Diabetes is a major cause of heart disease and stroke in U.S. adults, as well as the most common cause of blindness, kidney failure, and amputations not related to trauma. Type 2 diabetes is characterized by the resistance of target tissues to respond to insulin, which controls glucose levels in the blood; and a gradual failure of insulin-secreting cells in the pancreas.

"These new variants, along with other recent genetic findings, provide a window into disease causation that may be our best hope for the next generation of therapeutics. By pinpointing particular pathways involved in diabetes risk, these discoveries can empower new approaches to understanding environmental influences and to the development of new, more precisely targeted drugs," said NHGRI Director Francis S. Collins, M.D., Ph.D., who is a co-author of the study. Dr. Collins's laboratory is a participant in the FINRISK 2002 and Finland-United States Investigation of NIDDM Genetics (FUSION), which were among the studies that contributed data to the new analysis. FUSION is funded by NHGRI's Division of Intramural Research and the National Institute of Diabetes and Digestive and Kidney Diseases (NIDDK).

Researchers said more work is needed to understand the impact of their discovery that a genetic variant called JAZF1 appears to be involved in diabetes as well as prostate cancer. One of the study's lead authors, Eleftheria Zeggini, Ph.D., of the University of Oxford, said, "This is now the second example of a gene which affects both type 2 diabetes and prostate cancer. We don't yet know what the connections are, but this may have important implications for the future design of drugs for both of these conditions."

The research was conducted by the DIAbetes Genetics Replication And Meta-analysis (DIAGRAM) consortium, which brought together many groups active in the field of diabetes research. In the *Nature Genetics* paper, DIAGRAM researchers combined the data from three previously published genome-wide association studies in an effort to boost the statistical power of their searches—an approach that scientists refer to as meta-analysis. The strategy paid off, enabling researchers to identify six genetic variants associated with type 2 diabetes that had gone undetected in the smaller, individual studies.

Editor's note: Further research has indicated that changes in the JAZF1 gene affect risk for both type II diabetes and prostate cancer, but that they are not the same mutations. In other words, certain JAZF1 mutations increase diabetes risk, and certain other JAZF1 mutations increase prostate cancer risk, but there isn't a mutation that increases risk for both diseases. How the JAZF1 gene plays a role in these diseases remains under study.

While a number of genes that affect risk for type 2 diabetes have now been identified, only a small proportion of cases appear to be due to particular gene mutations. Current data suggest that diabetes risk is controlled by a number of genes acting in concert. No single gene will determine whether a person develops diabetes; it is the interaction of many different genes with each other and environmental factors.

Researchers Identify Genetic Elements Influencing the Risk of Type 2 Diabetes

A team led by researchers at the National Human Genome Research Institute (NHGRI), part of the National Institutes of Health (NIH), has captured the most comprehensive snapshot to date of deoxyribonucleic acid (DNA) regions that regulate genes in human pancreatic islet cells, a subset of which produces insulin.

The study highlights the importance of genome regulatory sequences in human health and disease, particularly type 2 diabetes, which affects more than twenty million people in the United States and two hundred million people worldwide. The findings appeared November 3, 2010, in *Cell Metabolism*.

"This study applies the power of epigenomics to a common disease with both inherited and environmental causes," said NHGRI Scientific Director Daniel Kastner, M.D., Ph.D. "Epigenomic studies are exciting new avenues for genomic analysis, providing the opportunity to peer deeper into genome function, and giving rise to new insights about our genome's adaptability and potential."

Epigenomic research focuses on the mechanisms that regulate the expression of genes in the human genome. Genetic information is written in the chemical language of DNA, a long molecule of nucleic acid wound around specialized proteins called histones. Together, they constitute chromatin, the DNA-protein complex that forms chromosomes during cell division. The researchers used DNA sequencing technology to search the chromatin of islet cells for specific histone modifications and other signals marking regulatory DNA. Computational analysis of the large amounts of DNA sequence data generated in this study identified different classes of regulatory DNA.

"This study gives us an encyclopedia of regulatory elements in islet cells of the human pancreas that may be important for normal function and whose potential dysfunction can contribute to disease," said senior author and NIH Director Francis S. Collins, M.D., Ph.D. "These elements represent an important component of the uncharted genetic underpinnings of type-2 diabetes that is outside of protein-coding genes."

Among the results, the researchers detected about eighteen thousand promoters, which are regulatory sequences immediately adjacent to the start of genes. Promoters are like molecular on-off switches and more than one switch can control a gene. Several hundred of these were previously unknown and found to be highly active in the islet cells.

"Along the way, we also hit upon some unexpected but fascinating findings," said co-lead author Praveen Sethupathy, Ph.D., NHGRI postdoctoral fellow. "For example, some of the most important regulatory DNA in the islet, involved in controlling hormones such as insulin, completely lacked typical histone modifications, suggesting an unconventional mode of gene regulation."

The researchers also identified at least thirty-four thousand distal regulatory elements, so called because they are farther away from the genes. Many of these were bunched together, suggesting they may cooperate to form regulatory modules. These modules may be unique to islets and play an important role in the maintenance of blood glucose levels.

"Genome-wide association studies have told us there are genetic differences between type 2 diabetic and nondiabetic individuals in specific regions of the genome, but substantial efforts are required to understand how these differences contribute to disease," said co-lead author Michael Stitzel, Ph.D., NHGRI postdoctoral fellow. "Defining regulatory elements in human islets is a critical first step to understanding the molecular and biological effects for some of the genetic variants statistically associated with type 2 diabetes."

The researchers also found that fifty single nucleotide polymorphisms, or genetic variants, associated with islet-related traits or diseases are located within or very close to nonpromoter regulatory elements. Variants associated with type 2 diabetes are present in six such elements that function to boost gene activity. These results suggest that regulatory elements may be a key component to understanding the molecular defects that contribute to type 2 diabetes.

Genetic association data pertaining to diabetes or other measures of islet function continue to be generated. The catalog of islet regulatory elements generated in the study provides an openly accessible resource for anyone to reference and ask whether newly emerging, statistically associated variants are falling within these regulatory elements. The raw data can be found at the National Center for Biotechnology Information's Gene Expression Omnibus using accession number GSE23784.

"These findings represent important strides that were not possible just five years ago, but that are now realized with advances in genome sequencing technologies," said NHGRI Director Eric D. Green, M.D., Ph.D. "The power of DNA sequencing is allowing us to go from studies of a few genes at a time to profiling the entire genome. The scale is tremendously expanded."

Chapter 55

Heart Disease and Genetics

Chapter Contents

Section 55.1

How Genetics Impact Heart Disease Risk

Genetics can influence the risk for heart disease in many ways. Genes control every aspect of the cardiovascular system, from the strength of the blood vessels to the way cells in the heart communicate. For many common conditions, such as coronary artery disease, stroke, atrial fibrillation, and diabetes, there are many risk factors—genetic, lifestyle, and environmental—that increase a person's risk of developing the disease.

Genetic tests do not currently exist to measure individual risk for most cardiovascular diseases because the specific genetic factors are not yet fully understood. This makes family history, along with information about patient lifestyle and environment, one of the most important tools doctors have for assessing individual risk. When a family member is diagnosed with cardiovascular disease, other family members may be encouraged to undergo screening to detect early stages of disease.

Aspects of family history that indicate a higher risk for heart disease include:

- early onset of cardiovascular disease, for instance coronary artery disease in men younger than fifty-five and women younger than sixty-five;

- cardiovascular disease in two or three relatives on the same side of the family;

- late onset of cardiovascular disease on both sides of the family;

- the loss of a family member to sudden cardiac death.

With the appropriate medical treatment, people at increased risk for heart disease can delay the onset and lessen the severity of the disease.

While coronary artery disease, stroke, and diabetes are common diseases with many contributing factors, other less common cardiac conditions have a stronger genetic component. Genetic testing can be used to diagnose conditions such as hypertrophic cardiomyopathy, long QT syndrome, and similar arrhythmia conditions that can run in families. A genetic variation (mutation) in a single gene can be detected in some patients and identify the underlying genetic cause of the disease.

Inherited conditions that lead to arrhythmias and sudden cardiac death are particularly well understood. These conditions fall into two categories. One group of conditions results from problems with the flow of certain molecules between the cells in the heart. An imbalance of these molecules can impair the electrical impulses that control the heartbeat. Examples of these conditions include:

- **Brugada syndrome:** A genetic disorder of the heart rhythm that can cause ventricular fibrillation and sudden cardiac arrest.

- **CPVT (catecholaminergic polymorphic ventricular tachycardia):** A disorder of the calcium channels in the heart muscle, resulting in problems with electrical signaling and irregular heartbeats, especially during exercise, and even sudden cardiac death.

- **Long QT syndrome:** A prolonged electrical recovery phase (QT interval) of the heartbeat that can result in rapid, chaotic beats and sudden cardiac death.

The second group of conditions results from changes in the structure of the heart. These conditions can also cause abnormal heart rhythms, but typically they are diagnosed due to changes in the size of the heart chambers or thickness of the heart muscle. Hypertrophic cardiomyopathy and arrhythmogenic right ventricular cardiomyopathy can both cause deadly arrhythmias.

Genetic testing is available for inherited arrhythmias. Patients with these conditions should be referred to a specialized clinic for expert evaluation and genetic counseling.

Action Tips

- Make sure your family doctor knows.

- Discuss risk and lifestyle with your children and siblings.

- As some diseases are more common in some families, your own risk may be higher than average. The higher risk may be caused by genes you have inherited. Or it may be because people in the same family tend to be alike in the choices they make about diet and healthy living. Having a family history means that you should try to make lifestyle changes to reduce your risk.

Section 55.2

Genetic Link to Aortic Valve Disease Discovered

Researchers at the Sainte-Justine University Hospital Center and University of Montreal have identified genetic origins in 10 percent of an important form of congenital heart diseases by studying the genetic variability within families. "This is more than the sum of the genes found to date in all previous studies, which explained only 1 percent of the disease," says Dr. Marc-Phillip Hitz, lead author of the study published in *PLoS Genetics*, under the direction of Dr. Gregor Andelfinger, pediatric cardiologist and principal investigator leading an international research team, who calls this study "a very important step towards a molecular catalog, which ultimately may explain the evolution of disease in individual patients and allow us to influence the progression of the disease."

Congenital heart malformations are at the forefront of all malformations in newborns, and one of the most important causes of infant mortality in Western countries. For their study, the researchers focused on malformations of the aortic valve, where familial clustering of cases often suggests a hereditary component. The researchers therefore decided to adopt a "family approach" and selected families with several members having a heart condition, in order to be able to establish a direct link with the disease. Using very strict filtering criteria to identify possible causal copy number variants—a structural form of variation of the genetic makeup that leads to an increase or decrease in the copy number of small parts of deoxyribonucleic acid (DNA) within the genome—the researchers retained only rare variants directly involved in the disease processes and causing severe adverse health effects. The variants had to be carried by the patients but not by healthy members of their family. Researchers then validated the identified genes by confirming that they were highly expressed in the developing mouse heart.

The study also noted that many affected patients carried more than one rare variant. This finding had already been made in the context of other congenital diseases. In addition, the study reveals that in the fifty-nine families analyzed, no copy number variants recurred between two families. "Despite the homogeneity of the French-Canadian population as compared to other populations and similarities seen within families, we realize that copy number variants are very different between families with no genealogical connection. From a genetic point of view, the diseases we looked at are a 'family affair.'"

Moreover, although the study focused on the aortic valve area, genes explaining associated conditions have been identified. "It is striking that the majority of the identified genes also play an important role in blood vessels, not just in the valves of the heart," says Dr. Andelfinger. Indeed, the images are of striking clarity: expression patterns of the genes identified selectively stain areas of the heart where lesions are observed. "Numerous patients continue to have problems after successful initial intervention on the aortic valve, such as aortic dilation. Our study sheds new light on the link between the two issues, something we always observed clinically but had a hard time to explain," he concludes.

Section 55.3

New Research on Genetic Ties to Heart Attack, Arrhythmia, and Coronary Artery Disease

Common Gene Variant May Increase Risk for a Type of Cardiac Arrhythmia

An international research team has identified a common gene variant associated with a form of the irregular heartbeat called atrial fibrillation. In their report in the journal *Nature Genetics*, published online, the investigators describe finding that variations affecting a protein that may help control the heart's electrical activity appear to increase the risk of what is called lone atrial fibrillation (AF), a type seen in younger individuals with no other form of heart disease.

"The genetic location we have identified could be a new drug target for the treatment of AF," says Patrick Ellinor, M.D., PhD, of the Massachusetts General Hospital (MGH) Cardiovascular Research Center and Cardiac Arrhythmia Service, a co-corresponding author of the report. "We also will be investigating whether these variants can help us predict patients' clinical outcomes or their response to the various treatments for AF."

The most common type of irregular heartbeat, atrial fibrillation affects more than 2.2 million people in the United States. In AF the upper chambers of the heart, called the atria, beat in a rapid and uncoordinated fashion, which can cause blood to pool within the heart. If blood clots form within the heart, they can break loose, travel to the brain, and cause a stroke. While AF is most commonly seen in older individuals with hypertension, heart failure, or other forms of heart disease, about 10 percent of AF patients begin having symptoms when they are younger and have no other known cardiovascular disease, a condition called lone AF.

Patients with lone AF are more likely to have overt symptoms and to require treatment, which includes the use of blood-thinning drugs to prevent clots and other medications that slow heart rhythm. If AF persists, procedures such as minimally invasive catheter ablation can inactivate the regions of the heart that trigger the arrhythmia.

Family history is known to increase the risk of AF and plays a larger role in lone AF. Several earlier genome-wide association studies (GWAS) linked gene variants on chromosomes 4 and 16 to increased risk for both forms of AF. To search for additional variants associated with the more heritable lone AF, the research team conducted a meta-analysis of five previous GWAS studies involving more than 1,300 individuals with lone AF—defined for this study as those with no other heart disease whose symptoms began before age sixty-five—and almost 13,000 unaffected participants.

The analysis associated lone AF with several common variants on a segment of chromosome 1. The most significant variants were found in the gene for KCNN3, a potassium channel protein that carries signals across cell membranes in organs including the brain and the heart. While the exact cardiac role of the protein is unknown, it may play a part in resetting the electrical activity of the atria, a process that goes awry in AF. Animal studies have suggested that a related protein, KCNN2, may help control signals originating in the atria and in the pulmonary veins, areas known to be involved in lone AF. The researchers replicated the association of KCNN3 variants with lone AF in data from two additional GWAS studies involving another 1,000 lone AF patients and 3,500 controls.

Ellinor, an assistant professor of medicine at Harvard Medical School, and his colleagues note that additional study is required to clarify exactly how variations in KCNN3 and associated genes may affect the risk for lone AF, whether these and other gene variants can predict how a patient's symptoms will progress, and to investigate their usefulness as treatment targets. The study was supported by a wide range of public and private funders, including the National Institutes of Health.

Common Gene Variants Influence Risk for Sudden Cardiac Death

A new study has identified several common genetic variants related to a risk factor for sudden cardiac death. The report receiving early online release in the journal *Nature Genetics* identifies variants in genes, some known and some newly discovered, that influence the QT interval measured on the electrocardiogram (EKG) performed routinely in doctors' offices. These findings could eventually help to prevent sudden cardiac death and arrhythmia by limiting the use of medications that affect QT interval in people with these variants.

The QT interval is the time from the beginning of electrical activation of the heart to the end of electrical relaxation. "It is well established that prolongation of the QT interval in the general population is a potent and heritable risk factor for sudden death. In addition, QT prolongation results from medications leading to drug-induced cardiac arrhythmias and sudden death. This is a cardiotoxic side effect of scores of medications in widespread use and has been a major barrier to the development of novel drugs. From studies of families with congenital long QT syndrome, we know that rare mutations with strong effects on ion channel function lead to QT prolongation and sudden death. But the common genetic basis for QT prolongation has been very difficult to establish," said Christopher Newton-Cheh, M.D., MPH, of the Massachusetts General Hospital Center for Human Genetic Research and Cardiovascular Research Center (CVRC) and lead author of the *Nature Genetics* article.

To search for QT-associated variants, the investigators formed the QTGEN consortium, assembling more than thirteen thousand individuals from three studies, including the National Heart, Lung and Blood Institute's and Boston University's Framingham Heart Study, the Rotterdam Study, and the Cardiovascular Health Study. All individuals had undergone testing of hundreds of thousands of common variations called single-nucleotide polymorphisms (SNPs).

By pooling results from the three studies, investigators identified fourteen common variants in ten different gene regions (some regions had more than one variant) that were related to QT interval duration. A separate companion paper from the QTSCD consortium published by *Nature Genetics* and led by Arne Pfeufer, M.D. (Technical University Munich) and Aravinda Chakravarti, PhD (Johns Hopkins) included more than fifteen thousand individuals from Europe and the United States. This independent study strongly confirmed twelve out of fourteen of the QTGEN variants, and identified two additional gene regions. "We were very reassured to see such strong replication in two independent studies," said Newton-Cheh.

The QTGEN investigators examined the effect of a genotype score comprised of all fourteen variants tested together. The top 20 percent of the population with the highest genotype scores had 160–210 percent higher risk of prolonged QT interval compared to the 20 percent of the population with the lowest scores. They also had ~10 millisecond longer QT intervals, which is approximately the degree of QT interval prolongation observed for some drugs pulled from the market for arrhythmias.

"While it is commonly a combination of risk factors that contributes to drug-induced arrhythmias—such as older age, female sex, use of other medications, or heart disease—it is certainly possible that common genetic variants will add incrementally to risk prediction," said Newton-Cheh. "It's currently premature to advocate screening gene variants for risk assessment, but someday it may be possible to identify individuals who are at particularly high risk and should avoid such medications."

Newton-Cheh adds, "It's likely that many more genes will be found to contribute to changes in QT interval, and the real challenge will be understanding the mechanism behind their effects. Five of the gene regions we identified had never before been implicated in QT interval physiology and these genetic observations may thus provide key insights into normal and abnormal human biology."

International Collaborative Identifies Thirteen New Heart-Disease-Associated Gene Sites

An international research collaboration has identified thirteen new gene sites associated with the risk of coronary artery disease and validated ten sites found in previous studies. Several of the novel sites discovered in the study, which is being published online in *Nature Genetics*, do not appear to relate to known risk factors, suggesting previously unsuspected mechanisms for cardiovascular disease.

"We now have identified twenty-three specific genetic 'letters' that appear to confer risk for myocardial infarction and other aspects of coronary artery disease," says Sekar Kathiresan, M.D., director of preventive cardiology at Massachusetts General Hospital and one of several co-lead authors of the report. "Knowing these sites lays the groundwork for isolating the genes responsible and developing new treatments based on those genes."

Although inherited factors may account for as much as 60 percent of the variation in risk for coronary artery disease, variants identified in genome-wide association studies (GWAS) account for only a small fraction of that risk. Since some of those previous studies may not have been large enough to identify genes with modest effect, 167 investigators at research centers around the world formed the Coronary ARtery DIsease Genome-wide Replication and Meta-analysis (CARDIoGRAM) Consortium.

The researchers first assembled data from fourteen previous GWAS for meta-analysis—a technique that combines results from several studies into a larger sample—which reviewed data from more than 22,000 individuals with heart disease and almost 65,000 controls. The most promising sites identified in the meta-analysis were then genotyped in another group of more than 56,600 individuals, about half with cardiac disease. The investigators also analyzed potential mechanisms and metabolic pathways by which newly identified variants might affect risk.

Results of the analyses confirmed ten of twelve previously reported gene variants associated with coronary artery disease and identified thirteen sites not previously reported. While most of these variants were most strongly associated with early-onset heart disease, the associations did not vary with the actual clinical condition for which patients were treated—heart attack or coronary artery disease requiring bypass surgery or angioplasty/stenting. Of the twenty-three variants validated in this study, seven are associated with low-density lipoprotein (LDL) cholesterol levels and one with hypertension, but the others have no relation to known cardiovascular risk factors.

"The lack of apparent association with the risk factors we know so well is the source of a lot of excitement concerning these results," Kathiresan explains. "If these variants do not act through known mechanisms, how do they confer risk for heart disease? It suggests there are new mechanisms we don't yet understand. Another good thing about these findings is that they are in human patients, not in cells or mice, which gives us a good starting point for figuring out new disease pathways."

International Study Identifies Gene Variants Associated with Early Heart Attack

The largest study ever completed of genetic factors associated with heart attacks has identified nine genetic regions—three not previously described—that appear to increase the risk for early-onset myocardial infarction. The report from the Myocardial Infarction Genetics Consortium, based on information from a total of twenty-six thousand individuals in ten countries, will appear in *Nature Genetics* and is receiving early online release.

"For several decades, it has been known that the risk for heart attack—the leading cause of death and disability in the United States—clusters in families and that some of this familial clustering is due to differences in deoxyribonucleic acid (DNA) sequence," says

Sekar Kathiresan, M.D., director of preventive cardiology at Massachusetts General Hospital (MGH) and corresponding author of the *Nature Genetics* report. "We set out to find specific, single-letter differences in the genome, what are called single-nucleotide polymorphisms (SNPs), that may be responsible for an increased familial risk for heart attack."

Groundwork for the current study was laid more than ten years ago when co-author Christopher O'Donnell, M.D., now based at the Framingham Heart Study, began to gather data on patients treated at the MGH for early-onset heart attack—men under fifty and women under sixty. Kathiresan soon joined the project, and in 2006 they formed the Myocardial Infarction Genetics Consortium along with David Altshuler, M.D., PhD, of the MGH Center for Human Genetic Research and the Broad Institute of the Massachusetts Institute of Technology (MIT) and Harvard, eventually involving six groups around the world that had collected samples on a total of about three thousand early-onset heart attack patients and three thousand healthy controls.

The current study took advantage of several scientific tools developed over the past decade. These include the International Haplotype Map, a comprehensive map of SNPs across the genome; genotyping arrays that allow screening of hundreds of thousands of SNPs at once; and a gene chip developed by Altshuler's team that can simultaneously screen for SNPs and for copy-number variants—deletions or duplications of gene segments, a type of change associated with several disease categories. After analysis of the consortium's samples identified SNPs that could be associated with heart attack risk, the researchers ran replication screens in three independent groups of samples, resulting in a total of thirteen thousand heart attack patients and thirteen thousand controls.

Significant associations with the risk of early-onset heart attacks were found for common SNPs in nine genetic regions. Three of those associations with heart attack risk were identified for the first time; and one of the novel regions also had been found, in a separate study by O'Donnell, to promote the buildup of atherosclerotic plaque in the coronary arteries. To analyze the effect of inheriting several risk-associated SNPs, participants were assigned a genotype score, which revealed that those with the highest number of risk-associated variants had more than twice the risk of an early-onset heart attack as those with the fewest. No risk associations were identified with copy-number variants.

Although the increased risk associated with individual SNPs is small, knowledge gained from the association could prove extremely valuable. "One of the known variants we identified is at a gene called

PCSK9, which was originally identified in 2003," explains Kathiresan, an assistant professor of medicine at Harvard Medical School. "Extensive study of that gene region has led to significant insight into the biology of atherosclerosis and heart attack and to efforts to develop targeted drugs. We are optimistic that investigating the mechanics of the newly mapped variants could yield similar insights. And since we already have effective ways to reduce heart-attack risk, individuals at higher genetic risk may benefit from earlier intervention, something that needs to be tested in future studies."

Chapter 56

Hypertension: Research Reveals Genetic Links

Chapter Contents

Section 56.1

Research Uncovers Genetic Clues to Blood Pressure

Excerpted from "Researchers Uncover Genetic Clues to Blood Pressure,"
an NIH News Release, National Institutes of Health, May 10, 2009.

An international research team has identified a number of unsuspected genetic variants associated with systolic blood pressure (SBP), diastolic blood pressure (DBP), and hypertension (high blood pressure), suggesting potential avenues of investigation for the prevention or treatment of hypertension. The research was funded in part by the National Heart, Lung, and Blood Institute (NHLBI) of the National Institutes of Health (NIH) and by several other NIH institutes and centers.

The analysis of over twenty-nine thousand participants was presented at the American Society of Hypertension, Inc. scientific meeting on May 8, 2009, and was published online in the journal *Nature Genetics* on May 10, 2009.

"This study provides important new insights into the biology of blood pressure regulation and, with continued research, may lead to the development of novel therapeutic approaches to combat hypertension and its complications," said NHLBI Director Elizabeth G. Nabel, M.D.

About one in three adults (approximately seventy-two million people) in the United States has high blood pressure. Hypertension can lead to coronary heart disease, heart failure, stroke, kidney failure, and other health problems, and causes over seven million deaths worldwide each year.

Blood pressure has a substantial genetic component, and hypertension runs in families. Previous attempts to identify genes associated with blood pressure, however, have met with limited success.

In a genome-wide association study (GWAS), researchers scanned millions of common genetic variants of individuals from the Cohorts for Heart and Aging Research in Genomic Epidemiology (CHARGE) consortium to find variants associated with blood pressure and hypertension. This extensive resource includes white men and women from the Framingham Heart Study, Atherosclerosis Risk in Communities study, Cardiovascular Health Study, the Rotterdam Study, the Rotterdam Extension Study, and the Age, Gene/Environment Susceptibility Reykjavik Study.

The investigators identified a number of genetic variants or single-nucleotide polymorphisms (SNPs) associated with SBP, DBP, and hypertension. When they jointly analyzed their findings with those from the GWAS of over thirty-four thousand participants in the Global BPgen Consortium (whose results are presented in an accompanying paper in the same issue of *Nature Genetics*), they identified eleven genes showing significant associations across the genome: four for SBP, six for DBP, and one for hypertension.

"Large-scale genome-wide association studies are providing a number of important insights into identifying genes that play a role in diseases with major public health impact," said Dr. Daniel Levy, first author of the study and director, the NHLBI's Framingham Heart Study and Center for Population Studies. "We have identified eight key genes, few of which would have been on anyone's short list of suspected blood pressure genes until now."

The international research team included Cornelia M. van Duijn, Ph.D., Erasmus Medical Center, Rotterdam, the Netherlands; Aravinda Chakravarti, Ph.D., Johns Hopkins University; Bruce Psaty, M.D., Ph.D., University of Washington; and Vilmundur Gudnason, M.D., Ph.D., Icelandic Heart Association, Kopayogur, Iceland.

The blood pressure genes include ATP2B1, which encodes PMCA1, a cell membrane enzyme that is involved in calcium transport; CACNB2, which encodes part of a calcium channel protein; and CYP17A1, which encodes an enzyme that is necessary for steroid production. One detected variant is within the gene SH2B3 and has been associated with autoimmune diseases, hinting that pathways involved with the immune response may influence blood pressure.

Blood pressure is measured in millimeters of mercury (mm Hg), and expressed with two numbers, for example, 120/80 mm Hg. The first number (systolic pressure) is the pressure when the heart beats while pumping blood. The second number (diastolic pressure) is the pressure in large arteries when the heart is at rest between beats.

Researchers found that the top ten gene variants, or SNPs, for systolic and diastolic blood pressure were each associated with around a 1 and 0.5 mm Hg increase in systolic and diastolic blood pressure, respectively. The prevalence of hypertension increased as the number of variants increased.

People who carry very few blood pressure genetic risk variants have blood pressure levels that are several mm Hg lower than those who carry multiple risk variants. In practical terms this is enough to increase the risk for cardiovascular disease. A prolonged increase in DBP of only 5 mm Hg is associated with a 34 percent increase in risk for stroke and a 21 percent increase of coronary heart disease.

Section 56.2

Study Identifies New Gene Targets for Hypertension Treatment

A new report from scientists at Massachusetts General Hospital (MGH) and their colleagues in centers around the world finds that common variants in twenty-eight regions of deoxyribonucleic acid (DNA) are associated with blood pressure in human patients. Of the identified regions, most were completely unsuspected, although some harbor genes suspected of influencing blood pressure based on animal studies. In the study receiving advance online publication in *Nature*, members of the International Consortium for Blood Pressure Genome-Wide Association Studies (ICBP-GWAS) analyzed genetic data from over 275,000 individuals from around the world. They also identified for the first time the involvement of an important physiologic pathway in blood pressure control, potentially leading to a totally new class of hypertension drugs.

"Identifying these novel pathways expands our current understanding of the determinants of blood pressure and highlights potential targets for new drugs to treat and prevent cardiovascular complications," says Christopher Newton-Cheh, MD, MPH, of the MGH Center for Human Genetic Research and the Cardiovascular Research Center, co-chair of the ICBP-GWAS Steering Committee and a senior and corresponding author on the *Nature* paper.

It is well known that hypertension can run in families and that some rare genetic syndromes raise blood pressure, but identifying genes associated with the common form of hypertension has been challenging. To get a study sample large enough to detect variants with modest effects, ICBP-GWAS researchers conducted a meta-analysis of thirty genome-wide association studies that included measurements of participants' blood pressures. Analysis of 2.5 million DNA sequence variants in more than 69,000 individuals of European ancestry identified several chromosomal regions where genes influencing blood pressure appeared to be located. To confirm the results of the first-stage analysis, the researchers genotyped the strongest variants in more than 133,000 additional individuals of European descent. Combining the results identified twenty-eight gene regions associated with both systolic and diastolic blood pressure, of which sixteen were novel. A second paper from the consortium also receiving online publication on September 11, 2011, in *Nature Genetics*, identified six additional novel variants.

Some of the new variants were already known to cause other diseases. "We were quite astonished to see that two common variants known for decades to cause hemochromatosis—an iron overload condition that affects as many as one in three hundred Americans—were also associated with higher blood pressure," says Newton-Cheh. "The hemochromatosis genes are part of a physiologic pathway that is also involved in pulmonary hypertension, but this finding opens our eyes to its potential involvement in systemic hypertension."

To test whether the blood pressure variants identified in Europeans were associated with blood pressure in other ethnicities, the consortium genotyped almost 74,000 individuals of either East Asian, South Asian, or African ancestries. Genetic risk scores incorporating all identified variants were strongly associated with blood pressure levels in each of those groups and also with the risk of stroke and coronary heart disease. "Seeing that the blood pressure variants in aggregate lead to stroke and heart attack was perhaps not surprising, given the evidence that blood pressure treatment lowers these risks," said Newton-Cheh.

But the most important finding may be identification of a new pathway central to blood pressure regulation. Three of the twenty-eight blood-pressure-associated regions include genes that are part of a pathway called the cyclic guanosine monophosphate (cGMP) system, which is involved in the relaxation of blood vessels and excretion of sodium by the kidneys, two fundamental mechanisms of hypertension treatment. Animal studies have suggested a role for this pathway in blood pressure control, and the current findings strongly support its relevance in human patients.

"We have previously shown that variants in natriuretic peptide genes, part of the cGMP system, influence blood pressure. We were therefore pleased but not surprised to see other genes that influence the cGMP system in this recent crop of discoveries," said Newton-Cheh, an assistant professor of Medicine at Harvard Medical School. "The greatest attention in blood pressure research has been focused on another pathway called the renin-angiotensin-aldosterone system (RAAS), which is targeted by several hypertension therapies. But only one common gene variant has been associated with genes in the RAAS pathway.

"Finding several independent associations that converge on cGMP points to its central importance in blood pressure control," he adds. "In fact, there are several drugs that target these systems in development to treat pulmonary hypertension and heart failure, but our findings suggest that they could have a much larger role in hypertension treatment in general. The next phase of our research will focus on finding additional genes and variants that influence blood pressure and on establishing how some of the cGMP-involved genes affect blood pressure in humans and respond to existing drugs and to those in development."

Section 56.3

Study Identifies Key Genetic Mechanisms That Help Control High Blood Pressure

"Breakthrough in Understanding the Genetics of High Blood Pressure," November 9, 2011. Reprinted with permission from the University of Leicester Press Office. © 2011 University of Leicester (http://www.le.ac.uk). All rights reserved.

A researcher from the University of Leicester's Department of Cardiovascular Sciences has been involved in a groundbreaking study into the causes of high blood pressure.

The study, published in the academic journal *Hypertension*, analyzed genetic material in human kidneys in a search for genes that might contribute to high blood pressure. The findings open up new avenues for future investigation into the causes of high blood pressure in humans.

The study identified key genes, messenger ribonucleic acids (RNAs) and micro RNAs present in the kidneys that may contribute to human hypertension. It also uncovered two microRNAs that contribute to the regulation of renin—a hormone long thought to play a part in controlling blood pressure.

Although scientists have long known that the kidneys play a role in regulating blood pressure, this is the first time that key genes involved in the process have been identified through a large, comprehensive gene expression analysis of the human kidneys. It is also the first time that researchers have identified micro RNAs that control the expression of the hormone renin.

The scientists studied tissue samples from the kidneys of fifteen male hypertensive patients (patients with high blood pressure) and seven male patients with normal blood pressure, and compared their messenger RNA (mRNA) and micro RNA (miRNA).

Messenger RNA (mRNA) is a single-stranded molecule that helps in the production of protein from deoxyribonucleic acid (DNA). Genetic information is copied from DNA to mRNA strands, which provide a template from which the cell can make new proteins. MicroRNA (miRNA) is a very small molecule that helps regulate the process of converting mRNA into proteins.

The study was co-authored by the University of Leicester's Dr. Maciej Tomaszewski, Senior Clinical Lecturer in Cardiovascular Medicine in the Department of Cardiovascular Sciences, and a Consultant Physician in Leicester Blood Pressure Clinic - European Centre of Excellence.

Dr. Tomaszewski commented: "I am very excited about this publication. Renin is one of the most important contributors to blood pressure regulation. The novel insights into its expression within the human kidney from this study open up new avenues for the development of new antihypertensive medications. The collection of hypertensive and normotensive kidneys is available for our studies in Leicester thanks to a long-term international collaboration. We will continue using this unique research resource in our further studies to decipher the genetic background of human hypertension."

Researchers described the discovery of these miRNAs as "the first real evidence to implicate renin" as a cause of high blood pressure. The findings also indicate which genes and miRNAs are involved in renin production. This increased understanding of the mechanisms underlying hypertension could lead to innovative new treatments for high blood pressure.

Researchers used samples of human kidneys stored in the Silesian Renal Tissue Bank (SRTB), all of which came from Polish males, individuals of white European ancestry. The SRTB stores human kidney samples for use in genetic research into cardiovascular diseases. Samples were selected from fifteen patients known to have high blood pressure, along with seven patients with normal blood pressure who were used as a control group for the study. The scientists used a range of techniques to study the genes, mRNAs, and miRNAs present in the medulla (the inner part of the kidney) and the cortex (the outer part).

Chapter 57

Heredity and Movement Disorders

Chapter Contents

Section 57.1

Genetics of
Essential Tremor

Excerpted from "Essential Tremor," Genetics Home Reference (http://ghr.nlm.nih.gov), February 2008. Reviewed by David A. Cooke, M.D., FACP, May 2013.

What is essential tremor?

Essential tremor is a disorder of the nervous system that causes involuntary, rhythmic shaking (tremor), especially in the hands. It involves tremor without any other signs or symptoms, and is distinguished from tremor that results from other disorders or known causes, such as tremors seen with Parkinson disease or head trauma.

Essential tremor usually occurs when the muscles are opposing gravity, such as when the hands are extended, and worsens with movement. This type of tremor is usually not evident at rest.

In addition to the hands and arms, muscles of the trunk, face, head, and neck may also exhibit tremor in this disorder; the legs and feet are not usually involved.

Head tremor may appear as a "yes-yes" or "no-no" movement while the affected individual is seated or standing. In some people with essential tremor, voice quality may be affected.

Essential tremor is not considered a dangerous or debilitating condition, and it does not shorten the lifespan. If severe, however, it may interfere somewhat with fine motor skills such as using eating utensils, writing, shaving, or applying makeup.

Symptoms of essential tremor may be aggravated by emotional stress, fatigue, hunger, caffeine, cigarette smoking, or extremes of temperature.

Essential tremor may appear at any age, but is most common in the elderly. Some studies have suggested that people with essential tremor may have a higher than average risk of developing Parkinson disease, sensory problems such as hearing loss, or other neurological conditions, while others suggest that essential tremor may be associated with increased longevity.

How common is essential tremor?

Essential tremor is a common disorder, affecting millions of people in the United States. Estimates of its prevalence vary widely because several other disorders, as well as certain medications and other factors, can result in similar tremors. Essential tremor may affect as many as 14 percent of people over the age of sixty-five.

What genes are related to essential tremor?

Essential tremor is a complex disorder. Several genes are believed to help determine an individual's risk of developing this condition. Environmental factors may also be involved.

Some studies have found the DRD3 gene to be associated with essential tremor. The DRD3 gene provides instructions for making a protein called dopamine receptor D3, which is found in the brain. This protein responds to a chemical messenger (neurotransmitter) called dopamine to trigger signals within the nervous system, including signals involved in producing physical movement. A variant of the DRD3 gene seen in some families affected by essential tremor may cause the corresponding dopamine receptor D3 protein to respond more strongly to the neurotransmitter, possibly causing the involuntary shaking seen in this condition.

In other studies, the gene HS1BP3 has also been associated with essential tremor. The HS1BP3 gene provides instructions for making a protein called hematopoietic-specific protein 1 binding protein 3. This protein is believed to help regulate chemical signaling in the brain region involved in coordinating movements (the cerebellum) and in specialized nerve cells in the brain and spinal cord that control the muscles (motor neurons). A variant of the HS1BP3 gene has been identified in some families affected by essential tremor, but it has also been found in unaffected people. It is unknown what relationship, if any, this genetic change may have to the signs and symptoms of this condition.

How do people inherit essential tremor?

Essential tremor can be passed through generations in families, but the inheritance pattern varies. In most affected families, essential tremor appears to be inherited in an autosomal dominant pattern, which means one copy of the altered gene in each cell is sufficient to cause the disorder. In other families, the inheritance pattern is unclear. Essential tremor may also appear in people with no previous history of the disorder in their family.

Section 57.2

Parkinson Disease: Genetic Links

Excerpted from "Learning about Parkinson's Disease," National Human Genome Research Institute (www.genome.gov), June 27, 2011.

What Do We Know about Heredity and Parkinson Disease?

Parkinson disease (PD) is a neurological condition that typically causes tremor and/or stiffness in movement. The condition affects about 1 to 2 percent of people over the age of sixty years, and the chance of developing PD increases as we age. Most people affected with PD are not aware of any relatives with the condition, but in a number of families there is a family history. When three or more people are affected in a family, especially if they are diagnosed at an early age (under fifty years) we suspect that there may be a gene making this family more likely to develop the condition.

Genetics: The Basics

Our genetic material is stored in the center of every cell in our bodies (skin cells, hair cells, blood cells). This genetic material comes in individual units called genes. We all have thousands of genes. Genes carry the information the body needs to make proteins, which are the substances in the body that actually carry out all the functions we need to live and grow. Our genes affect many things about us: our height, eye color, why we respond to some medications better than others, and our likelihood of developing certain conditions. We have two copies of every gene: we inherit one copy, one member of each pair, from our mother and the other from our father. We then pass only one copy of a gene from each pair of genes to the next generation. Whether we pass on the gene we got from our father or the one from our mother is purely by chance, like flipping a coin heads or tails.

We all have genes that don't work properly. In most cases the other copy of the gene makes up for the one that does not work properly and we are healthy. A problem only arises if we meet someone else who has a nonworking copy of the same gene and we have a child who inherits two nonworking copies of that gene. This is called recessive inheritance.

Sometimes if one of our genes is not working properly, the other copy of the gene cannot make up for it and that causes a condition or an increased risk of developing a condition. Each time we have a child we randomly pass on one copy of each gene. If the child inherits the copy that doesn't work properly, they too may develop the condition. This is called dominant inheritance.

What Genes Are Linked to Parkinson Disease?

In 1997, we studied a large family that came from a small town in Southern Italy in which PD was inherited from parent to child (dominant inheritance). We found the gene that caused their inherited Parkinson disease and it coded for a protein called alpha-synuclein. If one studies the brains of people with PD after they die, one can see tiny little accumulations of protein called Lewy bodies (named after the doctor who first found them). Research has shown that there is a large amount of alpha-synuclein protein in the Lewy bodies of people who have noninherited PD as well as in the brains of people who have inherited PD. This immediately told us that alpha-synuclein played an important role in all forms of PD, and we are still doing a lot of research to better understand this role.

Currently, seven genes that cause some form of Parkinson disease have been identified. Mutations (changes) in three known genes called SNCA (PARK1), UCHL1 (PARK 5), and LRRK2 (PARK8) and another mapped gene (PARK3) have been reported in families with dominant inheritance. Mutations in three known genes, PARK2 (PARK2), PARK7 (PARK7), and PINK1 (PARK6) have been found in affected individuals who had siblings with the condition but whose parents did not have Parkinson disease (recessive inheritance). There is some research to suggest that these genes are also involved in early-onset Parkinson disease (diagnosed before the age of thirty) or in dominantly inherited Parkinson disease but it is too early yet to be certain.

New research studies, called genome-wide association studies (GWAS) are an approach that involves rapidly scanning markers across the complete sets of DNA, or genomes, of many people to find genetic variations associated with a particular disease. GWAS have been able to identify genetic variations that contribute to common diseases, including Parkinson disease.

What Determines Who Gets Parkinson Disease?

In most cases inheriting a nonworking copy of a single gene will not cause someone to develop Parkinson disease. We believe that many other complicating factors, such as additional genes and environmental factors, determine who will get the condition, when they get it, and how it affects them. In the families we have studied, some people who inherit the gene develop the condition and others live their entire lives without showing any symptoms. There is a lot of research on genes and the environment that is attempting to understand how all these factors interact.

Genetic Testing in Parkinson Disease

Genetic testing has recently become available for the parkin and PINK1 genes. Parkin is a large gene and testing is difficult. At the current stage of understanding, testing is likely to give a meaningful result only for people who develop the condition before the age of thirty years. PINK1 appears to be a rare cause of inherited Parkinson disease. A small percentage (~2 percent) of those developing the condition at an early age appear to carry mutations in the PINK1 gene. Genetic testing for the PARK7, SNCA, and LRRK2 genes is also available.

Individuals and families who are interested in having genetic testing can learn more about their risk for Parkinson disease and the availability and accuracy of genetic testing for this disease by setting up an appointment with a genetics health professional. Genetic professionals work as members of health care teams providing information and support to individuals or families who have genetic disorders or may be at risk for inherited conditions. Genetic professionals can discuss the risks, benefits, and limitations of available genetic testing for Parkinson disease.

Chapter 58

Genetic Factors in Obesity

Chapter Contents

Section 58.1

Genes and Obesity: Basic Facts

Excerpted from "Genes and Obesity," Centers for Disease
Control and Prevention (www.cdc.gov), May 17, 2013.

What Do Genes Have to Do with Obesity?

Obesity is the result of chronic energy imbalance in a person who
consistently takes in more calories from food and drink than are needed
to power their body's metabolic and physical functions. The rapidly rising
population prevalence of obesity in recent decades has been attributed
to an "obesogenic" environment, which offers ready access to high-calorie
foods but limits opportunities for physical activity. The obesity epidemic
can be considered a collective response to this environment. Obesity
is an important public health problem because it increases the risk of
developing diabetes, heart disease, stroke, and other serious diseases.

Even in an obesogenic environment, not everyone becomes obese.
Before the genomic research era, studies of family members, twins,
and adoptees offered indirect scientific evidence that a sizable portion of the variation in weight among adults is due to genetic factors.
For example, a key study that compared the body mass index (BMI)
of twins reared either together or apart found that inherited factors
had more influence than childhood environment.

One Gene or Many?

Rarely, obesity occurs in families according to a clear inheritance
pattern caused by changes in a single gene. The most commonly implicated gene is MC4R, which encodes the melanocortin 4 receptor.
Changes in MC4R that diminish its function are found in a small
fraction (less than 5 percent) of obese people in various ethnic groups.
Affected children feel extremely hungry and become obese because of
consistent overeating (hyperphagia). So far, rare variants in at least
nine genes have been implicated in single-gene (monogenic) obesity.

In most obese people, no single genetic cause can be identified.
Since 2006, genome-wide association studies have found more than

fifty genes associated with obesity, most with very small effects. Several of these genes also have variants that are associated with monogenic obesity, a phenomenon that has been observed in many other common conditions. Most obesity seems to be multifactorial, that is, the result of complex interactions among many genes and environmental factors.

How Do Genes Control Energy Balance?

The brain regulates food intake by responding to signals received from fat (adipose) tissue, the pancreas, and the digestive tract. These signals are transmitted by hormones—such as leptin, insulin, and ghrelin—and other small molecules. The brain coordinates these signals with other inputs and responds with instructions to the body: either to eat more and reduce energy use, or to do the opposite. Genes are the basis for the signals and responses that guide food intake, and small changes in these genes can affect their levels of activity. Some genes with variants that have been associated with obesity are listed in Table 58.1.

Table 58.1. Selected genes with variants that have been associated with obesity

Gene symbol	Gene name	Gene product's role in energy balance
ADIPOQ	Adipocyte-, C1q-, and collagen domain-containing	Produced by fat cells, adiponectin promotes energy expenditure
FTO	Fat mass- and obesity-associated gene	Promotes food intake
LEP	Leptin	Produced by fat cells
LEPR	Leptin receptor	When bound by leptin, inhibits appetite
INSIG2	Insulin-induced gene 2	Regulation of cholesterol and fatty acid synthesis
MC4R	Melanocortin 4 receptor	When bound by alpha-melanocyte stimulating hormone, stimulates appetite
PCSK1	Proprotein convertase subtilisin/kexin type 1	Regulates insulin biosynthesis
PPARG	Peroxisome proliferator-activated receptor gamma	Stimulates lipid uptake and development of fat tissue

Energy is crucial to survival. Human energy regulation is primed to protect against weight loss, rather than to control weight gain. The "thrifty genotype" hypothesis was proposed to help explain this observation. It suggests that the same genes that helped our ancestors survive occasional famines are now being challenged by environments in which food is plentiful year round.

Some New Directions

Epigenetics: Environmental exposures during critical periods of human development can cause permanent changes in a gene's activity without changing the sequence of the gene itself. Studying these "epigenetic" effects involves measuring chemical modifications of deoxyribonucleic acid (DNA), ribonucleic acid (RNA), or associated proteins that influence gene expression. Although epigenetics might help explain how early exposures such as infant feeding influence adult obesity, epidemiologic studies using these techniques are still at an early stage.

References

Walley AJ, Asher JE, Froguel P. The genetic contribution to non-syndromic human obesity. *Nat Rev Genet.* 2009 Jul;10(7):431–42.

Choquet H, Meyre D. Genetics of Obesity: What have we learned? *Curr Genomics.* 2011 May;12(3):169–79.

Section 58.2

Obesity and Genetics: What We Know

"Obesity and Genetics: What We Know, What We Don't Know,
and What It Means," Centers for Disease Control and Prevention
(www.cdc.gov), January 20, 2011.

Introduction

Rising rates of obesity seem to be a consequence of modern life,
with access to large amounts of palatable, high-calorie food and limited
need for physical activity. However, this environment of plenty affects
different people in different ways. Some are able to maintain a reasonable balance between energy input and energy expenditure. Others
have a chronic imbalance that favors energy input, which expresses
itself as overweight and obesity. What accounts for these differences
between individuals?

What We Know

- Biological relatives tend to resemble each other in many ways,
  including body weight. Individuals with a family history of obesity may be predisposed to gain weight and interventions that
  prevent obesity are especially important.

- In an environment made constant for food intake and physical
  activity, individuals respond differently. Some people store more
  energy as fat in an environment of excess; others lose less fat in
  an environment of scarcity. The different responses are largely
  due to genetic variation between individuals.

- Fat stores are regulated over long periods of time by complex
  systems that involve input and feedback from fatty tissues, the
  brain, and endocrine glands like the pancreas and the thyroid.
  Overweight and obesity can result from only a very small positive energy input imbalance over a long period of time.

- Rarely, people have mutations in single genes that result in severe obesity that starts in infancy. Studying these individuals is

providing insight into the complex biological pathways that regulate the balance between energy input and energy expenditure.

- Pharmaceutical companies are using genetic approaches (pharmacogenomics) to develop new drug strategies to treat obesity.

- The tendency to store energy in the form of fat is believed to result from thousands of years of evolution in an environment characterized by tenuous food supplies. In other words, those who could store energy in times of plenty were more likely to survive periods of famine and to pass this tendency to their offspring.

What We Don't Know

- Why are biological relatives more similar in body weight? What genes are associated with this observation? Are the same genetic associations seen in every family? How do these genes affect energy metabolism and regulation?

- Why are interventions based on diet and exercise more effective for some people than others? What are the biological differences between these high and low responders? How do we use these insights to tailor interventions to specific needs?

- What elements of energy regulation feedback systems are different in individuals? How do these differences affect energy metabolism and regulation?

- Do additional obesity syndromes exist that are caused by mutations in single genes? If so, what are they? What are the natural history, management strategy, and outcome for affected individuals?

- Obese individuals have genetic similarities that may shed light on the biological differences that predispose to gain weight. This knowledge may be useful in preventing or treating obesity in predisposed people.

- How do genetic variations that are shared by obese people affect gene expression and function? How do genetic variation and environmental factors interact to produce obesity? What are the biological features associated with the tendency to gain weight? What environmental factors are helpful in countering these tendencies?

- Will pharmacologic approaches benefit most people affected with obesity? Will these drugs be accessible to most people?

- How can thousands of years of evolutionary pressure be countered? Can specific factors in the modern environment (other than the obvious) be identified and controlled to more effectively counter these tendencies?

What It Means

1. For people who are genetically predisposed to gain weight, preventing obesity is the best course. Predisposed persons may require individualized interventions and greater support to be successful in maintaining a healthy weight.

2. Obesity is a chronic lifelong condition that is the result of an environment of caloric abundance and relative physical inactivity modulated by a susceptible genotype. For those who are predisposed, preventing weight gain is the best course of action.

3. Genes are not destiny. Obesity can be prevented or can be managed in many cases with a combination of diet, physical activity, and medication.

Section 58.3

"Obesity Genes" May Influence Food Choices and Eating Habits

"'Obesity Genes' May Influence Food Choices, Eating Patterns,"
May 23, 2012. © 2012 Miriam Hospital (http://www.miriamhospital.org).
All rights reserved. Reprinted with permission.

Blame it on your genes? Researchers from the Miriam Hospital's Weight Control and Diabetes Research Center say individuals with variations in certain "obesity genes" tend to eat more meals and snacks, consume more calories per day, and often choose the same types of high-fat, sugary foods.

Their study, published online by the *American Journal of Clinical Nutrition* and appearing in the June 2012 issue, reveals certain variations within the FTO and BDNF genes—which have been previously linked to obesity—may play a role in eating habits that can cause obesity.

The findings suggest it may be possible to minimize genetic risk by changing one's eating patterns and being vigilant about food choices, in addition to adopting other healthy lifestyle habits, like regular physical activity.

"Understanding how our genes influence obesity is critical in trying to understand the current obesity epidemic, yet it's important to remember that genetic traits alone do not mean obesity is inevitable," said lead author Jeanne M. McCaffery, Ph.D., of the Miriam Hospital's Weight Control and Diabetes Research Center.

"Our lifestyle choices are critical when it comes to determining how thin or heavy we are, regardless of your genetic traits," she added. "However, uncovering genetic markers can possibly pinpoint future interventions to control obesity in those who are genetically predisposed."

Previous research has shown individuals who carry a variant of the fast mass and obesity-associated gene FTO and BDNF (or brain-derived neurotrophic factor gene) are at increased risk for obesity. The genes have also been linked with overeating in children and this is one of the first studies to extend this finding to adults. Both FTO and BDNF are expressed in the part of the brain that controls eating and appetite, although the mechanisms by which these gene variations influence obesity is still unknown.

As part of the Look AHEAD (Action in Health and Diabetes) trial, more than two thousand participants completed a questionnaire about their eating habits over the past six months and also underwent genotyping. Researchers focused on nearly a dozen genes that have been previously associated with obesity. They then examined whether these genetic markers influenced the pattern or content of the participants' diet.

Variations in the FTO gene specifically were significantly associated with a greater number of meals and snacks per day, greater percentage of energy from fat, and more servings of fats, oils, and sweets. The findings are largely consistent with previous research in children.

Researchers also discovered that individuals with BDNF variations consumed more servings from the dairy and the meat, eggs, nuts, and beans food groups. They also consumed approximately one hundred more calories per day, which McCaffery notes could have a substantial influence on one's weight.

"We show that at least some of the genetic influence on obesity may occur through patterns of dietary intake," she said. "The good news is that eating habits can be modified, so we may be able to reduce one's genetic risk for obesity by changing these eating patterns."

McCaffery says that while this research greatly expands their knowledge on how genetics may influence obesity, the data must be replicated before the findings can be translated into possible clinical measures.

The Look AHEAD trial, funded by the National Institutes of Diabetes and Digestive and Kidney Diseases, is a randomized, multisite clinical trial examining whether weight loss achieved through an intensive lifestyle intervention can reduce cardiovascular disease and cardiovascular disease-related death among overweight individuals with Type 2 diabetes. The program will be compared to a control condition involving a program of diabetes support and education.

Section 58.4

Genes Identified for Common Childhood Obesity

Genetics researchers have identified at least two new gene variants that increase the risk of common childhood obesity.

"This is the largest-ever genome-wide study of common childhood obesity, in contrast to previous studies that have focused on more extreme forms of obesity primarily connected with rare disease syndromes," said lead investigator Struan F.A. Grant, Ph.D., associate director of the Center for Applied Genomics at the Children's Hospital of Philadelphia. "As a consequence, we have definitively identified and characterized a genetic predisposition to common childhood obesity."

The study, by an international collaborative group, the Early Growth Genetics (EGG) Consortium, appeared online on April 9, 2012, in *Nature Genetics*.

Obesity Prevalence in Children on the Rise

As one of the major health issues affecting modern societies, obesity has increasingly received public attention, especially given a rising prevalence of the condition among children. Research indicates that obese adolescents tend to have higher risk of mortality as adults. Although environmental factors, such as food choices and sedentary habits, contribute to the increasing rates of obesity in childhood, twin studies and other family-based evidence have suggested a genetic component to the disease as well.

Previous studies have identified gene variants contributing to obesity in adults and in children with extreme obesity, but relatively little is known about genes implicated in regular childhood obesity.

Genome Study for Common Obesity

"The Center for Applied Genomics at the Children's Hospital of Philadelphia has recruited and genotyped the world's largest collection of deoxyribonucleic acid (DNA) from children with common obesity," said Grant. "However, in order to have sufficient statistical power to detect novel genetic signals, we needed to form a large international consortium to combine results from similar datasets from around the world."

The National Institutes of Health partly funded this research, which analyzed previous studies supported by many other European, Australian, and North American organizations.

The current meta-analysis included fourteen previous studies encompassing 5,530 cases of childhood obesity and 8,300 control subjects, all of European ancestry. The study team identified two novel loci, one near the OLFM4 gene on chromosome 13, the other within the HOXB5 gene on chromosome 17. They also found a degree of evidence for two other gene variants. None of the genes were previously implicated in obesity. "The known biology of three of the genes," added Grant, "hints at a role of the intestine, although their precise functional role in obesity is currently unknown."

"This work opens up new avenues to explore the genetics of common childhood obesity," said Grant. "Much work remains to be done, but these findings may ultimately be useful in helping to design future preventive interventions and treatments for children, based on their individual genomes."

Chapter 59

Stroke: Genetic Links

Genetics and Stroke

Stroke is a leading cause of death and a major cause of disability in the United States. A stroke occurs when the blood supply to part of the brain is blocked, or when a blood vessel in the brain bursts, causing damage to a part of the brain.

Some health conditions and behavioral and lifestyle factors can put individuals at a higher risk for stroke. Important risk factors include high blood pressure, heart disease, diabetes, and cigarette smoking.

Individuals can help prevent a stroke by making behavioral and lifestyle changes that lower their risk.

Genetics and Family History

Genes play a role in the development of risk factors that can lead to a stroke, such as high blood pressure, heart disease, diabetes, and vascular conditions. An increased risk for stroke within a family may also be due to common behavioral factors, such as a sedentary lifestyle or poor eating habits. Thus, family health history is an important tool for identifying people at increased risk for stroke because it reflects both an individual's genes and shared environmental risk factors.

"Genetics and Stroke" is reprinted from "Stroke Awareness," Centers for Disease Control and Prevention (www.cdc.gov), January 31, 2013. "Recent Research on Genetic Links to Stroke" is excerpted from "Researchers Discover New Genetic Variants Associated with Increased Risk of Stroke," an NIH News Release, National Institutes of Health, April 15, 2009.

In a 2003 study in Utah, 86 percent of all early strokes occurred in just 11 percent of families. This shows that a relatively small subset of families in the population with history of stroke account for the majority of cases. These families may benefit the most from screening and lifestyle interventions.[1]

Stroke also occurs as a complication of several genetic disorders, the most common of these being sickle cell disease. Other genetic disorders such as CADASIL (cerebral autosomal dominant arteriopathy with subcortical infarcts and leukoencephalopathy) have stroke as the primary feature, but these disorders are quite rare. Research in inherited diseases that include stroke is providing insights into how genes contribute to stroke risk with the goal of developing new approaches for prediction, prevention, and treatment of the disease.

Recent Research on Genetic Links to Stroke

Scientists have identified a previously unknown connection between two genetic variants and an increased risk of stroke, providing strong evidence for the existence of specific genes that help explain the genetic component of stroke. The research was funded by the National Heart, Lung, and Blood Institute (NHLBI) of the National Institutes of Health (NIH) and by several other NIH institutes and centers.

The analysis of over nineteen thousand participants was published online on April 15, 2009, by the *New England Journal of Medicine* and appeared in print on April 23, 2009.

The genetic variants were discovered by analyzing the genomes of individuals from the CHARGE (Cohorts for Heart and Aging Research in Genomic Epidemiology) consortium. This extensive resource includes participants from the Framingham Heart Study, Atherosclerosis Risk in Communities study, Cardiovascular Health Study, and Rotterdam Study.

"This study, which integrates longstanding observational trials such as Framingham with cutting edge genomic technologies, moves us closer to the era of personalized medicine," said NHLBI Director Elizabeth G. Nabel, M.D. "As we learn more about the role that an individual's unique genetic makeup plays in their overall health, we will ultimately be able to tailor care to better diagnose, prevent, and treat conditions such as stroke."

Stroke is the third leading cause of death in the United States and causes serious long-term disabilities for many Americans.

The research team included Sudha Seshadri, M.D., associate professor of neurology, and Philip A. Wolf, M.D., principal investigator of the

Framingham Heart Study and professor of neurology, Boston University School of Medicine, and involved investigators from numerous universities. Supported by a grant from the National Institute of Neurological Disorders and Stroke (NINDS), Dr. Wolf has studied the risk factors for stroke in the Framingham Heart Study over the past three decades.

The researchers discovered that two previously unsuspected common genetic variants or single-nucleotide polymorphisms (SNPs, pronounced "snips") were consistently associated with total stroke (all types) and ischemic stroke in white persons. The SNPs were located on chromosome 12p13 near the gene NINJ2, which encodes ninjurin2, a member of the ninjurin nerve-injury-induced protein family.

"Consistent with the discoveries from genome-wide association studies in many other common disorders, the risk of stroke associated with these SNPs is not sufficiently high to make an individual change their stroke prevention plan. However, the results will lead scientists to direct their attention to new, important biologic mechanisms and hopefully new treatments to prevent stroke," noted Walter Koroshetz, M.D., deputy director of NINDS.

The association of one of the genetic variants was replicated in two independent samples: North American black persons and Dutch white persons. The association held when the analyses were adjusted for systolic blood pressure, hypertension, diabetes, atrial fibrillation, and current smoking.

"This impressive report shows how the power of genome-wide association studies can be enhanced by pooling data from large, population-based studies that follow participants over long periods of time. It also underscores the value of replicating initial results in populations with different demographics," said National Human Genome Research Institute Acting Director Alan E. Guttmacher, M.D.

Genome-wide association studies (GWAS) are a relatively new tool that allow researchers to rapidly scan the complete set of deoxyribonucleic acid (DNA)—a genome—of many individuals in order to find genetic variations, or misspellings, associated with a particular disease or condition. This technique has revealed numerous relationships between genetic variations and conditions such as type 2 diabetes, obesity, and heart disorders. GWAS are possible due to the completion of the human genome in 2003 and the International HapMap Project in 2005, the advent of powerful information technology, and the participation of thousands of study volunteers whose confidentiality is safeguarded.

"Discovering genes for stroke has been a challenge in part because there are many different types of stroke. These results provide strong evidence for a previously unknown gene that may predispose to stroke and suggests that more genes will be discovered—improving our chances of reducing the toll from this important public health problem," said Christopher O'Donnell, M.D., M.P.H., senior advisor to the NHLBI director for genome research and associate director of the Framingham Heart Study.

There are two major types of stroke. The most common kind, ischemic stroke, is caused by a blood clot that blocks a blood vessel in the brain. The second type, hemorrhagic stroke, is caused by a blood vessel that breaks and bleeds into or around the brain. Stroke causes permanent brain injury. Stroke survivors suffer from disability that varies from mild to extremely severe.

Chapter 60

Genetics and Tourette Syndrome

What is Tourette syndrome?

Tourette syndrome is a complex disorder characterized by repetitive, sudden, and involuntary movements or noises called tics. Tics usually appear in childhood, and their severity varies over time. In most cases, tics become milder and less frequent in late adolescence and adulthood.

Tourette syndrome involves both motor tics, which are uncontrolled body movements, and vocal or phonic tics, which are outbursts of sound. Some motor tics are simple and involve only one muscle group. Simple motor tics, such as rapid eye blinking, shoulder shrugging, or nose twitching, are usually the first signs of Tourette syndrome. Motor tics also can be complex (involving multiple muscle groups), such as jumping, kicking, hopping, or spinning.

Vocal tics, which generally appear later than motor tics, also can be simple or complex. Simple vocal tics include grunting, sniffing, and throat clearing. More complex vocalizations include repeating the words of others (echolalia) or repeating one's own words (palilalia). The involuntary use of inappropriate or obscene language (coprolalia) is possible, but uncommon, among people with Tourette syndrome.

In addition to frequent tics, people with Tourette syndrome are at risk for associated problems including attention deficit hyperactivity disorder (ADHD), obsessive-compulsive disorder (OCD), anxiety, depression, and problems with sleep.

Excerpted from "Tourette Syndrome," Genetics Home Reference (http://ghr.nlm .nih.gov), May 2013.

How common is Tourette syndrome?

Although the exact incidence of Tourette syndrome is uncertain, it is estimated to affect one to ten in one thousand children. This disorder occurs in populations and ethnic groups worldwide, and it is more common in males than in females.

What genes are related to Tourette syndrome?

A variety of genetic and environmental factors likely play a role in causing Tourette syndrome. Most of these factors are unknown, and researchers are studying risk factors before and after birth that may contribute to this complex disorder. Scientists believe that tics may result from changes in brain chemicals (neurotransmitters) that are responsible for producing and controlling voluntary movements.

Mutations involving the SLITRK1 gene have been identified in a small number of people with Tourette syndrome. This gene provides instructions for making a protein that is active in the brain. The SLITRK1 protein probably plays a role in the development of nerve cells, including the growth of specialized extensions (axons and dendrites) that allow each nerve cell to communicate with nearby cells. It is unclear how mutations in the SLITRK1 gene can lead to this disorder.

Most people with Tourette syndrome do not have a mutation in the SLITRK1 gene. Because mutations have been reported in so few people with this condition, the association of the SLITRK1 gene with this disorder has not been confirmed. Researchers suspect that changes in other genes, which have not been identified, are also associated with Tourette syndrome.

How do people inherit Tourette syndrome?

The inheritance pattern of Tourette syndrome is unclear. Although the features of this condition can cluster in families, many genetic and environmental factors are likely to be involved. Among family members of an affected person, it is difficult to predict who else may be at risk of developing the condition.

Tourette syndrome was previously thought to have an autosomal dominant pattern of inheritance, which suggests that one mutated copy of a gene in each cell would be sufficient to cause the condition. Several decades of research have shown that this is not the case. Almost all cases of Tourette syndrome probably result from a variety of genetic and environmental factors, not changes in a single gene.

Part Five

Genetic Research

Chapter 61

The Human Genome Project

Chapter Contents

Section 61.1

Basic Facts about the Human Genome Project

"About the Human Genome Project," Oak Ridge National Laboratory (www.ornl.gov), September 19, 2011.

What is the Human Genome Project?

Begun formally in 1990, the U.S. Human Genome Project (HGP) was a thirteen-year effort coordinated by the U.S. Department of Energy and the National Institutes of Health. The project originally was planned to last fifteen years, but rapid technological advances accelerated the completion date to 2003. Project goals were as follows:

- To identify all the approximately twenty thousand to twenty-five thousand genes in human deoxyribonucleic acid (DNA)

- To determine the sequences of the three billion chemical base pairs that make up human DNA

- To store this information in databases

- To improve tools for data analysis

- To transfer related technologies to the private sector

- To address the ethical, legal, and social issues (ELSI) that may arise from the project.

To help achieve these goals, researchers also studied the genetic makeup of several nonhuman organisms. These include the common human gut bacterium *Escherichia coli*, the fruit fly, and the laboratory mouse.

A unique aspect of the U.S. Human Genome Project is that it was the first large scientific undertaking to address potential ELSI implications arising from project data.

Another important feature of the project was the federal government's long-standing dedication to the transfer of technology to the private sector. By licensing technologies to private companies and awarding grants for innovative research, the project catalyzed the multibillion-dollar U.S. biotechnology industry and fostered the development of new medical applications.

Landmark papers detailing sequence and analysis of the human genome were published in February 2001 and April 2003 issues of *Nature* and *Science*.

What's a genome? And why is it important?

A genome is all the DNA in an organism, including its genes. Genes carry information for making all the proteins required by all organisms. These proteins determine, among other things, how the organism looks, how well its body metabolizes food or fights infection, and sometimes even how it behaves.

DNA is made up of four similar chemicals (called bases and abbreviated A, T, C, and G) that are repeated millions or billions of times throughout a genome. The human genome, for example, has three billion pairs of bases.

The particular order of As, Ts, Cs, and Gs is extremely important. The order underlies all of life's diversity, even dictating whether an organism is human or another species such as yeast, rice, or fruit fly, all of which have their own genomes and are themselves the focus of genome projects. Because all organisms are related through similarities in DNA sequences, insights gained from nonhuman genomes often lead to new knowledge about human biology.

What are some practical benefits to learning about DNA?

Knowledge about the effects of DNA variations among individuals can lead to revolutionary new ways to diagnose, treat, and someday prevent the thousands of disorders that affect us. Besides providing clues to understanding human biology, learning about nonhuman organisms' DNA sequences can lead to an understanding of their natural capabilities that can be applied toward solving challenges in health care, agriculture, energy production, environmental remediation, and carbon sequestration.

What are some of the ethical, legal, and social challenges presented by genetic information, and what is being done to address these issues?

The Department of Energy and the National Institutes of Health Genome Programs set aside 3 percent to 5 percent of their respective annual HGP budgets for the study of the project's ethical, legal, and social issues (ELSI). Nearly $1 million was spent on HGP ELSI research.

Section 61.2

Insights Learned from the Human DNA Sequence

Reprinted from the Oak Ridge National Laboratory (www.ornl.gov), October 9, 2009.

By the Numbers

- The human genome contains 3.2 billion chemical nucleotide base pairs (A, C, T, and G).

- The average gene consists of 3,000 base pairs, but sizes vary greatly, with the largest known human gene being dystrophin at 2.4 million base pairs.

- The total number of genes is estimated at 25,000, much lower than previous estimates of 80,000 to 140,000 that had been based on extrapolations from gene-rich areas as opposed to a composite of gene-rich and gene-poor areas.

- The human genome sequence is almost exactly the same (99.9 percent) in all people.

- Functions are unknown for more than 50 percent of discovered genes.

The Wheat from the Chaff

- About 2 percent of the genome encodes instructions for the synthesis of proteins.

- Repeat sequences that do not code for proteins make up at least 50 percent of the human genome.

- Repeat sequences are thought to have no direct functions, but they shed light on chromosome structure and dynamics. Over time, these repeats reshape the genome by rearranging it, thereby creating entirely new genes or modifying and reshuffling existing genes.

- During the past fifty million years, a dramatic decrease seems to have occurred in the rate of accumulation of repeats in the human genome.

How It's Arranged

- The human genome's gene-dense "urban centers" are predominantly composed of the deoxyribonucleic acid (DNA) building blocks G and C.

- In contrast, the gene-poor "deserts" are rich in the DNA building blocks A and T. GC- and AT-rich regions usually can be seen through a microscope as light and dark bands on chromosomes.

- Genes appear to be concentrated in random areas along the genome, with vast expanses of noncoding DNA between.

- Particular gene sequences have been associated with numerous diseases and disorders, including breast cancer, muscle disease, deafness, and blindness.

- Stretches of up to thirty thousand C and G bases repeating over and over often occur adjacent to gene-rich areas, forming a barrier between the genes and the "junk DNA." These CpG islands are believed to help regulate gene activity.

- Chromosome 1 (the largest human chromosome) has the most genes (3,168), and Y chromosome has the fewest (344).

How the Human Genome Compares with That of Other Organisms

- Unlike the human's seemingly random distribution of gene-rich areas, many other organisms' genomes are more uniform, with genes evenly spaced throughout.

- Humans have on average three times as many kinds of proteins as the fly or worm because of messenger ribonucleic acid (mRNA) transcript "alternative splicing" and chemical modifications to the proteins. This process can yield different protein products from the same gene.

- Humans share most of the same protein families with worms, flies, and plants, but the number of gene family members has expanded in humans, especially in proteins involved in development and immunity.

- The human genome has a much greater portion (50 percent) of repeat sequences than the mustard weed (11 percent), the worm (7 percent), and the fly (3 percent).

- Over 40 percent of predicted human proteins share similarity with fruit fly or worm proteins.

- Although humans appear to have stopped accumulating repeated DNA over fifty million years ago, there seems to be no such decline in rodents. This may account for some of the fundamental differences between hominids and rodents, although gene estimates are similar in these species. Scientists have proposed many theories to explain evolutionary contrasts between humans and other organisms, including those of life span, litter sizes, inbreeding, and genetic drift.

Variations and Mutations

- Scientists have identified millions of locations where single-base DNA differences occur in humans. This information promises to revolutionize the processes of finding DNA sequences associated with such common diseases as cardiovascular disease, diabetes, arthritis, and cancers.

- The ratio of germline (sperm or egg cell) mutations is 2:1 in males versus females. Researchers point to several reasons for the higher mutation rate in the male germline, including the greater number of cell divisions required for sperm formation than for eggs.

What We Still Don't Understand: A Checklist for Future Research

- Exact gene number, exact locations, and functions
- Gene regulation
- DNA sequence organization
- Chromosomal structure and organization
- Noncoding DNA types, amount, distribution, information content, and functions
- Coordination of gene expression, protein synthesis, and post-translational events

- Interaction of proteins in complex molecular machines
- Predicted versus experimentally determined gene function
- Evolutionary conservation among organisms
- Protein conservation (structure and function)
- Proteomes (total protein content and function) in organisms
- Correlation of SNPs (single-base DNA variations among individuals) with health and disease
- Disease-susceptibility prediction based on gene sequence variation
- Genes involved in complex traits and multigene diseases
- Complex systems biology, including microbial consortia useful for environmental restoration
- Developmental genetics, genomics

Applications, Future Challenges

Deriving meaningful knowledge from the DNA sequence will define research through the coming decades to inform our understanding of biological systems. This enormous task will require the expertise and creativity of tens of thousands of scientists from varied disciplines in both the public and private sectors worldwide.

The draft sequence already is having an impact on finding genes associated with disease. Over thirty genes have been pinpointed and associated with breast cancer, muscle disease, deafness, and blindness. Additionally, finding the DNA sequences underlying such common diseases as cardiovascular disease, diabetes, arthritis, and cancers is being aided by the human variation maps (SNPs) generated in the Human Genome Project (HGP) in cooperation with the private sector. These genes and SNPs provide focused targets for the development of effective new therapies.

One of the greatest impacts of having the sequence may well be in enabling an entirely new approach to biological research. In the past, researchers studied one or a few genes at a time. With whole-genome sequences and new high-throughput technologies, they can approach questions systematically and on a grand scale. They can study all the genes in a genome, for example, or all the transcripts in a particular tissue or organ or tumor, or how tens of thousands of genes and proteins work together in interconnected networks to orchestrate the chemistry of life.

Postsequencing projects are well under way worldwide. These explorations will result in a profound, new, and more comprehensive understanding of complex living systems, with applications to agriculture, human health, energy, global climate change, and environmental remediation, among others.

Section 61.3

The Human Genome Project: Current Knowledge and Future Research Directions

"Human Genome Project," Research Portfolio Online Reporting Tools (RePORT), a service of the National Institutes of Health (www.nih.gov), March 29, 2013.

Yesterday

Just a half-century ago, very little was known about the genetic factors that contribute to human disease.

In 1953, James Watson and Francis Crick described the double helix structure of deoxyribonucleic acid (DNA), the chemical compound that contains the genetic instructions for building, running, and maintaining living organisms.

Methods to determine the order, or sequence, of the chemical letters in DNA were developed in the mid-1970s.

In 1990, the National Institutes of Health (NIH) and the Department of Energy joined with international partners in a quest to sequence all three billion letters, or base pairs, in the human genome, which is the complete set of DNA in the human body. This concerted, public effort was the Human Genome Project.

The Human Genome Project's goal was to provide researchers with powerful tools to understand the genetic factors in human disease, paving the way for new strategies for their diagnosis, treatment, and prevention.

From the start, the Human Genome Project supported an Ethical, Legal and Social Implications (ESLI) research program to address the many complex issues that might arise from this science.

All data generated by the Human Genome Project were made freely and rapidly available on the Internet, serving to accelerate the pace of medical discovery around the globe.

The Human Genome project spurred a revolution in biotechnology innovation around the world and played a key role in making the United States the global leader in the new biotechnology sector.

In April 2003, researchers successfully completed the Human Genome Project, under budget and more than two years ahead of schedule.

Today

The Human Genome Project has already fueled the discovery of more than 1,800 disease genes.

As a result of the Human Genome Project, today's researchers can find a gene suspected of causing an inherited disease in a matter of days, rather than the years it took before the genome sequence was in hand.

There are now more than two thousand genetic tests for human conditions. These tests enable patients to learn their genetic risks for disease and also help health care professionals to diagnose disease.

At least 350 biotechnology-based products resulting from the Human Genome Project are currently in clinical trials.

Having the complete sequence of the human genome is similar to having all the pages of a manual needed to make the human body. The challenge now is to determine how to read the contents of these pages and understand how all of these many, complex parts work together in human health and disease.

One major step toward such comprehensive understanding was the development in 2005 of the HapMap, which is a catalog of common genetic variation, or haplotypes, in the human genome. In 2010, the third phase of the HapMap project was published, with data from eleven global populations, the largest survey of human genetic variation performed to date. HapMap data have accelerated the search for genes involved in common human diseases, and have already yielded impressive results in finding genetic factors involved in conditions ranging from age-related blindness to obesity.

The tools created through the Human Genome Project continue to underlie efforts to characterize the genomes of important organisms used extensively in biomedical research, including fruit flies, roundworms, and mice.

NIH's Ethical, Legal and Social Implications program has become a model for other research efforts seeking to address ethical issues in a proactive manner.

With the drastic decline in the cost of sequencing whole exomes or genomes, groundbreaking comparative genomic studies are now identifying the causes of rare diseases such as Kabuki and Miller syndromes.

Much work still remains to be done. Despite many important genetic discoveries, the genetics of complex diseases such as heart disease are still far from clear.

Pharmacogenomics is a field that looks at how genetic variation affects an individual's response to a drug. Pharmacogenomic tests can already identify whether or not a breast cancer patient will respond to the drug Herceptin, whether an acquired immune deficiency syndrome (AIDS) patient should take the drug Abacavir, or what the correct dose of the blood-thinner Warfarin should be.

Tomorrow

An ambitious new initiative, The Cancer Genome Atlas, aims to identify all the genetic abnormalities seen in fifty major types of cancer.

Based on a deeper understanding of disease at the genomic level, we will see a whole new generation of targeted interventions, many of which will be drugs that are much more effective and cause fewer side effects than those available today.

NIH-supported access to high-throughput screening of small molecule libraries will provide academic researchers with powerful new research probes to explore the hundreds of thousands of proteins believed to be encoded by the approximately twenty-five thousand genes in the human genome, and will provide innovative techniques to spur development of new, more effective, types of drugs.

NIH is striving to cut the cost of sequencing an individual's genome to $1,000 or less. Having one's complete genome sequence will make it easier to diagnose, manage, and treat many diseases.

Individualized analysis based on each person's genome will lead to a powerful form of preventive, personalized, and preemptive medicine. By tailoring recommendations to each person's DNA, health care professionals will be able to work with individuals to focus efforts on the specific strategies—from diet to high-tech medical surveillance—that are most likely to maintain health for that particular individual.

The increasing ability to connect DNA variation with nonmedical conditions, such as intelligence and personality traits, will challenge society, making the role of ethical, legal, and social implications research more important than ever.

Chapter 62

Behavioral Genetics

What is behavioral genetics?

Sir Francis Galton (1822–1911) was the first scientist to study heredity and human behavior systematically. The term "genetics" did not even appear until 1909, only two years before Galton's death. With or without a formal name, the study of heredity always has been, at its core, the study of biological variation. Human behavioral genetics, a relatively new field, seeks to understand both the genetic and environmental contributions to individual variations in human behavior. This is not an easy task, for the following reasons:

- It often is difficult to define the behavior in question. Intelligence is a classic example. Is intelligence the ability to solve a certain type of problem? The ability to make one's way successfully in the world? The ability to score well on an intelligence quotient (IQ) test? During the late summer of 1999, a Princeton molecular biologist published the results of impressive research in which he enhanced the ability of mice to learn by inserting a gene that codes for a protein in brain cells known to be associated with memory. Because the experimental animals performed better than controls on a series of traditional tests of learning, the press dubbed this gene "the smart gene" and the "IQ gene,"

Excerpted from "Behavioral Genetics," Oak Ridge National Laboratory (www .ornl.gov), September 16, 2008. Reviewed by David A. Cooke, M.D., FACP, May 2013.

as if improved memory were the central, or even sole, criterion for defining intelligence. In reality, there is no universal agreement on the definition of intelligence, even among those who study it for a living.

- Having established a definition for research purposes, the investigator still must measure the behavior with acceptable degrees of validity and reliability. That is especially difficult for basic personality traits such as shyness or assertiveness, which are the subject of much current research. Sometimes there is an interesting conflation of definition and measurement, as in the case of IQ tests, where the test score itself has come to define the trait it measures. This is a bit like using batting averages to define hitting prowess in baseball. A high average may indicate ability, but it does not define the essence of the trait.

- Behaviors, like all complex traits, involve multiple genes, a reality that complicates the search for genetic contributions.

- As with much other research in genetics, studies of genes and behavior require analysis of families and populations for comparison of those who have the trait in question with those who do not. The result often is a statement of "heritability," a statistical construct that estimates the amount of variation in a population that is attributable to genetic factors. The explanatory power of heritability figures is limited, however, applying only to the population studied and only to the environment in place at the time the study was conducted. If the population or the environment changes, the heritability most likely will change as well. Most important, heritability statements provide no basis for predictions about the expression of the trait in question in any given individual.

What indications are there that behavior has a biological basis?

Behavior often is species specific. A chickadee, for example, carries one sunflower seed at a time from a feeder to a nearby branch, secures the seed to the branch between its feet, pecks it open, eats the contents, and repeats the process. Finches, in contrast, stay at the feeder for long periods, opening large numbers of seeds with their thick beaks. Some mating behaviors also are species specific. Prairie chickens, native to the upper Midwest, conduct an elaborate mating ritual, a sort of line dance for birds, with spread wings and synchronized group movements.

Some behaviors are so characteristic that biologists use them to help differentiate between closely related species.

Behaviors often breed true. We can reproduce behaviors in successive generations of organisms. Consider the instinctive retrieval behavior of a yellow Labrador or the herding posture of a border collie.

Behaviors change in response to alterations in biological structures or processes. For example, a brain injury can turn a polite, mild-mannered person into a foul-mouthed, aggressive boor, and we routinely modify the behavioral manifestations of mental illnesses with drugs that alter brain chemistry. More recently, geneticists have created or extinguished specific mouse behaviors—ranging from nurturing of pups to continuous circling in a strain called "twirler"—by inserting or disabling specific genes.

In humans, some behaviors run in families. For example, there is a clear familial aggregation of mental illness.

Behavior has an evolutionary history that persists across related species. Chimpanzees are our closest relatives, separated from us by a mere 2 percent difference in DNA sequence. We and they share behaviors that are characteristic of highly social primates, including nurturing, cooperation, altruism, and even some facial expressions. Genes are evolutionary glue, binding all of life in a single history that dates back some 3.5 billion years. Conserved behaviors are part of that history, which is written in the language of nature's universal information molecule—deoxyribonucleic acid (DNA).

How is behavioral genetics studied?

Traditional research strategies in behavioral genetics include studies of twins and adoptees, techniques designed to sort biological from environmental influences. More recently, investigators have added the search for pieces of DNA associated with particular behaviors, an approach that has been most productive to date in identifying potential locations for genes associated with major mental illnesses such as schizophrenia and bipolar disorder. Yet even here there have been no major breakthroughs, no clearly identified genes that geneticists can tie to disease. The search for genes associated with characteristics such as sexual preference and basic personality traits has been even more frustrating.

Genetics and molecular biology have provided some significant insights into behaviors associated with inherited disorders. For example, we know that an extra chromosome 21 is associated with the mental retardation that accompanies Down syndrome, although the processes that disrupt brain function are not yet clear. We also know the steps from gene to effect for a number of single-gene disorders that result in mental retardation, including phenylketonuria (PKU), a treatable metabolic disorder for which all newborns in the United States are tested.

In general, it is easier to discern the relationship between biology and behavior for chromosomal and single-gene disorders than for common, complex behaviors that are of considerable interest to specialist and nonspecialist alike. So the former are at the more informative end of a sliding scale of certainty with respect to our understanding of human behavior. At the other end of the scale are the hard-to-define personality traits, while somewhere in between are traits such as schizophrenia and bipolar disorder—organic diseases whose biological roots are undeniable yet unknown and whose unpredictable onset teaches us about the importance of environmental contributions, even as it reminds us of our ignorance.

What implications does behavioral genetics research have for society?

Researchers in the field of behavioral genetics have asserted claims for a genetic basis of numerous physical behaviors, including homosexuality, aggression, impulsivity, and nurturing. A growing scientific and popular focus on genes and behavior has contributed to a resurgence of behavioral genetic determinism—the belief that genetics is the major factor in determining behavior.

Are behaviors inbred, written indelibly in our genes as immutable biological imperatives, or is the environment more important in shaping our thoughts and actions? Such questions cycle through society repeatedly, forming the public nexus of the "nature vs. nurture controversy," a strange locution to biologists, who recognize that behaviors exist only in the context of environmental influence. Nonetheless, the debate flares anew every few years, reigniting in response to genetic analyses of traits such as intelligence, criminality, or homosexuality, characteristics weighted with social, political, and legal meaning.

What social consequences would genetic diagnoses of such traits as intelligence, criminality, or homosexuality have on society? What effect would the discovery of a behavioral trait associated with increased criminal activity have on our legal system? If we find a "gay gene," will it mean greater or lesser tolerance? Will it lead to proposals that those affected by the "disorder" should undergo treatment to be "cured" and that measures should be taken to prevent the birth of other individuals so afflicted?

There are several scientific obstacles to correlating genotype (an individual's genetic endowment) and behavior. One problem is in defining a specific endpoint that characterizes a condition, be it schizophrenia or intelligence. Another problem is in identifying and excluding other possible causes of the condition, thereby permitting a determination of the significance of a supposed correlation. Much current research on genes and behavior also engenders very strong feelings because of the potential social and political consequences of accepting these supposed truths. Thus, more than any other aspect of genetics, discoveries in behavioral genetics should not be viewed as irrefutable until there has been substantial scientific corroboration.

How do genes influence behavior?

No single gene determines a particular behavior. Behaviors are complex traits involving multiple genes that are affected by a variety of other factors. This fact often gets overlooked in media reports hyping scientific breakthroughs on gene function, and, unfortunately, this can be very misleading to the public.

For example, a study published in 1999 claimed that overexpression of a particular gene in mice led to enhanced learning capacity. The popular press referred to this gene as "the learning gene" or the "smart gene." What the press didn't mention was that the learning enhancements observed in this study were short-term, lasting only a few hours to a few days in some cases.

Dubbing a gene as a "smart gene" gives the public a false impression of how much scientists really know about the genetics of a complex trait like intelligence. Once news of the "smart gene" reaches the public, suddenly there is talk about designer babies and the potential of genetically engineering embryos to have intelligence and other desirable traits, when in reality the path from genes to proteins to development of a particular trait is still a mystery.

With disorders, behaviors, or any physical trait, genes are just a part of the story, because a variety of genetic and environmental factors are involved in the development of any trait. Having a genetic variant doesn't necessarily mean that a particular trait will develop. The presence of certain genetic factors can enhance or repress other genetic factors. Genes are turned on and off, and other factors may be keeping a gene from being turned "on." In addition, the protein encoded by a gene can be modified in ways that can affect its ability to carry out its normal cellular function.

Genetic factors also can influence the role of certain environmental factors in the development of a particular trait. For example, a person may have a genetic variant that is known to increase his or her risk for developing emphysema from smoking, an environmental factor. If that person never smokes, then emphysema will not develop.

Chapter 63

Nutrigenomics: Developing Personalized Diets for Disease Prevention

Personal health recommendations and diets tailored to better prevent diseases may be in our future, just by focusing on genetics.

Researchers at Kansas State University recently published an academic journal article discussing the potential for nutrigenomics, a field that studies the effects of food on gene expression. The researchers discussed the possibility of using food to prevent an individual's genes from expressing disease. The researchers said nutrigenomics could completely change the future of public health and the food and culinary industries.

"Nutrigenomics involves tailoring diets to someone's genetic makeup," said Koushik Adhikari, K-State assistant professor of sensory analysis. "I speculate that in five to ten years, you would go to a genetic counselor or a physician who could help you understand your genetic makeup, and then a nutritional professional could customize your diet accordingly."

Adhikari collaborated with Denis Medeiros, professor and department head of human nutrition, and Jean Getz, former K-State graduate student in human nutrition, for an article on nutrigenomics that was published in the January 2010 issue of *Food Technology*. Getz, now a student at the School of Osteopathic Medicine at Michigan State University, wrote the article while at K-State.

Nutrigenomics is a fast-moving field of research that combines molecular biology, genetics, and nutrition to regulate gene expression through specific nutrients. Nutrients have been shown to affect gene expression through transcription factors, which are biochemical entities that bind to deoxyribonucleic acid (DNA) and either promote or inhibit transcription of genes. By understanding the roles of specific nutrients and how they might cause diseases, scientists could recommend specific foods for an individual based on his or her genetics.

"Scientists are looking at the molecular mechanisms in the body," Adhikari said. "At the molecular level, you can look at what specific nutrients can do to your body that would trigger genes to act properly, in a healthy way."

Medeiros said K-State researchers in human nutrition are doing these kinds of studies. Some are studying the impact plant chemicals have on different types of cancers in terms of their potential prevention effects. Other researchers are looking at how wolfberry, a Chinese fruit, could be used to improve vision.

"These studies not only answer whether the concerned nutrients prevent a disease, but also how they exert their health benefits," Medeiros said.

Current health recommendations for people in the United States are general for the overall population. However, with nutrigenomics research, health recommendations could be better modified to individuals.

"That is where I think the main focus of nutrigenomics is going to be in the future," Adhikari said. "It could tell you that you have the propensity for certain chronic diseases so that you could modify your diet accordingly. With a better understanding of how nutrients alter gene expression, there is a potential that food could be used instead of medication to combat problems like high cholesterol."

Adhikari said this kind of personalized health care is in the near future since the human genome has been mapped. Now scientists are focusing on identifying single-nucleotide polymorphisms, which are a small change in a person's DNA sequence like sensitivity to bitterness. Polymorphisms could determine if a person has a propensity for different chronic diseases. At K-State, Adhikari and Mark Haub, associate professor of human nutrition, are leading a study of the genotypes of diabetic and nondiabetic individuals to determine if there is a link between the risk for type-2 diabetes and bitter-taste sensitivity.

Nutrigenomics would require a collaborative effort from people in genetics and the industries of public health, food science, and culinary. Adhikari said more options should be available so that consumers can make the healthiest choice. He said the food industry should collaborate with the culinary industry to create more healthful and appealing foods.

"This is one of the major issues with the food industry," he said. "It's very easy to make good-tasting food. Put some lard or butter in it, and it's going to taste good. The challenge is how to take the fat out and create healthful but also good-tasting food."

Consumer education also will be an important factor for the future of nutrigenomics and public health. Adhikari said consumers are often skeptical of genetically modified foods, where scientists modify a food's DNA by splicing and adding genes. However, this practice is different from nutrigenomics, which focuses on using foods' natural components to promote better health.

The researchers said a shift in public health is greatly needed, and with an increasing incidence of obesity and chronic diseases such as types 2 diabetes, nutrigenomics might prove to be the panacea in the future.

Chapter 64

Pharmacogenomics

What is pharmacogenomics?

Pharmacogenomics is the study of how an individual's genetic inheritance affects the body's response to drugs. The term comes from the words "pharmacology" and "genomics" and is thus the intersection of pharmaceuticals and genetics.

Pharmacogenomics holds the promise that drugs might one day be tailor-made for individuals and adapted to each person's own genetic makeup. Environment, diet, age, lifestyle, and state of health all can influence a person's response to medicines, but understanding an individual's genetic makeup is thought to be the key to creating personalized drugs with greater efficacy and safety.

Pharmacogenomics combines traditional pharmaceutical sciences such as biochemistry with annotated knowledge of genes, proteins, and single nucleotide polymorphisms.

What are the anticipated benefits of pharmacogenomics?

More powerful medicines: Pharmaceutical companies will be able to create drugs based on the proteins, enzymes, and ribonucleic acid (RNA) molecules associated with genes and diseases. This will facilitate drug discovery and allow drug makers to produce a therapy

Reprinted from the Oak Ridge National Laboratory (www.ornl.gov), September 19, 2011.

more targeted to specific diseases. This accuracy not only will maximize therapeutic effects but also decrease damage to nearby healthy cells.

Better, safer drugs the first time: Instead of the standard trial-and-error method of matching patients with the right drugs, doctors will be able to analyze a patient's genetic profile and prescribe the best available drug therapy from the beginning. Not only will this take the guesswork out of finding the right drug, it will speed recovery time and increase safety as the likelihood of adverse reactions is eliminated. Pharmacogenomics has the potential to dramatically reduce the estimated one hundred thousand deaths and two million hospitalizations that occur each year in the United States as the result of adverse drug response.[1]

More accurate methods of determining appropriate drug dosages: Current methods of basing dosages on weight and age will be replaced with dosages based on a person's genetics—how well the body processes the medicine and the time it takes to metabolize it. This will maximize the therapy's value and decrease the likelihood of overdose.

Advanced screening for disease: Knowing one's genetic code will allow a person to make adequate lifestyle and environmental changes at an early age so as to avoid or lessen the severity of a genetic disease. Likewise, advance knowledge of a particular disease susceptibility will allow careful monitoring, and treatments can be introduced at the most appropriate stage to maximize their therapy.

Better vaccines: Vaccines made of genetic material, either deoxyribonucleic acid (DNA) or RNA, promise all the benefits of existing vaccines without all the risks. They will activate the immune system but will be unable to cause infections. They will be inexpensive, stable, easy to store, and capable of being engineered to carry several strains of a pathogen at once.

Improvements in the drug discovery and approval process: Pharmaceutical companies will be able to discover potential therapies more easily using genome targets. Previously failed drug candidates may be revived as they are matched with the niche population they serve. The drug approval process should be facilitated as trials are targeted for specific genetic population groups—providing greater degrees of success. The cost and risk of clinical trials will be reduced by targeting only those persons capable of responding to a drug.

Decrease in the overall cost of health care: Decreases in the number of adverse drug reactions, the number of failed drug trials, the time it takes to get a drug approved, the length of time patients are on medication, the number of medications patients must take to find an effective therapy, the effects of a disease on the body (through early detection), and an increase in the range of possible drug targets will promote a net decrease in the cost of health care.

Is pharmacogenomics in use today?

To a limited degree. The cytochrome P450 (CYP) family of liver enzymes is responsible for breaking down more than thirty different classes of drugs. DNA variations in genes that code for these enzymes can influence their ability to metabolize certain drugs. Less active or inactive forms of CYP enzymes that are unable to break down and efficiently eliminate drugs from the body can cause drug overdose in patients. Today, clinical trials researchers use genetic tests for variations in cytochrome P450 genes to screen and monitor patients. In addition, many pharmaceutical companies screen their chemical compounds to see how well they are broken down by variant forms of CYP enzymes.[2]

Another enzyme called TPMT (thiopurine methyltransferase) plays an important role in the chemotherapy treatment of a common childhood leukemia by breaking down a class of therapeutic compounds called thiopurines. A small percentage of Caucasians have genetic variants that prevent them from producing an active form of this protein. As a result, thiopurines elevate to toxic levels in the patient because the inactive form of TMPT is unable to break down the drug. Today, doctors can use a genetic test to screen patients for this deficiency, and the TMPT activity is monitored to determine appropriate thiopurine dosage levels.[3]

What are some of the barriers to pharmacogenomics progress?

Pharmacogenomics is a developing research field that is still in its infancy. Several of the following barriers will have to be overcome before many pharmacogenomics benefits can be realized.

Complexity of finding gene variations that affect drug response: Single nucleotide polymorphisms (SNPs) are DNA sequence variations that occur when a single nucleotide (A, T, C, or G) in the genome sequence is altered. SNPs occur every one hundred to three hundred bases along the three-billion-base human genome, therefore millions of SNPs must be identified and analyzed to determine their involvement (if any) in drug response. Further complicating the process is our limited knowledge of which genes are involved with each drug response. Since many genes are likely to influence responses, obtaining the big picture on the impact of gene variations is highly time-consuming and complicated.

Limited drug alternatives: Only one or two approved drugs may be available for treatment of a particular condition. If patients have gene variations that prevent them using these drugs, they may be left without any alternatives for treatment.

Disincentives for drug companies to make multiple pharmacogenomic products: Most pharmaceutical companies have been successful with their "one size fits all" approach to drug development. Since it costs hundreds of millions of dollars to bring a drug to market, will these companies be willing to develop alternative drugs that serve only a small portion of the population?

Educating healthcare providers: Introducing multiple pharmacogenomic products to treat the same condition for different population subsets undoubtedly will complicate the process of prescribing and dispensing drugs. Physicians must execute an extra diagnostic step to determine which drug is best suited to each patient. To interpret the diagnostic accurately and recommend the best course of treatment for each patient, all prescribing physicians, regardless of specialty, will need a better understanding of genetics.

References

1. J. Lazarou, B. H. Pomeranz, and P. N. Corey. Incidence of adverse drug reactions in hospitalized patients: a meta-analysis of prospective studies. *JAMA.* Apr 15, 1998. 279(15):1200–1205.

2. J. Hodgson, and A. Marshall. Pharmacogenomics: will the regulators approve? *Nature Biotechnolgy.* 16: 243–46. 1998.

3. S. Pistoi. Facing your genetic destiny, part II. *Scientific American.* February 25, 2002.

Chapter 65

Gene Therapy

Chapter Contents

Section 65.1

What Is Gene Therapy?

Excerpted from "Gene Therapy," Genetics Home Reference
(http://ghr.nlm.nih.gov), June 3, 2013.

What is gene therapy?

Gene therapy is an experimental technique that uses genes to treat or prevent disease. In the future, this technique may allow doctors to treat a disorder by inserting a gene into a patient's cells instead of using drugs or surgery. Researchers are testing several approaches to gene therapy, including the following:

- Replacing a mutated gene that causes disease with a healthy copy of the gene

- Inactivating, or "knocking out," a mutated gene that is functioning improperly

- Introducing a new gene into the body to help fight a disease.

Although gene therapy is a promising treatment option for a number of diseases (including inherited disorders, some types of cancer, and certain viral infections), the technique remains risky and is still under study to make sure that it will be safe and effective. Gene therapy is currently being tested only for the treatment of diseases that have no other cures.

How does gene therapy work?

Gene therapy is designed to introduce genetic material into cells to compensate for abnormal genes or to make a beneficial protein. If a mutated gene causes a necessary protein to be faulty or missing, gene therapy may be able to introduce a normal copy of the gene to restore the function of the protein.

A gene that is inserted directly into a cell usually does not function. Instead, a carrier called a vector is genetically engineered to deliver the gene. Certain viruses are often used as vectors because they can deliver the new gene by infecting the cell. The viruses are modified so they can't cause disease when used in people. Some types of virus, such as retroviruses, integrate their genetic material (including the new gene) into a chromosome in the human cell. Other viruses, such as adenoviruses, introduce their deoxyribonucleic acid (DNA) into the nucleus of the cell, but the DNA is not integrated into a chromosome.

The vector can be injected or given intravenously (by intravenous [IV] line) directly into a specific tissue in the body, where it is taken up by individual cells. Alternately, a sample of the patient's cells can be removed and exposed to the vector in a laboratory setting. The cells containing the vector are then returned to the patient. If the treatment is successful, the new gene delivered by the vector will make a functioning protein.

Researchers must overcome many technical challenges before gene therapy will be a practical approach to treating disease. For example, scientists must find better ways to deliver genes and target them to particular cells. They must also ensure that new genes are precisely controlled by the body.

Is gene therapy safe?

Gene therapy is under study to determine whether it could be used to treat disease. Current research is evaluating the safety of gene therapy; future studies will test whether it is an effective treatment option. Several studies have already shown that this approach can have very serious health risks, such as toxicity, inflammation, and cancer. Because the techniques are relatively new, some of the risks may be unpredictable; however, medical researchers, institutions, and regulatory agencies are working to ensure that gene therapy research is as safe as possible.

Comprehensive federal laws, regulations, and guidelines help protect people who participate in research studies (called clinical trials). The U.S. Food and Drug Administration (FDA) regulates all gene therapy products in the United States and oversees research in this area. Researchers who wish to test an approach in a clinical trial must first obtain permission from the FDA. The FDA has the authority to reject or suspend clinical trials that are suspected of being unsafe for participants.

The National Institutes of Health (NIH) also plays an important role in ensuring the safety of gene therapy research. NIH provides guidelines for investigators and institutions (such as universities and hospitals) to follow when conducting clinical trials with gene therapy. These guidelines state that clinical trials at institutions receiving NIH funding for this type of research must be registered with the NIH Office of Biotechnology Activities. The protocol, or plan, for each clinical trial is then reviewed by the NIH Recombinant DNA Advisory Committee

(RAC) to determine whether it raises medical, ethical, or safety issues that warrant further discussion at one of the RAC's public meetings.

An Institutional Review Board (IRB) and an Institutional Biosafety Committee (IBC) must approve each gene therapy clinical trial before it can be carried out. An IRB is a committee of scientific and medical advisors and consumers that reviews all research within an institution. An IBC is a group that reviews and approves an institution's potentially hazardous research studies. Multiple levels of evaluation and oversight ensure that safety concerns are a top priority in the planning and carrying out of gene therapy research.

What are the ethical issues surrounding gene therapy?

Because gene therapy involves making changes to the body's set of basic instructions, it raises many unique ethical concerns. The ethical questions surrounding gene therapy include the following:

- How can "good" and "bad" uses of gene therapy be distinguished?

- Who decides which traits are normal and which constitute a disability or disorder?

- Will the high costs of gene therapy make it available only to the wealthy?

- Could the widespread use of gene therapy make society less accepting of people who are different?

- Should people be allowed to use gene therapy to enhance basic human traits such as height, intelligence, or athletic ability?

Current gene therapy research has focused on treating individuals by targeting the therapy to body cells such as bone marrow or blood cells. This type of gene therapy cannot be passed on to a person's children. Gene therapy could be targeted to egg and sperm cells (germ cells), however, which would allow the inserted gene to be passed on to future generations. This approach is known as germline gene therapy.

The idea of germline gene therapy is controversial. While it could spare future generations in a family from having a particular genetic disorder, it might affect the development of a fetus in unexpected ways or have long-term side effects that are not yet known. Because people who would be affected by germline gene therapy are not yet born, they can't choose whether to have the treatment. Because of these ethical concerns, the U.S. government does not allow federal funds to be used for research on germline gene therapy in people.

Section 65.2

Gene Therapy and Children

Gene therapy carries the promise of cures for many diseases and for types of medical treatment most of us would not have thought possible. With its potential to eliminate and prevent hereditary diseases such as cystic fibrosis and hemophilia and its use as a possible cure for heart disease, acquired immunodeficiency syndrome (AIDS), and cancer, gene therapy is a potential medical miracle-worker.

But what about gene therapy for children? There's a fair amount of risk involved in trials of this kind of therapy, and to date, only kids who are seriously ill or have illnesses incurable by conventional means have been involved in clinical trials using gene therapy.

For those with serious illnesses that aren't responsive to conventional therapies, however, gene therapy may soon offer hope that didn't exist just a short time ago.

About Genes

Our genes are part of what makes us unique. Inherited from our parents, they go far in determining our physical traits—like the color of our eyes and the color and texture of our hair. They also determine things like whether babies will be male or female, the amount of oxygen blood can carry, and intelligence quotient (IQ).

Genes are composed of strands of a molecule called deoxyribonucleic acid (DNA) and are located in single file within the chromosomes. The genetic message is encoded by the building blocks of the DNA, which are called nucleotides. Approximately three billion pairs of nucleotides are in the chromosomes of a human cell, and each person's genetic makeup has a unique sequence of nucleotides. This is mainly what makes us different from one another.

Scientists believe that every human has about twenty-five thousand genes per cell. A mutation, or change, in any one of these genes can result in a disease, physical disability, or shortened lifespan. These mutations can be passed from one generation to another, inherited just like a mother's red hair or a father's brown eyes. Mutations also can occur spontaneously in some cases, without having been passed on by a parent. With gene therapy, the treatment or elimination of inherited diseases or physical conditions due to these mutations could become a reality.

Gene therapy involves the manipulation of genes to fight or prevent diseases. Put simply, it introduces a "good" gene into a person who has a disease caused by a "bad" gene.

Two Types of Gene Therapy

The two forms of gene therapy are:

1. Somatic gene therapy involves introducing a "good" gene into targeted cells to treat the patient — but not the patient's future children because these genes do not get passed along to offspring. In other words, even though some of the patient's genes may be altered to treat a disease, it won't change the chance that the disease will be passed on to the patient's children. This is the more common form of gene therapy being done.

2. Germline gene therapy involves modifying the genes in egg or sperm cells, which will then pass any genetic changes to future generations. In experimenting with this type of therapy, scientists injected fragments of DNA into fertilized mouse eggs. The mice grew into adults and their offspring had the new gene. Scientists found that certain growth and fertility problems could be corrected with this therapy, which led them to think that the same could be true for humans. However, although it has potential for preventing inherited disease, this type of therapy is controversial and very little research is being done in this area, both for technical and ethical reasons.

Possible Effects of Gene Therapy

Gene therapy is done only through clinical trials, which often take years to complete. After new drugs or procedures are tested in laboratories, clinical trials are conducted with human patients under strictly controlled circumstances. Such trials usually last two to four years and go through several phases of research. In the United States, the U.S. Food and Drug Administration (FDA) must then approve the new therapy for the marketplace, which can take another two years.

The most active research being done in gene therapy for kids has been for genetic disorders such as cystic fibrosis. Other gene therapy trials involve children with severe immunodeficiencies, such as adenosine deaminase (ADA) deficiency (a rare genetic disease that makes kids prone to serious infection), and those with familial hypercholesterolemia (extremely high levels of serum cholesterol).

Gene therapy does have risks and limitations. The viruses and other agents used to deliver the "good" genes can affect more than the cells for which they're intended. If a gene is added to DNA, it could be put in the wrong place, which could potentially cause cancer or other damage.

Genes also can be "overexpressed," meaning they can drive the production of so much of a protein that they can be harmful. Another risk is that a virus introduced into one person could be transmitted to others or into the environment.

Although the National Cancer Institute reports that such problems have not occurred in any of the human gene therapy trials to date, not everyone is excited about this new kind of treatment.

Gene therapy trials in children present an ethical dilemma, according to some gene therapy experts. Kids with an altered gene may have mild or severe effects, and the severity often can't be determined in infants. So just because some kids appear to have a genetic problem doesn't mean they'll be substantially affected by it, but they'll have to live with the knowledge of that problem.

Kids could be tested for disorders if there is a medical treatment or a lifestyle change that could be beneficial—or if knowing they don't carry the gene reduces the medical surveillance needed. For example, finding out a child doesn't carry the gene for a disorder that runs in the family might mean that he or she doesn't have to undergo yearly screenings or other regular exams.

The Future of Gene Therapy

To cure genetic diseases, scientists must first determine which gene or set of genes causes each disease. The Human Genome Project and other international efforts have completed the initial work of sequencing and mapping virtually all of the twenty-five thousand to thirty-five thousand genes in the human cell. This research will provide new strategies to diagnose, treat, cure, and possibly prevent human diseases.

Although this information will help scientists determine the genetic basis of many diseases, it will be a long time before diseases actually can be treated through gene therapy.

Gene therapy's potential to revolutionize medicine in the future is exciting, and hopes are high for its role in curing and preventing childhood diseases. One day it may be possible to treat an unborn child for a genetic disease even before symptoms appear.

Scientists hope that the human genome mapping will help lead to cures for many diseases and that successful clinical trials will create new opportunities. For now, however, it's a wait-and-see situation, calling for cautious optimism.

Section 65.3

Gene Therapy for Advanced Parkinson Disease Shows Promise

An experimental surgical treatment for Parkinson disease (PD)—which involves inserting the human gene known as GAD deep into a brain structure—improved motor symptoms in people with a moderately advanced stage of Parkinson. The results were reported in the March 17, 2011, online issue of *The Lancet Neurology*.

Gene therapy is a method which delivers a therapeutic substance, made by a gene, directly to a specific area of the body. In the new study, scientists used an inactivated virus to deliver the gene called glutamic acid decarboxylase (GAD) into brain cells. GAD makes a neurotransmitter called gamma-aminobutyric acid (GABA) which can suppress overactivity in the brain's subthalamic nucleus—overactivity that contributes to the movement symptoms and complications of Parkinson, such as dyskinesia. An earlier study showed that the use of this virus to deliver the GAD gene into the brain was a safe approach in people with PD.

Investigators at seven U.S. research centers led by Andrew Feigin, M.D., of the Feinstein Institute for Medical Research, North Shore University Hospital, Manhasset, New York, surgically inserted catheters into the brains of sixteen study participants to carry the GAD gene to the subthalamic nucleus on both sides of the brain. An additional twenty-one participants underwent sham surgery, a simulated injection procedure in which the skull is not opened and participants do not receive the GAD gene. Sham surgery is important for research design and helps to maintain "blinding" of the study, meaning neither the participants nor medical personnel knew which participants had gene therapy.

Results

Six months after the surgery, motor symptoms in participants who received gene therapy improved by an average of 23 percent, as measured by a standard rating scale, the Unified Parkinson's Disease Rating Scale (UPDRS); symptoms in participants who had sham surgery improved by an average of 13 percent.

Participants experienced mild to moderate side effects, mainly headache and nausea, but no other adverse consequences.

What Does It Mean?

The idea of injecting a gene into the brain to make a protein to treat PD has long been discussed in the scientific community. This study is the first rigorously designed clinical trial to test that hypothesis, and it is the first double-blinded study to show a positive benefit. As a proof of principle, this study confirmed that gene therapy can be performed safely. In terms of its larger impact, this study serves as encouragement to researchers and people with Parkinson, and confirms the need for more study. It is important to note that the gene injected into the brain—GAD—resulted in benefits in movement problems in the range of the effects of deep brain stimulation. GAD is not a therapy that slows down the progression of PD, an important goal for future gene therapies.

Section 65.4

Gene Therapy for Cancer: Questions and Answers

Excerpted from "Gene Therapy for Cancer: Questions and Answers,"
National Cancer Institute (www.cancer.gov), August 31, 2006.
Reviewed by David A. Cooke, M.D., FACP, May 2013.

What are genes?

Genes are the biological units of heredity. Genes determine obvious traits, such as hair and eye color, as well as more subtle characteristics, such as the ability of the blood to carry oxygen. Complex characteristics, such as physical strength, may be shaped by the interaction of a number of different genes along with environmental influences.

Genes are located on chromosomes inside cells and are made of deoxyribonucleic acid (DNA), which is a type of biological molecule. Humans have between thirty thousand and forty thousand genes. Genes carry the instructions that allow cells to produce specific proteins, such as enzymes.

To make proteins, a cell must first copy the information stored in genes into another type of biological molecule called ribonucleic acid (RNA). The cell's protein synthesizing machinery then decodes the information in the RNA to manufacture specific proteins. Only certain genes in a cell are active at any given moment. As cells mature, many genes become permanently inactive. The pattern of active and inactive genes in a cell and the resulting protein composition determine what kind of cell it is and what it can and cannot do. Flaws in genes can result in disease.

What is gene therapy?

Advances in understanding and manipulating genes have set the stage for scientists to alter a person's genetic material to fight or prevent disease. Gene therapy is an experimental treatment that involves introducing genetic material (DNA or RNA) into a person's cells to fight disease. Gene therapy is being studied in clinical trials (research studies with people) for many different types of cancer and for other diseases. It is not currently available outside a clinical trial.

How is gene therapy being studied in the treatment of cancer?

Researchers are studying several ways to treat cancer using gene therapy. Some approaches target healthy cells to enhance their ability to fight cancer. Other approaches target cancer cells, to destroy them or prevent their growth. Some gene therapy techniques under study are described below:

- In one approach, researchers replace missing or altered genes with healthy genes. Because some missing or altered genes (e.g., p53) may cause cancer, substituting "working" copies of these genes may be used to treat cancer.

- Researchers are also studying ways to improve a patient's immune response to cancer. In this approach, gene therapy is used to stimulate the body's natural ability to attack cancer cells. In one method under investigation, researchers take a small blood sample from a patient and insert genes that will cause each cell to produce a protein called a T-cell receptor (TCR). The genes are transferred into the patient's white blood cells (called T lymphocytes) and are then given back to the patient. In the body, the white blood cells produce TCRs, which attach to the outer surface of the white blood cells. The TCRs then recognize and attach to certain molecules found on the surface of the tumor cells. Finally, the TCRs activate the white blood cells to attack and kill the tumor cells.

- Scientists are investigating the insertion of genes into cancer cells to make them more sensitive to chemotherapy, radiation therapy, or other treatments. In other studies, researchers remove healthy blood-forming stem cells from the body, insert a gene that makes these cells more resistant to the side effects of high doses of anticancer drugs, and then inject the cells back into the patient.

- In another approach, researchers introduce "suicide genes" into a patient's cancer cells. A pro-drug (an inactive form of a toxic drug) is then given to the patient. The pro-drug is activated in cancer cells containing these "suicide genes," which leads to the destruction of those cancer cells.

- Other research is focused on the use of gene therapy to prevent cancer cells from developing new blood vessels (angiogenesis).

How are genes transferred into cells so that gene therapy can take place?

In general, a gene cannot be directly inserted into a person's cell. It must be delivered to the cell using a carrier, or "vector." The vectors most commonly used in gene therapy are viruses. Viruses have a unique ability to recognize certain cells and insert genetic material into them.

In some gene therapy clinical trials, cells from the patient's blood or bone marrow are removed and grown in the laboratory. The cells are exposed to the virus that is carrying the desired gene. The virus enters the cells and inserts the desired gene into the cells' DNA. The cells grow in the laboratory and are then returned to the patient by injection into a vein. This type of gene therapy is called ex vivo because the cells are grown outside the body. The gene is transferred into the patient's cells while the cells are outside the patient's body.

In other studies, vectors (often viruses) or liposomes (fatty particles) are used to deliver the desired gene to cells in the patient's body. This form of gene therapy is called in vivo, because the gene is transferred to cells inside the patient's body.

What types of viruses are used in gene therapy, and how can they be used safely?

Many gene therapy clinical trials rely on retroviruses to deliver the desired gene. Other viruses used as vectors include adenoviruses, adeno-associated viruses, lentiviruses, poxviruses, and herpes viruses. These viruses differ in how well they transfer genes to the cells they recognize and are able to infect, and whether they alter the cell's DNA permanently or temporarily. Thus, researchers may use different vectors, depending on the specific characteristics and requirements of the study.

Scientists alter the viruses used in gene therapy to make them safe for humans and to increase their ability to deliver specific genes to a patient's cells. Depending on the type of virus and the goals of the research study, scientists may inactivate certain genes in the viruses to prevent them from reproducing or causing disease. Researchers may also alter the virus so that it better recognizes and enters the target cell.

What risks are associated with current gene therapy trials?

Viruses can usually infect more than one type of cell. Thus, when viral vectors are used to carry genes into the body, they might infect healthy cells as well as cancer cells. Another danger is that the new gene might be inserted in the wrong location in the DNA, possibly causing harmful mutations to the DNA or even cancer.

In addition, when viruses or liposomes are used to deliver DNA to cells inside the patient's body, there is a slight chance that this DNA could unintentionally be introduced into the patient's reproductive cells. If this happens, it could produce changes that may be passed on if a patient has children after treatment.

Other concerns include the possibility that transferred genes could be "overexpressed," producing so much of the missing protein as to be harmful; that the viral vector could cause inflammation or an immune reaction; and that the virus could be transmitted from the patient to other individuals or into the environment. Scientists use animal testing and other precautions to identify and avoid these risks before any clinical trials are conducted in humans.

What major problems must scientists overcome before gene therapy becomes a common technique for treating disease?

Scientists need to identify more efficient ways to deliver genes to the body. To treat cancer and other diseases effectively with gene therapy, researchers must develop vectors that can be injected into the patient and specifically focus on the target cells located throughout the body. More work is also needed to ensure that the vectors will successfully insert the desired genes into each of these target cells.

Researchers also need to be able to deliver genes consistently to a precise location in the patient's DNA, and ensure that transplanted genes are precisely controlled by the body's normal physiologic signals.

Although scientists are working hard on these problems, it is impossible to predict when they will have effective solutions.

The first disease approved for treatment with gene therapy was adenosine deaminase (ADA) deficiency. What is this disease and why was it selected?

ADA deficiency is a rare genetic disease. The normal ADA gene produces an enzyme called adenosine deaminase, which is essential to the body's immune system. Patients with ADA deficiency do not have normal ADA genes and do not produce functional ADA enzymes. ADA-deficient children are born with severe immunodeficiency and are prone to repeated serious infections, which may be life threatening. Although ADA deficiency can be treated with a drug called PEG-ADA, the drug is extremely costly and must be taken for life by injection into a vein.

ADA deficiency was selected for the first approved human gene therapy trial for several reasons:

- The disease is caused by a defect in a single gene, which increases the likelihood that gene therapy will succeed.

- The gene is regulated in a simple, "always-on" fashion, unlike many genes whose regulation is complex.

- The amount of ADA present does not need to be precisely regulated. Even small amounts of the enzyme are known to be beneficial, while larger amounts are also tolerated well.

How do gene therapy trials receive approval?

A proposed gene therapy trial, or protocol, must be approved by at least two review boards at the scientists' institution. Gene therapy protocols must also be approved by the U.S. Food and Drug Administration (FDA), which regulates all gene therapy products. In addition, trials that are funded by the National Institutes of Health (NIH) must be registered with the NIH Recombinant DNA Advisory Committee (RAC). The NIH, which includes twenty-seven institutes and centers, is the federal focal point for biomedical research in the United States.

Why are there so many steps in this process?

Any studies involving humans must be reviewed with great care. Gene therapy in particular is potentially a very powerful technique, is relatively new, and could have profound implications. These factors make it necessary for scientists to take special precautions with gene therapy.

What are some of the social and ethical issues surrounding human gene therapy?

In large measure, the issues are the same as those faced whenever a powerful new technology is developed. Such technologies can accomplish great good, but they can also result in great harm if applied unwisely.

Gene therapy is currently focused on correcting genetic flaws and curing life-threatening disease, and regulations are in place for conducting these types of studies. But in the future, when the techniques of gene therapy have become simpler and more accessible, society will need to deal with more complex questions.

One such question is related to the possibility of genetically altering human eggs or sperm, the reproductive cells that pass genes on to future generations. (Because reproductive cells are also called germ cells, this type of gene therapy is referred to as germ-line therapy.) Another question is related to the potential for enhancing human capabilities—for example, improving memory and intelligence—by genetic intervention. Although both germ-line gene therapy and genetic enhancement have the potential to produce benefits, possible problems with these procedures worry many scientists.

Germ-line gene therapy would forever change the genetic makeup of an individual's descendants. Thus, the human gene pool would be permanently affected. Although these changes would presumably be for the better, an error in technology or judgment could have far-reaching consequences. The NIH does not approve germ-line gene therapy in humans.

In the case of genetic enhancement, there is concern that such manipulation could become a luxury available only to the rich and powerful. Some also fear that widespread use of this technology could lead to new definitions of "normal" that would exclude individuals who are, for example, of merely average intelligence. And, justly or not, some people associate all genetic manipulation with past abuses of the concept of "eugenics," or the study of methods of improving genetic qualities through selective breeding.

What is being done to address these social and ethical issues?

Scientists working on the Human Genome Project (HGP), which completed mapping and sequencing all of the genes in humans, recognized that the information gained from this work would have profound implications for individuals, families, and society. The Ethical, Legal, and Social Implications (ELSI) Research Program was established in 1990 as part of the HGP to address these issues. The ELSI Research Program fosters basic and applied research on the ethical, legal, and social implications of genetic and genomic research for individuals, families, and communities. The ELSI Research Program sponsors and manages studies and supports workshops, research consortia, and policy conferences on these topics.

Part Six

Information for
Parents of Children
with Genetic Disorders

Chapter 66

When Your Baby Has a Birth Defect

We see happy images of and tend to hear about only healthy babies. But many babies are born with a birth defect. These are abnormalities of structure, function, or body chemistry that will require medical or surgical care or could have some effect on a child's development.

About 150,000 babies are born in the United States each year with birth defects, according to the March of Dimes. There is a wide range of birth defects, from mild to severe, and they can be inherited or caused by something in the environment. In many cases, the cause is unknown. Doctors may detect a birth defect during prenatal testing.

If you've just found out that your child has a birth defect, you're probably experiencing many emotions. Parents in your situation often say they feel overwhelmed and uncertain about whether they'll be able to care for their child properly.

Steps to Take

Fortunately, you aren't alone—you'll find that many people and resources are available to help you. As the parent of a child with a birth defect, it's important for you to:

"When Your Baby Has a Birth Defect," September 2012, reprinted with permission from www.kidshealth.org. This information was provided by KidsHealth®, one of the largest resources online for medically reviewed health information written for parents, kids, and teens. For more articles like this, visit www.KidsHealth.org, or www.TeensHealth.org. Copyright © 1995–2012 The Nemours Foundation. All rights reserved.

- **Acknowledge your emotions:** Parents of children with birth
  defects experience shock, denial, grief, and even anger. Acknowledge your feelings and give yourself permission to mourn the loss
  of the healthy child you thought you'd have. Talk about your
  feelings with your spouse or partner and with other family members. You might also consider seeing a counselor. Your doctor
  might be able to recommend a social worker or psychologist in
  the area.

- **One of the best things you can do for yourself and your
  child is to seek support:** Getting in touch with someone who's
  been through the same thing can be helpful; ask your doctor or
  a social worker at your hospital if there are other parents in
  the area who have children with the same condition. Joining a
  support group may also help—ask the doctors or specialists for
  advice on finding a local or national support group or search
  online.

- **Celebrate your child:** Remember to let yourself enjoy your
  child the same way any parent would—by cuddling or playing,
  watching for developmental milestones (even if they're different from those in children without a birth defect), and sharing
  your joy with family members and friends. Many parents of kids
  with birth defects wonder if they should send out birth announce-
  ments. This is a personal decision—the fact that your child has a
  health problem doesn't mean you shouldn't be excited about the
  new addition to your family.

Getting Help and Information

Seek information: The amount each person would like to learn
varies from parent to parent, but try to educate yourself as much and
as soon as you are able. Start by asking your doctors lots of questions. Record the answers as best you can. If you're not satisfied
with the answers—or if a doctor is unable to answer your questions
thoroughly—don't be afraid to seek second opinions.

Other places to get information include:

- books written for parents of children with birth defects;

- national organizations such as the March of Dimes, the National
  Information Center for Children and Youth With Disabilities, or
  those representing a specific birth defect;

- support groups or other parents.

Keep a file with a running list of questions and the answers you find, as well as suggestions for further reading and any materials your child's doctor gives you. In addition, keep an updated list of all health care providers and their phone numbers, as well as emergency numbers, so you're able to reach them quickly and efficiently.

Part of this process of collecting information should involve exploring options for paying for treatment and ongoing care for your child. There can be extra medical and therapeutic costs associated with caring for a child with a birth defect. Besides health insurance, other resources are available, including nonprofit disability organizations, private foundations, Medicaid, and state and local programs. One of the hospital social workers should be able to help you learn more about these.

Seek early intervention: Early intervention is usually the best strategy. Designed to bring a team of experts together to assess your child's needs and establish a program of treatment, early intervention services include feeding support, identification of assistive technology that may help your child, occupational therapy, physical therapy, speech therapy, nutrition services, and social work services.

Besides identifying, evaluating, and treating your child's needs, early intervention programs will:

- tell you where you can get information about the disability;

- help you to learn how to care for your child at home;

- help you determine your payment options and tell you where you can find services for free;

- help you make important decisions about your child's care;

- provide counseling.

Your child's doctor or a social worker at the hospital where you gave birth should be able to connect you with the early intervention program in your area.

Use a team approach: Most children with birth defects require a team of professionals to treat them. Even if your child needs to see only one specialist, that person will need to coordinate care with your primary doctor. Although some hospitals already have teams ready to deal with problems such as heart defects, cleft lip and palate, or cerebral palsy, you may find yourself having to serve as both the main point of contact between the different care providers and the coordinator of your child's appointments. As soon as you are able, get to know the different team members. Make sure they know who else will be caring for your child and that you intend to play a key role.

The Future of Birth Defects

Research into the environmental and genetic causes of birth defects is ongoing. Technology contributes to understanding and preventing defects in various ways—for example, prenatal testing is growing increasingly sophisticated.

Safer and more accurate tests include:

- results of ultrasound tests and magnetic resonance imaging (MRI), which are sometimes combined with information from blood tests to determine the risk of having a child with certain birth defects;

- maternal blood screening to determine risk of chromosomal abnormalities;

- amniocentesis and chorionic villi sampling;

- pre-conception counseling to help you understand any risks for having a child with a birth defect.

Although none of these tests can prevent birth defects, they give a clearer, safer, and more accurate diagnosis at an earlier stage of pregnancy—giving parents more time to seek advice and consider their options.

Genetics research is advancing quickly. The Human Genome Project is working on identifying all of the genes in the human body, including gene mutations that are associated with a high risk for birth defects.

Early surgery is becoming an option in the treatment of some birth defects—and can take place even before a child is born. Surgeons now operate on fetuses to repair structural defects, such as hernias of the diaphragm, spina bifida, and lung malformations. These treatments can be controversial, however, because they can cause premature labor. And it's still a bit unclear as to whether they ultimately improve the child's outcome.

To get information on specific research about your child's disability, contact the national organization for that disability. Also, the March of Dimes and the National Information Center for Children and Youth With Disabilities and the National Organization for Rare Disorders, Inc. (NORD) may have information about current research.

Chapter 67

Tips for Parenting a Child with a Disability

If you have a child with a disability, you are not alone. Millions of parents in the United States are raising children with disabilities. Many resources (including fellow parents) can help you along the way. Here are some tips for parents:

- Learn as much as you can about your child's disability.
- Find programs to help your child.
- Talk to your family about how you're feeling.
- Talk to other parents of children with disabilities.
- Join a support group.
- Stick to a daily routine.
- Take it one day at a time.
- Take good care of yourself.

An important quality that you will need to nurture in your child is called "self-determination." Children who develop this quality have a sense of control over their lives and can set goals and work to attain them. Self-determination is important for all children, but researchers have found that students with disabilities who also have high levels of self-determination are more likely to become adults who are:

"Parenting a Child with a Disability," U.S. Department of Health and Human Services, Office on Women's Health, September 22, 2009.

- employed;

- satisfied with their lives; and

- living independently, or with support, outside of their family homes.

Here are some tips to help your child become self-determined:

- As early as possible, give your child opportunities to make choices and encourage your child to express wants and wishes. For instance, these could be choices about what to wear, what to eat, and how much help with doing things your child wants from you.

- Strike a balance between being protective and supporting risk taking. Learn to let go a little and push your child out into the world, even though it may be a little scary.

- Guide children toward solving their own problems and making their own choices. For instance, if your child has a problem at school, offer a listening ear and together brainstorm possible solutions. To the extent that your child can, let your child decide on the plan and the back-up plan.

Programs and Services

Every state has programs and services that can help you meet your child's and your family's needs:

- Early intervention services try to address the needs of children with disabilities and the needs of their families as early as possible. Often, the sooner issues are addressed, the better the outcome. Examples include nutrition counseling for parents, physical therapy for a baby with cystic fibrosis, or sign language lessons for a deaf child. Services vary by state.

- Special education and related services ensure that each child is given a free public education that accommodates his or her special needs. The law requires that every student with a disability have an Individualized Education Program (IEP), which is a plan for that child's education. The IEP includes a list of the services, accommodations, and assistive technology your child will need to succeed in school. Parents of a child with a disability are an important part of the team that writes the IEP. To the extent that they can, children with disabilities should also be encouraged to take part in writing the IEP.

596

- Parent Training and Information (PTI) centers provide parents with information about disabilities and legal rights under laws involving children with disabilities. PTIs can also tell you about resources in the community, state, and nation. PTI centers conduct workshops, conferences, and seminars for parents. And many have libraries where you can borrow books and videos. Every state has at least one PTI. Some states also have Community Parent Resource Centers (CPRCs). CPRCs do the same work as the PTIs, but they focus on reaching underserved parents of children with disabilities. Underserved parents include low-income parents, parents with limited ability to speak and write English, and parents with disabilities.

- Parent to Parent is a program that provides information and one-to-one emotional support to parents of children with disabilities. Trained and experienced parents are carefully matched in one-to-one relationships with parents who are new to the program. The matches are based upon similarities in disability and family issues.

Chapter 68

Early Intervention: An Overview

Early intervention services are concerned with all the basic and brand new skills that babies typically develop during the first three years of life, such as the following:

- Physical (reaching, rolling, crawling, and walking)

- Cognitive (thinking, learning, solving problems)

- Communication (talking, listening, understanding)

- Social/emotional (playing, feeling secure and happy)

- Self-help (eating, dressing)

Early intervention services are designed to meet the needs of infants and toddlers who have a developmental delay or disability. Sometimes it is known from the moment a child is born that early intervention services will be essential in helping the child grow and develop. Often this is so for children who are diagnosed at birth with a specific condition or who experience significant prematurity, very low birth weight, illness, or surgery soon after being born. Even before heading home from the hospital, this child's parents may be given a referral to their local early intervention office.

Some children have a relatively routine entry into the world, but may develop more slowly than others, experience setbacks, or develop in ways that seem very different from other children. For these children,

Excerpted from "Overview of Early Intervention," National Dissemination Center for Children with Disabilities (http://nichcy.org), September 2011.

a visit with a developmental pediatrician and a thorough evaluation may lead to an early intervention referral. However a child comes to be referred, assessed, and determined eligible—early intervention services provide vital support so that children with developmental needs can thrive and grow. Eligible children can receive early intervention services from birth through the third birthday.

Let's take a closer look at the early intervention process, beginning with "so you're concerned about your child's development." This overview will discuss actions you can take to find help for your child, including contacting the early intervention program in your community.

Part 1: So You're Concerned about Your Child's Development

It's not uncommon for parents and family members to become concerned when their beautiful baby or growing toddler doesn't seem to be developing according to the normal schedule of "baby" milestones—"He hasn't rolled over yet," or "the little girl next door is already sitting up on her own!" or "she should be saying a few words by now." And while it's true that children develop differently, at their own pace, and that the range of what's "normal" development is quite broad, it's hard not to worry and wonder.

If you think that your child is not developing at the same pace or in the same way as most children his or her age, it is often a good idea to talk first to your child's pediatrician. Explain your concerns. Tell the doctor what you have observed with your child. Your child may have a disability or a developmental delay, or he or she may be at risk of having a disability or delay. You can also get in touch with your community's early intervention program, and ask to have your little one evaluated to see if he or she has a developmental delay or disability. This evaluation is free of charge, won't hurt your child, and looks at his or her basic skills. Based on that evaluation, your child may be eligible for early intervention services, which will be designed to address your child's special needs or delays.

Where Do I Go for Help?

How might you find out about early intervention services in your community? Here are two ways:

- Ask your child's pediatrician to put you in touch with the early intervention system in your community or region.

- Contact the pediatrics branch in a local hospital and ask where you should call to find out about early intervention services in your area.

It is very important to write down the names and phone numbers of everyone you talk to. Having this information available will be helpful to you later on.

What Do I Say to the Early Intervention Contact Person?

Explain that you are concerned about your child's development. Say that you think your child may need early intervention services. Explain that you would like to have your child evaluated under the Individuals with Disabilities Education Act (IDEA—the nation's special education law). Write down any information the contact person gives you.

The person may refer you to what is known as Child Find. One of Child Find's purposes is to identify children who need early intervention services. Child Find operates in every state and conducts screenings to identify children who may need early intervention services. These screenings are provided free of charge.

Each state has one agency that is in charge of the early intervention system for infants and toddlers with special needs. This agency is known as the lead agency. It may be the state education agency or another agency, such as the health department. Each state decides which agency will serve as the lead agency.

What Happens Next?

Once you are in contact with the early intervention system, the system will assign someone to work with you and your child through the evaluation and assessment process. This person will be your temporary service coordinator. He or she should have a background in early childhood development and ways to help young children who may have developmental delays. The service coordinator should also know the policies for early intervention programs and services in your state.

The early intervention system will need to determine if your child is eligible for early intervention services. To do this, the staff will set up and carry out a multidisciplinary evaluation and assessment of your child. Read on for more information about this process.

Part 2: Your Child's Evaluation

What Is a Multidisciplinary Evaluation and Assessment?

The law IDEA requires that your child receive a timely, comprehensive, multidisciplinary evaluation and assessment. The purposes of the evaluation and assessment are to find out the following things:

- The nature of your child's strengths, delays, or difficulties

- Whether or not your child is eligible for early intervention services

Multidisciplinary means that the evaluation group is made up of qualified people who have different areas of training and experience. Together, they know about children's speech and language skills, physical abilities, hearing and vision, and other important areas of development. They know how to work with children, even very young ones, to discover if a child has a problem or is developing within normal ranges. Group members may evaluate your child together or individually.

Evaluation refers to the procedures used by these professionals to find out if your child is eligible for early intervention services. As part of the evaluation, the team will observe your child, ask your child to do things, talk to you and your child, and use other methods to gather information. These procedures will help the team find out how your child functions in five areas of development: cognitive development, physical development, communication, social-emotional development, and adaptive development.

Following your child's evaluation, you and a team of professionals will meet and review all of the data, results, and reports. The people on the team will talk with you about whether your child meets the criteria under IDEA and state policy for having a developmental delay, a diagnosed physical or mental condition, or being at risk for having a substantial delay. If so, your child is generally found to be eligible for services.

If found eligible, he or she will then be assessed. Assessment refers to the procedures used throughout the time your child is in early intervention. The purposes of these ongoing procedures are as follows:

- To identify your child's unique strengths and needs

- To determine what services are necessary to meet those needs

With your consent, your family's needs will also be identified. This process, which is family-directed, is intended to identify the resources, priorities, and concerns of your family. It also identifies the supports and services you may need to enhance your family's capacity to meet your child's developmental needs. The family assessment is usually conducted through an interview with you, the parents.

When conducting the evaluation and assessment, team members may get information from some or all of the following:

- Doctor's reports

- Results from developmental tests and performance assessments given to your child

- Your child's medical and developmental history
- Direct observations and feedback from all members of the multi-disciplinary team, including you, the parents
- Interviews with you and other family members or caretakers
- Any other important observations, records, and/or reports about your child

Who Pays for the Evaluation and Assessment?

Under IDEA, evaluations and assessments are provided at no cost to parents. They are funded by state and federal monies.

Who Is Eligible for Services?

Under the IDEA, "infants and toddlers with disabilities" are defined as children from birth to the third birthday who need early intervention services because they are experiencing developmental delays, as measured by appropriate diagnostic instruments and procedures, in one or more of the following areas:

- Cognitive development
- Physical development, including vision and hearing
- Communication development
- Social or emotional development
- Adaptive development

... or who have a diagnosed physical or mental condition that has a high probability of resulting in developmental delay.

The term may also include, if a state chooses, "children from birth through age two who are at risk of having substantial developmental delays if early intervention services are not provided." (34 Code of Federal Regulations §303.16)

My Child Has Been Found Eligible for Services. What's Next?

If your child and family are found eligible, you and a team will meet to develop a written plan for providing early intervention services to your child and, as necessary, to your family. This plan is called the Individualized Family Service Plan, or IFSP. It is a very important document, and you, as parents, are important members of the team that develops it.

Part 3: Your Child's Early Intervention Services

What Is an Individualized Family Service Plan, or IFSP?

The IFSP is a written document that, among other things, outlines the early intervention services that your child and family will receive. One guiding principal of the IFSP is that the family is a child's greatest resource, that a young child's needs are closely tied to the needs of his or her family. The best way to support children and meet their needs is to support and build upon the individual strengths of their family. So, the IFSP is a whole-family plan, with the parents as major contributors in its development. Involvement of other team members will depend on what the child needs. These other team members could come from several agencies and may include medical people, therapists, child development specialists, social workers, and others.

Your child's IFSP must include the following:

- Your child's present physical, cognitive, communication, social/ emotional, and adaptive development levels and needs

- Family information (with your agreement), including the resources, priorities, and concerns of you, as parents, and other family members closely involved with the child

- The major results or outcomes expected to be achieved for your child and family

- The specific services your child will be receiving

- Where in the natural environment (e.g., home, community) the services will be provided (if the services will not be provided in the natural environment, the IFSP must include a statement justifying why not)

- When and where your son or daughter will receive services

- The number of days or sessions he or she will receive each service and how long each session will last

- Whether the service will be provided on a one-on-one or group basis

- Who will pay for the services

- The name of the service coordinator overseeing the implementation of the IFSP

- The steps to be taken to support your child's transition out of early intervention and into another program when the time comes

The IFSP may also identify services your family may be interested in, such as financial information or information about raising a child with a disability. The IFSP is reviewed every six months and is updated at least once a year. The IFSP must be fully explained to you, the parents, and your suggestions must be considered. You must give written consent before services can start. If you do not give your consent in writing, your child will not receive services. Each state has specific guidelines for the IFSP. Your service coordinator can explain what the IFSP guidelines are in your state.

What's Included in Early Intervention Services?

Under IDEA, early intervention services must include a multidisciplinary evaluation and assessment, a written Individualized Family Service Plan, service coordination, and specific services designed to meet the unique developmental needs of the child and family. Early intervention services may be simple or complex, depending on the child's needs. They can range from prescribing glasses for a two-year-old to developing a comprehensive approach with a variety of services and special instruction for a child, including home visits, counseling, and training for his or her family. Depending on your child's needs, his or her early intervention services may include the following:

- Family training, counseling, and home visits
- Special instruction
- Speech-language pathology services (sometimes referred to as speech therapy)
- Audiology services (hearing impairment services)
- Occupational therapy
- Physical therapy
- Psychological services; medical services (only for diagnostic or evaluation purposes)
- Health services needed to enable your child to benefit from the other services
- Social work services
- Assistive technology devices and services
- Transportation
- Nutrition services
- Service coordination services

How Are Early Intervention Services Delivered?

Early intervention services may be delivered in a variety of ways and in different places. Sometimes services are provided in the child's home with the family receiving additional training. Services may also be provided in other settings, such as a clinic, a neighborhood daycare center, hospital, or the local health department. To the maximum extent appropriate, the services are to be provided in natural environments or settings. Natural environments, broadly speaking, are where the child lives, learns, and plays. Services are provided by qualified personnel and may be offered through a public or private agency.

Will I Have to Pay for Services?

Whether or not you, as parents, will have to pay for any services for your child depends on the policies of your state. Under IDEA, the following services must be provided at no cost to families:

- Child Find services

- Evaluations and assessments

- The development and review of the Individualized Family Service Plan

- Service coordination

Depending on your state's policies, you may have to pay for certain other services. You may be charged a "sliding-scale" fee, meaning the fees are based on what you earn. Check with the contact person in your area or state. Some services may be covered by your health insurance, by Medicaid, or by Indian Health Services. Every effort is made to provide services to all infants and toddlers who need help, regardless of family income. Services cannot be denied to a child just because his or her family is not able to pay for them.

Chapter 69

Assistive Technology for Young Children

Research shows that assistive technology (AT) can help young children with disabilities to learn developmental skills.[1] Its use may help infants and toddlers to improve in many areas:

- Social skills including sharing and taking turns

- Communication skills

- Attention span

- Fine and gross motor skills

- Self-confidence and independence

The right type of assistive technology can improve a child's ability to communicate. This in turn may help reduce some negative behaviors. Examples of common assistive technology devices include wheel chairs, computers, computer software, and communication devices.

What types of assistive technology devices can infants and toddlers use?

There are two types of AT devices most commonly used by infants and toddlers—switches and augmentative communication devices:

Excerpted from "Assistive Technology for Infants, Toddlers, and Young Children with Disabilities." Reprinted with permission from PACER Center, Minneapolis, MN (952) 838-9000. www.pacer.org, © 2006. All rights reserved. Despite the older date of this material, the information describing the various types of assistive technologies is still relevant to parents of children with disabilities.

- There are many types of switches, and they can be used in many different ways. Switches can be used with battery-operated toys to give infants opportunities to play with them. For example, a switch might be attached directly to a stuffed pig. Then, every time an infant touches the toy, it wiggles and snorts. Switches can also be used to turn things off and on. Toddlers can learn to press a switch to turn on a device or to use interactive software. Children who have severe disabilities can also use switches. For example, a switch could be placed next to an infant's head so that every time she moved her head to the left a musical mobile hanging overhead would play.

- Augmentative communication materials and devices allow young children who cannot speak to communicate with the world around them. These devices can be simple, such as pointing to a photo on a picture board. Or, they can be more complicated—such as pressing message buttons on a device that activate pre-recorded messages such as "I'm hungry."

Why is assistive technology important?

Many of the skills learned in life begin in infancy: AT can help infants and toddlers with disabilities learn many of these crucial developmental skills. With assistive technology they can often learn the same things that nondisabled peers learn at the same age, only in a different way. Communication skills at this age are especially important since most of what an infant or toddler learns is through interacting with other people. This is especially true with family members and other primary caregivers.

Sometimes parents are reluctant to begin using an AT device. They may believe it will discourage their child from learning important skills. In truth, the opposite may be true. Research has shown that using AT devices, especially augmentative communication devices, may encourage a child to increase communication efforts and skills. The earlier a child is taught to use an AT device, the more easily the child will learn to accept and use it.

Assistive technology is also important because expectations for a child increase as he or she grows. Those around the child learn to say, "This is what the baby can do, with supports," instead of, "This is what the baby can't do." With assistive technology, parents learn that the dreams they had for their child don't necessarily end when he or she is diagnosed with a disability. The dreams may change a little, but they can still come true.

How can a family obtain AT devices for their infant or toddler?

There are two ways. First, infants and toddlers who have a disability may be eligible for early intervention services under Part C of a federal law called the Individuals with Disabilities Education Act (IDEA). If the child meets eligibility criteria for early intervention services, he or she may receive assistive technology devices and services as part of the services provided. The Individual Family Services Plan (IFSP) team, including the parents, makes the decision whether those services are needed based on assessment information. If so, these services are provided to the child through a written Individualized Family Services Plan, or IFSP.

Some infants and toddlers have delays that are not severe enough for them to be eligible for early intervention services. Many of these infants and toddlers may still benefit from using an AT device. In some cases, private insurance or medical assistance will pay for a device. Or, parents may choose to purchase a device directly for their child.

Many schools and communities have special lending libraries where parents can borrow toys with switches, computer software, and other devices. These libraries, such as the Tech Tots libraries sponsored by United Cerebral Palsy chapters around the country, give parents an opportunity to try various devices before deciding whether to purchase them.

If my young child is not eligible for early intervention services under IDEA, how will I know if she could still benefit from using an AT device?

Asking certain questions may help you make that decision. Some examples:

- Compared to other children of the same age, can my child play with toys independently?
- Can my child communicate effectively?
- How does my child move from place to place?
- Can my child sit, stand, or walk independently?
- Is my child able to feed himself or herself?

If you answer "No" to these questions, then assistive technology may help. In some cases, children with behavior problems actually have a communication impairment. They are frustrated that they cannot tell someone how they feel, and act out instead.

What is assistive technology for children who are eligible for early intervention under IDEA?

IDEA defines an assistive technology device as "any item, piece of equipment, or product system, whether acquired commercially off the shelf, modified, or customized, that is used to increase, maintain, or improve functional capabilities of a child with a disability." Under IDEA, assistive technology services are any services that directly assist a child with a disability to select, acquire, or use a device. AT services include:

- finding and paying for an assistive technology device;
- selecting and making a device work (modifying, customizing, etc.) for a child;
- repairing or replacing a device;
- coordinating and using other therapies or services with AT devices;
- evaluating the needs of a child with a disability, including a functional evaluation of in the child's natural learning environment;
- training or technical assistance for a child or that child's family; and
- training or technical assistance for professionals.

How does a parent request an AT evaluation under IDEA?

An AT evaluation should be included as part of an early intervention evaluation if there is reason to believe the child may need an AT device or service. However, parents may request AT evaluation at any time. Parents and family members, such as siblings or grandparents, if appropriate, should be involved in the entire process. Families have important information about their infant or toddler. When parents and family members are actively involved it is more likely that the child will get the right device and that it will be used properly.

What is the most effective way to evaluate an infant or toddler for an AT device or services?

Ideally, a multidisciplinary team will do an AT evaluation. Often this team will include an assistive technology specialist. This person should have a broad understanding about different kinds of technology, adapted toys, learning tools, communication devices, and other adapted equipment. A member of the team should also understand how technology may be used in all areas of a child's life to support developmental outcomes. This person should also have knowledge about infant and toddler development. Some early intervention programs have AT specialists on staff. Other programs may use a physical, occupational, or educational speech pathologist that has had additional training as their AT specialist. If an early intervention program does not have a technology expert, it can contract with a provider, a school district, or a community agency.

Before the evaluation takes place, team members should gather information about the child's interests, abilities, and family routines. This will help to determine what type of AT devices might be used during the evaluation. The evaluation is usually done in the environment where the child spends the most time. For infants and toddlers, this may be the family home or a childcare setting.

When the evaluation is finished, the evaluator will recommend any devices or services that will help the child reach the expected outcomes. Any devices recommended should be easy for the family and other caregivers to use.

An important part of the evaluation is its focus on a child's strengths and abilities. For example, if an infant with cerebral palsy can only wiggle her left foot, then being able to wiggle that foot is considered a strength. Any AT device should build on this strength. In this case, a switch could be positioned so that every time the infant wiggled her foot a music box would play. Creativity is a must when thinking about AT for children who have significant impairments! Parents and other primary caretakers are great resources.

Under IDEA, where can assistive technology devices and services be provided?

Early intervention services must be provided in natural environments to the extent appropriate. This would include the child's home, childcare setting, or other community settings where children without disabilities are found. It is the responsibility of the IFSP team to determine—based on evaluations and assessments—what services will meet the child's needs. These services, including assistive technology, will be written in the child's IFSP.

As a part of the decision-making process around assistive technology, the team will discuss where AT devices and services will best meet the child's needs (home, childcare, etc.). As children move from one service to another, everyone involved with the child should know what AT devices the child is using and how to obtain and use them. For example, if a two-and-a-half-year-old child is receiving early intervention services and will move to preschool at age three, the need for AT should be discussed at the transition planning conference. This will help to ensure that the child's access to assistive technology does not have gaps.

Under IDEA, who pays for assistive technology devices and services?

All early intervention services, including AT devices and services, must be provided at no cost to the family unless a state has established a system of payment for early intervention services.

What types of training can be provided under IDEA?

In general, parents, service providers, childcare provider and others who work with infants and toddlers and their families should be trained to use the AT device. Training could include:

- Basic information about the device, how to set it up, and how it works.

- How the device can be used in all parts of the child's life.

- How to know when something is wrong and how to fix minor problems.

- What to do or where to take the device if there is a major problem.

- How to change or adapt the device for a child as he grows or as activities become more complex. Parents and service providers who are trained and comfortable with the device are more likely to find creative ways to use it in all areas of a child's life. The need for training, including who will provide the training, should be included in the child's IFSP.

Where can parents get more information about assistive technology or IDEA?

Parents may call the Parent Center that serves their area.

Reference

1. Research cited in this article is from the Early Childhood Comprehensive Technology System (Project ECCTS) study, funded by the U.S. Department of Education's Office of Special Education Programs, under IDEA's Technology, Demonstration, and Utilization and Media Services Program.

Chapter 70

Education of Children with Special Needs

Chapter Contents

Section 70.1

Individualized Education Programs

What's an Individualized Education Program (IEP)?

Kids with delayed skills or other disabilities might be eligible for special services that provide individualized education programs in public schools, free of charge to families. Understanding how to access these services can help parents be effective advocates for their kids.

The passage of the updated version of the Individuals with Disabilities Education Act (IDEA 2004) made parents of kids with special needs even more crucial members of their child's education team.

Parents can now work with educators to develop a plan—the individualized education program (IEP)—to help kids succeed in school. The IEP describes the goals the team sets for a child during the school year, as well as any special support needed to help achieve them.

Who Needs an IEP?

A child who has difficulty learning and functioning and has been identified as a special needs student is the perfect candidate for an IEP.

Kids struggling in school may qualify for support services, allowing them to be taught in a special way, for reasons such as:

- learning disabilities;
- attention deficit hyperactivity disorder (ADHD);
- emotional disorders;
- cognitive challenges;
- autism;

- hearing impairment;

- visual impairment;

- speech or language impairment;

- developmental delay.

How Are Services Delivered?

In most cases, the services and goals outlined in an IEP can be provided in a standard school environment. This can be done in the regular classroom (for example, a reading teacher helping a small group of children who need extra assistance while the other kids in the class work on reading with the regular teacher) or in a special resource room in the regular school. The resource room can serve a group of kids with similar needs who are brought together for help.

However, kids who need intense intervention may be taught in a special school environment. These classes have fewer students per teacher, allowing for more individualized attention.

In addition, the teacher usually has specific training in helping kids with special educational needs. The children spend most of their day in a special classroom and join the regular classes for nonacademic activities (like music and gym) or in academic activities in which they don't need extra help.

Because the goal of IDEA is to ensure that each child is educated in the least restrictive environment possible, effort is made to help kids stay in a regular classroom. However, when needs are best met in a special class, then kids might be placed in one.

The Referral and Evaluation Process

The referral process generally begins when a teacher, parent, or doctor is concerned that a child may be having trouble in the classroom, and the teacher notifies the school counselor or psychologist.

The first step is to gather specific data regarding the student's progress or academic problems. This may be done through:

- a conference with parents;

- a conference with the student;

- observation of the student;

- analysis of the student's performance (attention, behavior, work completion, tests, classwork, homework, etc.).

615

This information helps school personnel determine the next step. At this point, strategies specific to the student could be used to help the child become more successful in school. If this doesn't work, the child would be tested for a specific learning disability or other impairment to help determine qualification for special services.

It's important to note, though, that the presence of a disability doesn't automatically guarantee a child will receive services. To be eligible, the disability must affect functioning at school.

To determine eligibility, a multidisciplinary team of professionals will evaluate the child based on their observations; the child's performance on standardized tests; and daily work such as tests, quizzes, classwork, and homework.

Who's on the Team?

The professionals on the evaluation team can include:

- a psychologist;
- a physical therapist;
- an occupational therapist;
- a speech therapist;
- a special educator;
- a vision or hearing specialist;
- others, depending on the child's specific needs.

As a parent, you can decide whether to have your child assessed. If you choose to do so, you'll be asked to sign a permission form that will detail who is involved in the process and the types of tests they use. These tests might include measures of specific school skills, such as reading or math, as well as more general developmental skills, such as speech and language. Testing does not necessarily mean that a child will receive services.

Once the team members complete their individual assessments, they develop a comprehensive evaluation report (CER) that compiles their findings, offers an educational classification, and outlines the skills and support the child will need.

The parents then have a chance to review the report before the IEP is developed. Some parents will disagree with the report, and they will have the opportunity to work together with the school to come up with a plan that best meets the child's needs.

Developing an IEP

The next step is an IEP meeting at which the team and parents decide what will go into the plan. In addition to the evaluation team, a regular teacher should be present to offer suggestions about how the plan can help the child's progress in the standard education curriculum.

At the meeting, the team will discuss your child's educational needs—as described in the CER—and come up with specific, measurable short-term and annual goals for each of those needs. If you attend this meeting, you can take an active role in developing the goals and determining which skills or areas will receive the most attention.

The cover page of the IEP outlines the support services your child will receive and how often they will be provided (for example, occupational therapy twice a week). Support services might include special education, speech therapy, occupational or physical therapy, counseling, audiology, medical services, nursing, vision or hearing therapy, and many others.

If the team recommends several services, the amount of time they take in the child's school schedule can seem overwhelming. To ease that load, some services may be provided on a consultative basis. In these cases, the professional consults with the teacher to come up with strategies to help the child but doesn't offer any hands-on instruction. For instance, an occupational therapist may suggest accommodations for a child with fine-motor problems that affect handwriting, and the classroom teacher would incorporate these suggestions into the handwriting lessons taught to the entire class.

Other services can be delivered right in the classroom, so the child's day isn't interrupted by therapy. The child who has difficulty with handwriting might work one-on-one with an occupational therapist while everyone else practices their handwriting skills. When deciding how and where services are offered, the child's comfort and dignity should be a top priority.

The IEP should be reviewed annually to update the goals and make sure the levels of service meet your child's needs. However, IEPs can be changed at any time on an as-needed basis. If you think your child needs more, fewer, or different services, you can request a meeting and bring the team together to discuss your concerns.

Your Legal Rights

Specific timelines ensure that the development of an IEP moves from referral to providing services as quickly as possible. Be sure to ask about this time frame and get a copy of your parents' rights when your child is referred. These guidelines (sometimes called procedural safeguards) outline your rights as a parent to control what happens to your child during each step of the process.

The parents' rights also describe how you can proceed if you disagree with any part of the CER or the IEP—mediation and hearings both are options. You can get information about low-cost or free legal representation from the school district or, if your child is in early intervention (for kids ages three to five), through that program.

Attorneys and paid advocates familiar with the IEP process will provide representation if you need it. You also may invite anyone who knows or works with your child whose input you feel would be helpful to join the IEP team.

A Final Word

Parents have the right to choose where their kids will be educated. This choice includes public or private elementary schools and secondary schools, including religious schools. It also includes charter schools and home schools.

However, it is important to understand that the rights of children with disabilities who are placed by their parents in private elementary schools and secondary schools are not the same as those of kids with disabilities who are enrolled in public schools or placed by public agencies in private schools when the public school is unable to provide a free appropriate public education (FAPE).

Two major differences that parents, teachers, other school staff, private school representatives, and the kids need to know about are:

1. Children with disabilities who are placed by their parents in private schools may not get the same services they would receive in a public school.

2. Not all kids with disabilities placed by their parents in private schools will receive services.

The IEP process is complex, but it's also an effective way to address how your child learns and functions. If you have concerns, don't hesitate to ask questions about the evaluation findings or the goals recommended by the team. You know your child best and should play a central role in creating a learning plan tailored to his or her specific needs.

Section 70.2

Three Ways Parents Can Help Their Disabled Child Stay in School

Children with disabilities, especially those with emotional behavior disorders and learning disabilities, are at significantly greater risk of dropping out of school than are their peers without disabilities. Parents, however, can increase the likelihood that their children will remain in school and graduate. Here are three ways you can help your child stay in school.

Stay Involved with Your Child

You and your extended family members have a tremendous influence on your child's desire to stay in school. It is important for you to talk frequently with your child about the importance of education. Let your child know that you care about how he or she is doing in school. Help your child understand school rules and expectations. Support your child's learning styles, habits, and skills in ways that help him or her succeed.

Work with the School to Encourage Learning Success

You can work with the school in many ways to encourage your child's learning success. Help teachers understand your child's strengths and unique needs by communicating regularly. You could explore alternative school placements, assistive technology, extracurricular activities, and school modifications and accommodations. If your child is frustrated or discouraged with school, ask for an Individualized Education Program (IEP) team meeting to discuss your child's struggles and investigate options and solutions.

Encourage Success Outside of School

Children who are engaged in extracurricular athletics and after-school activities are more likely to stay in school, according to education experts. The IEP team should discuss ways to include such activities in your child's IEP. You also may want to explore options outside of school, including volunteering, employment, mentoring relationships, youth groups, and community sports. Such activities can provide positive experiences that support success.

Section 70.3

Preparing for College: What Students with Disabilities Need to Know

Excerpted from "Transition of Students with Disabilities to Postsecondary Education: A Guide for High School Educators," U.S. Department of Education, March 2011.

Are students with disabilities entitled to changes in standardized testing conditions on entrance exams for institutions of postsecondary education?

In general, tests may not be selected or administered in a way that tests the disability rather than the achievement or aptitude of the individual. In addition, federal law requires changes to the testing conditions that are necessary to allow a student with a disability to participate as long as the changes do not fundamentally alter the examination or create undue financial or administrative burdens. In general, in order to request one or more changes in standardized testing conditions, which test administrators may also refer to as "testing accommodations," the student will need to contact the institution of postsecondary education or the entity that administers the exam and provide documentation of a disability and the need for a change in testing conditions.

Are institutions of postsecondary education permitted to ask an applicant if he or she has a disability before an admission decision is made?

Generally, institutions of postsecondary education are not permitted to make what is known as a "preadmission inquiry" about an applicant's disability status. Preadmission inquiries are permitted only if the institution of postsecondary education is taking remedial action to correct the effects of past discrimination or taking voluntary action to overcome the effects of conditions that limited the participation of individuals with disabilities.

After admission, in response to a student's request for "academic adjustments," reasonable modifications or auxiliary aids and services, institutions of postsecondary education may ask for documentation regarding disability status.

May institutions of postsecondary education deny an applicant admission because he or she has a disability?

No. If an applicant meets the essential requirements for admission, an institution may not deny that applicant admission simply because he or she has a disability. An institution may, however, require an applicant to meet any essential technical or academic standards for admission to, or participation in, the institution and its program. An institution may deny admission to any student, disabled or not, who does not meet essential requirements for admission or participation.

Are students obligated to inform institutions that they have a disability?

No. A student has no obligation to inform an institution of postsecondary education that he or she has a disability; however, if the student wants an institution to provide an academic adjustment or assign the student to accessible housing or other facilities, or if a student wants other disability-related services, the student must identify himself or herself as having a disability. The disclosure of a disability is always voluntary. For example, a student who has a disability that does not require services may choose not to disclose his or her disability.

What are academic adjustments and auxiliary aids and services?

Academic adjustments are defined in the Section 504 regulations at 34 C.F.R. § 104.44(a) as:

[S]uch modifications to [the] academic requirements as are necessary to ensure that such requirements do not discriminate or have the effect of discriminating, on the basis of [disability] against a qualified ... applicant or student [with a disability]. Academic requirements that the recipient can demonstrate are essential to the instruction being pursued by such student or to any directly related licensing requirement will not be regarded as discriminatory within the meaning of this section. Modifications may include changes in the length of time permitted for the completion of degree requirements, substitution of specific courses required for the completion of degree requirements, and adaptation of the manner in which specific courses are conducted.

Academic adjustments also may include a reduced course load, extended time on tests and the provision of auxiliary aids and services. Auxiliary aids and services include note-takers, readers, recording devices, sign language interpreters, screen-readers, voice recognition and other adaptive software or hardware for computers, and other devices designed to ensure the participation of students with impaired sensory, manual or speaking skills in an institution's programs and activities. Institutions are not required to provide personal devices and services such as attendants, individually prescribed devices, such as eyeglasses, readers for personal use or study, or other services of a personal nature, such as tutoring. If institutions offer tutoring to the general student population, however, they must ensure that tutoring services also are available to students with disabilities.

In general, what kind of documentation is necessary for students with disabilities to receive academic adjustments from institutions of postsecondary education?

Institutions may set their own requirements for documentation so long as they are reasonable and comply with Section 504 and Title II. It is not uncommon for documentation standards to vary from institution to institution; thus, students with disabilities should research documentation standards at those institutions that interest them. A student must provide documentation, upon request, that he or she has a disability, that is, an impairment that substantially limits a major life activity and that supports the need for an academic adjustment. The documentation should identify how a student's ability to function is limited as a result of her or his disability. The primary purpose of the documentation is to establish a disability in order to help the institution work interactively with the student to identify appropriate services. The focus should be on whether the information adequately documents the existence of a current disability and need for an academic adjustment.

Who is responsible for obtaining necessary testing to document the existence of a disability?

The student. Institutions of postsecondary education are not required to conduct or pay for an evaluation to document a student's disability and need for an academic adjustment, although some institutions do so. If a student with a disability is eligible for services through the state VR Services program, he or she may qualify for an evaluation at no cost. If students with disabilities are unable to find other funding sources to pay for necessary evaluation or testing for postsecondary education, they are responsible for paying for it themselves.

If students want to request academic adjustments, what must they do?

Institutions may establish reasonable procedures for requesting academic adjustments; students are responsible for knowing these procedures and following them. Institutions usually include information on the procedures and contacts for requesting an academic adjustment in their general information publications and websites. If students are unable to locate the procedures, they should contact an institution official, such as an admissions officer or counselor.

When should students notify the institution of their intention to request an academic adjustment?

As soon as possible. Although students may request academic adjustments at any time, students needing services should notify the institution as early as possible to ensure that the institution has enough time to review their request and provide an appropriate academic adjustment. Some academic adjustments, such as interpreters, may take time to arrange. In addition, students should not wait until after completing a course or activity or receiving a poor grade to request services and then expect the grade to be changed or to be able to retake the course.

How do institutions determine what academic adjustments are appropriate?

Once a student has identified him- or herself as an individual with a disability, requested an academic adjustment, and provided appropriate documentation upon request, institution staff should discuss with the student what academic adjustments are appropriate in light of the student's individual needs and the nature of the institution's program. Students with disabilities possess unique knowledge of their individual disabilities and should be prepared to discuss the functional challenges they face and, if applicable, what has or has not worked for them in the past. Institution staff should be prepared to describe the barriers students may face in individual classes that may affect their full participation, as well as to discuss academic adjustments that might enable students to overcome those barriers.

Who pays for auxiliary aids and services?

Once the needed auxiliary aids and services have been identified, institutions may not require students with disabilities to pay part or all of the costs of such aids and services, nor may institutions charge students with disabilities more for participating in programs or activities than they charge students who do not have disabilities. Institutions generally may not condition their provision of academic adjustments on the availability of funds, refuse to spend more than a certain amount to provide academic adjustments, or refuse to provide academic adjustments because they believe other providers of such services exist. In many cases, institutions may meet their obligation to provide auxiliary aids and services by assisting students in either obtaining them or obtaining reimbursement for their cost from an outside agency or organization. Such assistance notwithstanding, institutions retain ultimate responsibility for providing necessary auxiliary aids and services and for any costs associated with providing such aids and services or utilizing outside sources. However, as noted above, if the institution can demonstrate that providing a specific auxiliary aid or service would result in undue financial or administrative burdens, considering the institution's resources as a whole, it can opt to provide another effective one.

Chapter 71

Transition Planning for Children with Special Needs

Chapter Contents

Section 71.1

Parent Tips for Transition Planning

Successful and meaningful transition services are the result of careful planning. This planning is driven by a young person's dreams, desires, and abilities. It builds a youth's participation in school, home, and community living.

Transition planning helps to prepare young people for their futures. It helps them to develop skills they need to go on to other education programs after high school. It builds skills to live, work, and play in the community. It helps to build independence. Youth learn important adult decision-making roles when they participate in this school-based planning.

Must transition planning be part of the Individualized Education Program (IEP)?

Transition planning is required in the IEP for students by age sixteen. Many students will begin this planning at age fourteen or earlier so that they have the time to build skills they will need as adults. Parents should feel comfortable asking for transition planning to start earlier than age sixteen if they believe it is needed. Transition planning, goals, and services will be different for each student.

Transition services include instruction, community experiences, and building employment skills. They include post-school adult living objectives and, if needed, daily living skills training and functional vocational evaluations. All of these services must be provided in a manner that is sensitive to a student's cultural background and native language.

Transition services are based on a student's strengths as well as needs. They consider a young person's preferences and interests. Activities that are part of transition services must be results-oriented. This means that they are focused on building specific skills.

626

Must students be involved in transition planning?

Schools are required to invite students to participate in their IEP meetings whenever transition goals or services are considered. Transition services are a required component of IEPs for students age sixteen and older, and should be routinely discussed at IEP meetings. These services may become part of discussion and planning as early as the IEP team finds is needed for an individual student. (Some states require transition planning beginning at age fourteen.)

What if my child does not attend his or her IEP meeting?

If a youth is unable to participate in his or her IEP meeting or chooses not to attend, school personnel must take steps to ensure that the youth's preferences and interests are considered in developing the IEP.

The best transition plans are those that help youth achieve their dreams and aspirations. Youth should be included in all aspects of planning and goal setting, and encouraged to participate at IEP meetings. This participation helps keep team members focused on the young person's individual needs and desires. It also helps the youth to develop the skills for making decisions and becoming a self-advocate. Preparing young people for their role in transition planning helps them to become knowledgeable members of the IEP team.

How can I be sure that the IEP meets my child's transition needs?

Transition services begin with age-appropriate transition assessments. They include student and parent interviews, interest and skill inventories, and other tools.

In order for an IEP to meet a student's transition needs, both parents and school personnel participate in the assessment. The school does this through assessments and observations. Parents do it through day-to-day knowledge and talks with their child about his or her goals and dreams.

Answering the following questions may help guide how parents and students prepare for and participate in an effective IEP meeting that is focused on transition planning:

- What does the young person want to do with his or her life? What are his or her dreams, aspirations, or goals? The youth's answers should be incorporated into all aspects of transition planning. If a young person is nonverbal or has difficulty communicating, parents can still use their knowledge of their child to be sure that transition planning and services reflect the youth's preferences and choices.

- What are the young person's needs, abilities, and skills? Parents should be familiar with how much assistance their child needs or does not need to accomplish tasks.

- What are the outcomes that the youth and parents want? Parents and their child should bring suggestions to the transition planning meeting. Suggestions might include the kind of services, actions, or planning they believe is needed to achieve desired goals in the transition section of the IEP.

- Will the young person attend the transition IEP conference? Parents can help by encouraging their son or daughter to attend. He or she will be invited. Together, parents and youth can prepare for the meeting. If the youth does not attend, parents may represent their desires and wishes.

- How do young people develop self-advocacy skills? Parents and school staff should encourage self-advocacy in young people. Staff should direct questions to the youth, even when it is the parents who may provide answers. It is important to encourage young people to have and state (by any means available to them) their own opinions. It is important for students to understand their disability and to ask for the accommodations they may need.

- What are the programs, services, accommodations, or modifications the young person wants or needs? Parents and their youth need to think about and be clear on what they want or need. IEP team discussions address these topics, but often parents and young people have had conversations at home that will be useful in planning.

- What kinds of accommodations will students need when they go on to higher education or employment? Parents and youth need to think what accommodations will be needed after high school and how the youth will obtain them.

- Who will be responsible for what part of the transition plan in the IEP? It is wise for parents and youth to know who is responsible for each transition goal. Each task should have a specific timeline that is included in the IEP.

- Should the educational and transition programs emphasize practical or academic goals? Does the young person need a combination of both? This will depend on the goals of each individual student.

- What are the community-based training opportunities the school provides? Parents and their child should decide how much to participate in those activities.

- If a student plans on going to college, is he or she taking the courses needed to meet college entrance requirements?

- When will the young person graduate? What kind of diploma option is the best choice?

- Are work experience classes appropriate to reach employment goals? Research suggests that youth have more successful employment outcomes after high school if they have had hands-on, work-based learning experiences as students.

- How could the educational and transition program be more integrated into the regular program?

- Who will attend the IEP meeting? Parents and the youth should become familiar with the roles and functions of team members. They should also know what community agencies might be present (vocational rehabilitation, etc.). Parents may request that a specific community agency be invited to the IEP meeting if the youth is or may be using services from that agency. Becoming familiar with adult service systems or agencies now can be helpful in making future decisions. At times parents may want a family member, friend, or advocate to go to planning meetings with them for support or to take notes.

Parents and youth will want to have a copy of the daily school schedule each quarter or semester. It is important to have information on all classes available so that their child can participate in selecting classes and the scheduling process.

A final tip: Parents will need to start thinking about their child's legal status before he or she turns eighteen. If a youth is not able to make informed decisions about major issues (medical treatment, living accommodations, financial arrangements, etc.), the family may need to learn more about guardianship or conservatorship. The Individuals with Disabilities Education Act (IDEA) 2004 requires that students be notified at least one year in advance of the rights that will transfer to the student upon reaching the age of majority (becoming a legal adult in that state). These rights include being the responsible person for planning and agreeing or disagreeing with services in the IEP. It is important that parents understand what this means for them and their role in planning. The age of majority is eighteen in most states.

By learning as much as possible about the options available for transition planning, a parent can ensure that their young person's rights are protected while they are learning the skills needed to develop independence.

Section 71.2

Assisting Disabled Youth with Job Search and Retention

"Tapping into the Powers of Families: How Families of Youth with Disabilities Can Assist in Job Search and Retention," April 2011. © National Collaborative on Workforce and Disability for Youth (www.ncwd-youth .info). Reprinted with permission.

Families and other caring adults play a vital, yet unrecognized role in helping young people with disabilities explore careers, build work skills, and be successful in employment. Reasons why families are unrecognized in the career development process vary. Families themselves may not see the connection between work skills and everyday activities in the home. They may not realize that their knowledge of their son or daughter can contribute to the employment-related transition goals of their child's Individualized Education Program (IEP). They may think that schools, youth development professionals, or state vocational rehabilitation (VR) programs don't need their help, or may be unaware of how they might partner with such programs. Perhaps they simply have not been asked.

While many school, youth employment, and vocational rehabilitation professionals value family involvement and understand that involving families in their son's or daughter's program can lead to more positive career development experiences and successful employment results, this has not always been the case. Past models of case management placed the professional in a position of power and input from family members was not welcomed. Families who are seeking to maintain high expectations for their family member's future may be discouraged from actively participating in the work preparation, exploration, and placement processes.

The purpose of this section is to give families and other caring adults information on how their involvement can make a positive impact on a youth's work readiness, career exploration, and workplace success. Educators and other youth service professionals can also use this information to consider how to involve family members in a young person's work readiness and career development.

Families are often the first, most knowledgeable, and most consistent "case manager" youth with disabilities have. Families possess valuable information about a youth's strengths, interests, and needs. In a time of dwindling resources, family involvement can help professionals, such as teachers, social workers, and mentors, to streamline their assessment process, access personal networks for job opportunities, and build work readiness skills in the home.

The Changing Definition of "Family"

A young person may live in any number of family constructs, including ones in which couples are married, cohabitating, or the same sex, or in single-parent, blended, grandparent-led, foster care, or group home. A youth's "family" may not always include a mother and father. Rather, a sibling, aunt/uncle, grandparent, neighbor, teacher, peer, or other influential adult may play a guiding role for a young person. The National Collaborative on Workforce and Disability for Youth defines family this way in its Family Guideposts: "Family is defined broadly as adults and children related biologically, emotionally, or legally, including single parents, blended families, unrelated individuals living cooperatively, and partnered couples who live with biological, adopted, and foster children." It is important that professionals working to help youth prepare for and find employment acknowledge the many forms "family" can take, and allow input and participation from a wider variety of adults who have a positive influence on a youth.

Work Goals Start at Home

All families want their sons and daughters to be employed. This desire needs to hold true for youth with disabilities as well. Families can begin youth on the path towards successful employment by helping youth create goals for themselves. Even at a young age, youth begin to think about what types of jobs they may want. "I want to grow up and do what mommy does." or "When I get bigger, I'm going to be a policeman." Families can use this common curiosity to begin instilling an expectation that their family member will be employed as an adult. If the expectation of employment is there from an early age, it will be easier to build more specific skills and higher expectations as the youth gets older.

Families Can Build Work Skills at Home

Where do people learn the skills needed to be successful in the workplace? How does a person learn to be responsible, problem solve, appropriately interact with others, or take work direction? Does it come naturally? For some youth it might. However, many youth need opportunities to learn and practice these skills. Entry-level jobs have been a traditional way young people learn work skills, but recently the number of entry-level jobs available to youth has drastically decreased. Youth with disabilities may have greater difficulties finding work experience opportunities. Given these barriers, how do families help youth build the "soft skills" needed to be successful in the workplace?

Interacting Appropriately with Others

No matter what job a person has, it is necessary to interact with co-workers, suppliers, customers, or the community in an appropriate way. Employers are more likely to fire an employee if they have trouble interacting with others in workplace.

From an early age, families can have their youth practice appropriate interactions with family members, friends, relatives, teachers, and workers in stores they frequent. Families can reinforce that interacting appropriately with people does not mean that they have to like them. Discuss the different types of communication one might use in different environments such as on the street, in a professional setting, and with peers, family, and co-workers. Doing so would help youth understand what might be acceptable and expected in one setting may not be appropriate in another. Youth who are given the opportunity to practice how to deal with people in a variety of situations may respond better if conflict should arise.

Maintaining Personal Appearance for Work

Youth often express themselves through the clothes they like to wear. Being asked to wear dress clothes or a uniform can be seen as disrespectful to their individuality However, there are very few jobs that don't expect some level of appropriate appearance from their employees.

Families are in a position to teach youth the difference between times when proper dress is called for and times when they can choose what to wear. Situations like school, church, weddings, or certain family functions can be used to practice dressing appropriately for different occasions. Families can schedule times once a month where the family will dress up and eat at a restaurant. During these outings, have youth cover up any visible tattoos, leave baseball caps at home, forgo gum chewing, and make sure pants are pulled up. Consider it a dress rehearsal and draw the correlation between dressing up for certain situations and dressing appropriately for work so youth understand the similarities.

This same concept carries over to other aspects of personal appearance. Youth should be encouraged to shower at least every other day, and to have a hairstyle that helps maintain personal appearance. Hygiene basics like teeth brushing, body odor awareness, and clean clothes are expected in the workplace, and for some youth this may not be obvious. Family members are in the best position to give specific guidance to their son or daughter on these issues.

Responsibility

Employers want workers who are responsible enough to show up on time and do the tasks they are assigned. Chores in the home are an excellent way to help youth build a sense of responsibility that can carry over onto a job.

Assign tasks in the home that are the sole responsibility of the youth. For example, parents can make it the responsibility of their son or daughter to collect the trash from around the house and to bring the garbage can to the curb on collection day. Parents should check their youth's work and give feedback on how well the task was completed. It may be necessary to create a system of rewards initially so the youth has an incentive. Other ways to build responsibility could include tasks such as waking up and getting ready for school independently, caring for a pet, helping plan a family menu for the week, maintaining a clean room, being responsible for certain aspects of yard work, or babysitting.

Parents may already have these expectations in place for youth, so the value comes in relating the responsibilities a youth has at home with potential responsibilities a youth may encounter on the job. Jobs need to get done both at home and at work. A youth who recognizes this is better prepared for the world of work.

Problem Solving

The ability to solve problems as they arise is a skill desired by employers. What do you do if a customer is unhappy? How do you overcome barriers to finish an assigned task? When should you ask for help if needed? Eventually, youth will learn that things won't always happen as planned. Fortunately, family life presents plenty of opportunities to practice problem solving. Families can give youth the opportunity to give input to solve common problems such as cleaning the house, accommodating guests, budgeting, making decisions on recreational activities, or finding a needed service. If a problem has already been addressed, families can explain how they handled the situation and relate the situation to the workplace. For example, if the family needs a new dentist, the young person could do the research, develop some recommendations, and discuss it with the family. As the family discussion occurs, an analogy can be made to doing similar research in an office environment to locate a graphic artist, an editor, or a printer. Instead of jumping in to solve a problem a youth might have, families can ask the youth to list all the possible solutions and consider them together to find a good one.

Working as Part of a Team

Teamwork is required in most workplaces. Even in a job where most tasks are completed independently, there is still a strong expectation that people will work together to meet the goals of the company. Families can work with their youth so they understand the importance of working as part of a team. Volunteering is a wonderful way for families to build this skill. Find a volunteer activity that requires teamwork to complete a task and sign up as a family to help. For example, a local food bank may need help taking donations, placing them into categories, and stocking shelves. This would be hard for one person to complete, but easy for a group of people. Families can also encourage youth to participate in school- or community-based activities, such as sports or fine arts, that require teamwork to produce a finished product.

Taking Work Direction

Most workplaces have goals, whether it's to serve food quickly, manufacture something correctly, or provide a service that meets customer requirements. A major expectation of employers is that an employee is able to take directions from somebody else. The inability to take work direction is often a cause for youth to be dismissed from jobs or to quit jobs. Many youth have a hard time with this concept, especially if they have little exposure to the world of work. Taking work direction may be difficult during adolescence because it's a time that identities are forged and self-images are fragile. Families are the best source of support to help youth understand that they should not be offended when they are given directions in the home, at school, or at work. Families can remind them that taking direction is an important part of being an employee and helping a business get its work done.

Families Play a Role in Career Exploration

Career exploration is the process youth engage in to identify which jobs they may be interested in, to learn about the education and skill requirements of those jobs, and to participate in activities that allow them to experience what it is like to do those jobs. Families support youth in this process in many ways.

Inform Planning Tools

Most services for people with disabilities involve the creation of a plan that drives activities and outcomes, including needed supports and accommodations. For students in special education, the plan is the Individualized Education Program (IEP), which drives the educational supports and services for that student. For students with disabilities who are not in special education but who may need accommodations, the plan is known as a 504 Plan. If a young person is involved with vocational rehabilitation (VR), the plan is an Individual Plan for Employment (IPE) that addresses training, supports and accommodations, and services needed to move the young person into a job. And many school districts are adopting individual learning plans (known under many names) that ask all students to plan a course towards graduation and life after high school. There are even family service plans. Who writes these plans? Ideally they are written as a partnership between the professionals, families, and students/youth.

So, for example, a high school student with a visual impairment or a learning disability may have language in his/her IEP in school to receive digital textbooks and specialized software for a computer. When developing an IPE with the vocational rehabilitation counselor, the student will need to understand what technology (e.g. scanner, closed-circuit television [CCTV], specialized software, etc.) the student will need for the job the youth intends to do and make sure that specialized equipment is in place when he/she starts the job. Some of the equipment may be similar to what the student used in school, and some may be updated versions. The student and his/her family will need to understand what VR can pay for and what the employer is reasonably expected to pay for.

Families can use their knowledge of a youth's strengths, interests, and needs to help streamline the assessment and planning process and the creation of a service plan. Without family input, a professional has to engage in a long process of getting to know the youth before being able to plan for him or her. Additionally, families often can provide information about their youth so a plan can be crafted to avoid situations that pose barriers for their family members. Often, youth with disabilities will have several service plans in place at once. Families are in an ideal position to make sure there is consistency across all the plans, make sure they reflect high expectations, and ensure that all responsible parties are working towards the same goal.

Seek Multiple Work Experiences

Youth benefit from having as many opportunities to practice work and explore different careers as possible. Sadly, youth with disabilities are often not offered many work experiences. Schools and other service providers can only do so much to provide these opportunities. Families who understand the importance of multiple work experiences can help their youth find such things as volunteer opportunities, job shadowing, informational interviews, and workplace mentoring programs. Families can also advocate that career exploration and work experiences be incorporated into a student's IEP or IPE. The more opportunities to practice work a youth has, the better their employment outcomes as adults are likely to be.

Use Personal Networks

The majority of people secure employment through word of mouth and personal networks. A person's "personal network" is the informal system of family, friends, co-workers, neighbors, and other people one associates with in life. The term sounds technical, but everyone has some sort of personal network. Families can access their own networks to help find job and work experience opportunities for their youth. For example, let's say a youth is interested in learning more about landscaping careers. Families can ask people in their personal network if they know anybody who works in landscaping and see if they can arrange a job shadowing or summer job opportunity. If people consider how they found past jobs, they may discover that they have already used the power of personal networks.

Families Can Support Success in the Workplace

Once a youth finds a job, families can play an important role in helping the youth understand, keep, and grow in the job.

Transportation

A job doesn't do a person much good if the employee cannot get to the job and transportation isn't available. Families need to consider how a young person will travel to and from a job site. If a youth does not drive, this can pose a challenge. In fact, transportation remains a significant barrier to people with disabilities finding and maintaining jobs. Families can ask that a youth explore public transportation options or work toward achieving a driver's license as part of their IEP, or seek transportation training (sometimes called travel training or orientation and mobility training) at a local disability service organization, such as an independent living center or visual services center. In rural areas, it may be necessary for families to be the main mode of transportation for youth. Families may also explore community or nonprofit transportation options or organize a system of volunteers to help.

Understand the Role of Benefits and Supports

Many people with disabilities receive supplemental income or medical supports through public programs. In fact, many families may rely on a youth's financial benefits to supplement their overall family income. A common misperception is that people will lose their benefits if they are employed. Though it is true that many of these programs do have income restrictions, it is also true that several programs assist people with disabilities so they can remain employed while maintaining benefits. Families should learn about the impact work income will have on their youth's benefits. Fortunately, there are people at the national, state, and local level who can help interpret work incentive and benefits planning rules.

Families can also explore programs like Individual Development Accounts (IDA) that allow a person with low income to build assets through matching funds from a variety of sources. IDAs typically provide the ability to build funds towards postsecondary education, the purchase of the first home, or the starting of a small business. Families whose youth don't qualify for an IDA can also consider other asset building tools like supplemental needs trusts (sometimes referred to as a special needs trust) that allow for assets to be accumulated without impact to government benefits.

Identify and Solve Challenging Workplace Situations

There may be times when challenging behavioral, medical, or logistical situations arise for a youth in the workplace. The last thing anybody wants is for these situations to lead to a youth losing the job. Families can use their knowledge of the youth to help identify and address workplace issues. For example, if a youth has challenging behaviors, families can work with employment providers to create a plan to respond to any potential situations. Instead of an automatic dismissal from employment, the employer can engage the plan and resolve the issue.

Maintain High Expectations

We all have hopes and dreams for our children. Part of those dreams is the expectation that our children will achieve great things. The presence of a disability should not automatically lessen the expectations parents have for their son or daughter. Families are the perfect advocate for maintaining the expectation that their youth can and will be employed. Families often provide the baseline for what others will expect of a youth. If a family member expresses doubt that a child can achieve something, then others such as educators or employment counselors may follow suit. High expectations benefit youth and set the stage for others to expect great things as well.

Guideposts for Families

The National Collaborative on Workforce and Disability for Youth (NCWD/Youth), in collaboration with the Office of Disability Employment Policy, U.S. Department of Labor, developed the Guideposts for Success. Based on thirty years of research, the Guideposts identify what all youth, including youth with disabilities, need to make a successful transition to adulthood. The Guideposts are organized using the following five categories:

- School-based preparatory experiences
- Career preparation and work-based learning experiences
- Youth development and leadership
- Connecting activities
- Family involvement and supports

The National Collaborative on Workforce and Disability for Youth's Guideposts for Success outlines the following issues related to family involvement and engagement. Families and other caring adults need to have:

- high expectations which build upon the young person's strengths, interests, and needs and foster their ability to achieve independence and self-sufficiency;

- been involved in their lives and assisting them toward adulthood;

- access to information about employment, further education, and community resources;

- taken an active role in transition planning with schools and community partners;

- access to medical, professional, and peer support networks;

- an understanding of their youth's disability and how it affects his or her education, employment, and/or daily living options;

- knowledge of rights and responsibilities under various disability-related legislation;

- knowledge of and access to programs, services, supports, and accommodations available for young people with disabilities; and

- an understanding of how individualized planning tools can assist youth in achieving transition goals and objectives.

As families are exploring these issues, they may want to ask themselves three basic questions: Am I informed? Am I supportive of my youth? And, am I involved and engaged in helping him/her and or the school and other service providers?

In Closing

Youth with disabilities benefit from many supports and experiences to explore careers and build work skills. School programs and workforce development efforts are seen as the main suppliers of these supports, but families play a vital role as well. It is important that families and other caring adults leverage the school years, learn the expectations of employers, use everyday activities in the home to build work skills, and understand that they are partners in helping youth prepare for and maintain employment. Families who are knowledgeable about employment, who are willing to provide needed supports and experiences, and who maintain high expectations for success give youth a much better chance to be successful in the job search and in the workplace.

Chapter 72

Government Benefits for Children and Adults with Disabilities

Supplemental Security Income (SSI) Payments for Children with Disabilities

SSI makes monthly payments to people with low income and limited resources who are sixty-five or older, or blind or disabled. Your child younger than age eighteen can qualify if he or she meets Social Security's definition of disability for children, and if his or her income and resources fall within the eligibility limits. The amount of the SSI payment is different from one state to another because some states add to the SSI payment. Your local Social Security office can tell you more about your state's total SSI payment.

SSI Rules about Income and Resources

When we decide if your child can get SSI, we consider your child's income and resources. We also consider the income and resources of family members living in the child's household. These rules apply if your child lives at home. They also apply if he or she is away at school but returns home from time to time and is subject to your control.

If your child's income and resources, or the income and resources of family members living in the child's household, are more than the amount allowed, we will deny the child's application for SSI payments.

Excerpted from "Benefits for Children with Disabilities," U.S. Social Security Administration (www.ssa.gov), October 12, 2012.

We limit the monthly SSI payment to $30 when a child is in a medical facility where health insurance pays for his or her care.

SSI Rules about Disability

Your child must meet all of the following requirements to be considered disabled and therefore eligible for SSI:

- The child must not be working and earning more than $1,010 a month in 2012. (This earnings amount usually changes every year.) If he or she is working and earning that much money, we will find that your child is not disabled.

- The child must have a physical or mental condition, or a combination of conditions, that results in "marked and severe functional limitations." This means that the condition(s) must very seriously limit your child's activities.

- The child's condition(s) must have been disabling, or be expected to be disabling, for at least twelve months; or must be expected to result in death.

If your child's condition(s) results in "marked and severe functional limitations" for at least twelve continuous months, we will find that your child is disabled. But if it does not result in those limitations, or does not result in those limitations for at least twelve months, we will find that your child is not disabled.

Providing Information about Your Child's Condition

When you apply for benefits for your child, we will ask you for detailed information about the child's medical condition and how it affects his or her ability to function on a daily basis. We also will ask you to give permission for the doctors, teachers, therapists, and other professionals who have information about your child's condition to send the information to us.

If you have any of your child's medical or school records, please bring them with you. This will help speed up the decision on your application.

What Happens Next?

We send all of the information you give us to the Disability Determination Services in your state. Doctors and other trained staff in that state agency will review the information, and will request your child's medical and school records, and any other information needed to decide if your child is disabled.

If the state agency cannot make a disability decision using only the medical information, school records and other facts they have, they may ask you to take your child for a medical examination or test. We will pay for the exam or test.

We May Make Immediate SSI Payments to Your Child

It can take three to five months for the state agency to decide if your child is disabled. However, for some medical conditions, we make SSI payments right away and for up to six months while the state agency decides if your child is disabled.

Following are some conditions that may qualify:

- Human immunodeficiency virus (HIV) infection

- Total blindness

- Total deafness

- Cerebral palsy

- Down syndrome

- Muscular dystrophy

- Severe intellectual disorder (child age seven or older)

- Birth weight below 2 pounds, 10 ounces

If your child has one of the qualifying conditions, he or she will get SSI payments right away. However, the state agency may finally decide that your child's disability is not severe enough for SSI. If that happens, you will not have to pay back the SSI payments that your child got.

SSI Disability Reviews

Once your child starts receiving SSI, the law requires that we review your child's medical condition from time to time to verify that he or she is still disabled. This review must be done:

- at least every three years for children younger than age eighteen whose conditions are expected to improve; and

- by age one for babies who are getting SSI payments because of their low birth weight, unless we determine their medical condition is not expected to improve by their first birthday and we schedule the review for a later date.

We may perform a disability review even if your child's condition is not expected to improve. When we do a review, you must present evidence that your child is and has been receiving treatment that is considered medically necessary for your child's medical condition.

What Happens When Your Child Turns Age Eighteen

For disability purposes in the SSI program, a child becomes an adult at age eighteen, and we use different medical and nonmedical rules when deciding if an adult can get SSI disability payments. For example, we do not count the income and resources of family members when deciding whether an adult meets the financial limits for SSI. We count only the adult's income and resources. We also use the disability rules for adults when deciding whether an adult is disabled.

If your child is already receiving SSI payments, we must review the child's medical condition when he or she turns age eighteen. We usually do this review during the one-year period that begins on your child's eighteenth birthday. We will use the adult disability rules to decide whether your eighteen-year-old is disabled.

If your child was not eligible for SSI before his or her eighteenth birthday because you and your spouse had too much income or resources, he or she may become eligible for SSI at age eighteen.

Social Security Disability Insurance (SSDI) Benefits for Adults Disabled Since Childhood

The SSDI program pays benefits to adults who have a disability that began before they became twenty-two years old. We consider this SSDI benefit as a "child's" benefit because it is paid on a parent's Social Security earnings record.

For a disabled adult to become entitled to this "child" benefit, one of his or her parents:

- must be receiving Social Security retirement or disability benefits; or

- must have died and have worked long enough under Social Security.

These benefits also are payable to an adult who received dependents benefits on a parent's Social Security earnings record prior to age eighteen, if he or she is disabled at age eighteen. We make the disability decision using the disability rules for adults.

SSDI disabled adult "child" benefits continue as long as the individual remains disabled. Your child does not need to have worked to get these benefits.

How We Decide If Your "Child" Is Disabled for SSDI Benefits

If your child is age eighteen or older, we will evaluate his or her disability the same way we would evaluate the disability for any adult. We send the application to the Disability Determination Services in your state that makes the disability decision for us.

Employment Support Programs for Young People with Disabilities

We have many ways to encourage young people who are receiving SSI payments or SSDI benefits and who want to go to work.
Under SSI:

- When we figure your child's monthly SSI payment, we do not count most of your child's income. If your child is younger than age twenty-two and a student who regularly attends school, we exclude even more of his or her earnings each month. In 2012, disabled students younger than age twenty-two may exclude $1,700 of their monthly earnings, with an annual limit of $6,840, when counting their income for SSI purposes. These limits may increase each year.

- With a Plan to Achieve Self-Support (PASS), a child who is age fifteen or older can save some income and resources to pay for education and other things needed to be able to work. We do not count the saved income when we figure your child's income for SSI purposes. We do not count the saved income and resources when we figure the amount of your child's payment.

- Because of a medical condition(s), your child may need certain items and services in order to work, such as a wheelchair or a personal assistant. When figuring your child's SSI payment, we will not count some or all of the amount paid for these items and services in your child's earnings.

- Your child older than age fifteen may get help with rehabilitation and training.

- Medicaid coverage will continue even if your child's earnings are high enough to stop the monthly SSI payment as long as the earnings are under a certain amount.

Under SSDI:

- An adult disabled before age twenty-two can get the same help with work expenses explained above for an SSI child, and help with rehabilitation and training.

- Cash benefits may continue until the individual can work on a regular basis.

- Medicare may continue for up to ninety-three months (seven years, nine months).

Medicaid and Medicare

Medicaid is a health care program for people with low incomes and limited resources. In most states, children who get SSI payments qualify for Medicaid. In many states, Medicaid comes automatically with SSI eligibility. In other states, you must sign up for it. And some children can get Medicaid coverage even if they do not qualify for SSI. Check with your local Social Security office, your state Medicaid agency, or your state or county social services office for more information.

Medicare is a federal health insurance program for people age sixty-five or older and for people who have been getting Social Security disability benefits for at least two years.

There are two exceptions to this rule. Your child can get Medicare immediately if he or she:

- has a chronic renal disease and needs a kidney transplant or maintenance dialysis; or

- has Lou Gehrig disease (amyotrophic lateral sclerosis).

Chapter 73

Estate Planning for Families of Children with Special Needs

Chapter Contents

Section 73.1

Estate Planning: The First Five Things to Do

"Estate planning" is one of those things most parents of children
with special needs know they need to think about, but actually getting around to it is another story. To give us all a little jump-start on
this important step to ensuring our children's future, I asked Mary
Browning, an attorney who focuses her practice on estate planning,
including special-needs planning, to tell us the first five things to do.
Her recommendations:

1. **Write a letter of intent:** "A letter of intent is a letter that will
   act as a guideline for the caretakers of your child with special
   needs after your death," Browning explains. "The letter includes
   a wide range of information including contact information for
   doctors, teachers, and other professionals. The letter also contains the likes and dislikes of your child as well as any other
   information that you believe is important for the caretakers to
   know about your child. This letter should be updated on an annual basis and kept with your other important documents."

2. **Set up a special needs trust:** "Consult an attorney and have
   wills and/or a stand-alone special needs trust drafted for you,"
   suggests Browning. "Any assets passing to your child with special needs at your death should go into a special needs trust
   in order to protect your child's eligibility for governmental
   benefits. A special needs trust can be drafted within a will, or
   can be drafted as a stand-alone special needs trust, which can
   become the recipient of lifetime gifts or bequests to your child
   from you or other family members." To get started: Find an expert qualified to help you with a special needs trust; Browning
   suggests using the referral service offered by the National Alliance on Mental Illness (NAMI).

3. **Consider life insurance:** "Take a look at your current financial situation and estimate how much money your child with special needs will need in the future," Browning says. "Think about whether you should obtain life insurance to make sure that your child has sufficient assets at your death. There are many life-insurance agents that specialize in helping families with children with special needs. I recommend consulting with a life-insurance expert to determine if this is an affordable option for you. If you do acquire life insurance, make sure that whatever portion of the policy is allocated to the special-needs child is allocated to the special needs trust for that child."
   To get started: Find a life-insurance company with a special-needs division—Browning mentions Guardian, MetLife, The Hartford, and Mass Mutual as four that do.

4. **Remove your child's name from assets:** "Make sure that your child with special needs does not own assets in his or her own name," warns Browning. "Assets held in a child's name can disqualify such a child from governmental benefits. One option is to transfer the assets to a first-party special needs trust for that child's benefit. This type of trust allows the money to be used for the child's benefit and does not disqualify him or her from governmental benefits. However, unlike the third-party special needs trust discussed above, in a first-party special needs trust, at the child's death, Medicaid must be paid back from the trust assets. You should consult an attorney to discuss your options." To get started: The NAMI lawyer referral service can help you find a qualified attorney in your area.

5. **Seek legal guardianship of your adult child:** "If your child is not able to handle his or her own medical or financial decisions as a result of his or her special needs, you as a parent should apply to become legal guardian of the child," Browning advises. "Without that, once your child obtains the age of eighteen, you will have no legal right to make decisions on his or her behalf. The process of applying for guardianship differs in each state; therefore, you should consult an attorney in your state who has expertise in this area. If guardianship is appropriate for your child, it is important to start the process as soon as possible." To get started: If you're not already working with an attorney, see if the agency in your state that helps people with developmental disabilities offers assistance with guardianship.

Section 73.2

Supplemental Needs Trusts

A special needs trust—sometimes called a "supplemental needs
trust"—provides for the needs of a disabled person without disquali-
fying him or her from benefits received from government programs
such as Social Security and Medicaid. A special needs trust makes it
possible to appoint a trustee to maintain assets and retain or qualify
for public assistance benefits.

The first thing that may come to mind for most families who have
had experience with government benefits is that the government says
that a person with a disability cannot have a trust. Correct. However,
the special needs trust does not belong to the person with a disability. The
trust is established and administered by someone else—the trustee.
The person with the disability does not have a trust. He or she is nom-
inated as a beneficiary of the trust and is usually the only one who receives
the benefits. Furthermore, the trustee (manager) is given the absolute
discretion to determine when and how much the person should receive.

What the Social Security Administration Has to Say about Special Needs Trusts

The Social Security Administration's (1990) publication *Understanding SSI* discusses special needs trusts as follows:

- How do resources in this type of trust count in the Supplemental
  Security Income (SSI) program?

  - Money or property in this type of trust for an SSI beneficiary
    does not count toward the SSI resource limits of $2,000 for
    an individual.

- How does money from the trust affect the individual's SSI payments?

  - Money paid directly to the providers for items other than
    the person's food, clothing, and shelter does not reduce SSI

payments. (Items that are not "food, clothing, or shelter" include medical care, telephone bills, education, entertainment.)

- Money paid directly to the providers for food, clothing, and shelter does not reduce the individual's SSI payments—but only up to a limit. No matter how much money is spent for these items, no more than $155.66 (in 1991) is subtracted from the individual's SSI check.

- Money paid directly to the individual from the trust reduces the SSI payment. (U.S. Department of Health and Human Services, 1990, p. 46)

There are Three Types of Special Needs Trusts

Family-Type Special Needs Trusts

The parents provide the money for the trust, often by will, and sometimes by purchasing life insurance payable to the trust.

Some parents place their property in a "living" or "inter vivos" trust, and provide in the trust that the disabled son or daughter is the beneficiary. With that type of trust, there is no need to wait for the parents to die. The trust becomes effective immediately. This is a good idea for families where aunts, uncles, and grandparents might want to leave money for the trust. Anyone can give money to the trust, by either writing a check or writing a will.

The key to a family-type special needs trust is that the money *cannot* be used for housing, food, or clothing. Those are considered "basic needs" under SSI and Medicaid laws. If the disabled person is receiving free housing, food, or clothing from someone else, including a family member or a trust, then the government benefits will be reduced or eliminated.

The parents can provide the money for this type of trust, and so can other family members, such as grandparents, aunts, and uncles. The only person who cannot place money into this type of trust is the disabled person.

Court-Ordered Special Needs Trust

A court-ordered trust, also called a Type "A" special needs trust, is used only for special circumstances, such as where the person with a disability has inherited money, or received a court settlement.

Because the disabled person actually owns the money, the funds cannot be put into the usual special needs trust such as parents usually set up.

651

The "A" comes from the last letter of the federal statute, 42 U.S.C. § 1396p (d) (4) (A).

Only certain people are allowed to set up this type of trust:

- The disabled person's parent

- The disabled person's grandparent

- The legal guardian

- A court

To qualify, the disabled person has to be under sixty-five years old and meet the medical standards of Social Security, in terms of the disability. Someone who is not disabled enough to qualify for Social Security cannot have this type of trust.

The trust has to specify that after the disabled person has died, anything left over will pay back the state of residence for whatever medical assistance the government provided to the individual after the trust was set up.

Pooled Special Needs Trust

This trust has to be established through a nonprofit association. Anyone can put money into pooled trust—parents, grandparents, or even the individual with a disability (the "beneficiary"). The trusts pool the funds of many beneficiaries to invest and manage. Although the funds are pooled, each beneficiary still has his or her own account. A big advantage of pooled trusts is that they are willing to handle much smaller accounts than a bank or trust company, so people of modest means can have access to sophisticated trust services.

The nonprofit agency that administers the trust takes care of all the tax preparation, investment decisions, and serves as trustee.

Any money left in the trust after the beneficiary dies stays in the trust to help other persons with disabilities. The money does not go to the state.

A pooled trust can purchase a home for the beneficiary, and rent it to him or her. Before the pooled trust is set up, the parents and other family members explain what they want the trust to pay for, and who should be consulted about these matters.

In addition, you have to be considered physically or mentally "disabled" the same as anyone who receives Social Security or SSI.

Special needs trusts are complicated legally binding documents. Please consult a qualified trust attorney that has experience establishing these types of trusts.

Part Seven

Additional Help and Information

Chapter 74

Glossary of Terms Related to Human Genetics

allele: One of two or more versions of a gene. An individual inherits two alleles for each gene, one from each parent. If the two alleles are the same, the individual is homozygous for that gene. If the alleles are different, the individual is heterozygous.

amino acids: A set of twenty different molecules used to build proteins. Proteins consist of one or more chains of amino acids called polypeptides. The sequence of the amino acid chain causes the polypeptide to fold into a shape that is biologically active. The amino acid sequences of proteins are encoded in the genes.

anticodon: A trinucleotide sequence complementary to that of a corresponding codon in a messenger RNA (mRNA) sequence. An anticodon is found at one end of a transfer RNA (tRNA) molecule. During protein synthesis, each time an amino acid is added to the growing protein, a tRNA forms base pairs with its complementary sequence on the mRNA molecule, ensuring that the appropriate amino acid is inserted into the protein.

antisense: The non-coding DNA strand of a gene. A cell uses antisense DNA strand as a template for producing messenger RNA (mRNA) that directs the synthesis of a protein. Antisense can also refer to a method

The terms in this glossary were excerpted from the "Talking Glossary of Genetic Terms," National Human Genome Research Institute, National Institutes of Health. The complete text of this document is available online at http://www.genome.gov/glossary/index.cfm. Accessed June 6, 2013.

for silencing genes. To silence a target gene, a second gene is introduced that produces an mRNA complementary to that produced from the target gene. These two mRNAs can interact to form a double-stranded structure that cannot be used to direct protein synthesis.

apoptosis: The process of programmed cell death. It is used during early development to eliminate unwanted cells. In adults, apoptosis is used to rid the body of cells that have been damaged beyond repair. Apoptosis also plays a role in preventing cancer. If apoptosis is for some reason prevented, it can lead to uncontrolled cell division and the subsequent development of a tumor.

autosomal dominance: A pattern of inheritance characteristic of some genetic diseases. "Autosomal" means that the gene in question is located on one of the numbered, or non-sex, chromosomes. "Dominant" means that a single copy of the disease-associated mutation is enough to cause the disease.

autosome: Any of the numbered chromosomes, as opposed to the sex chromosomes. Humans have twenty-two pairs of autosomes and one pair of sex chromosomes (the X and Y). Autosomes are numbered roughly in relation to their sizes. That is, Chromosome 1 has approximately 2,800 genes, while chromosome 22 has approximately 750 genes.

base pair: Two chemical bases bonded to one another forming a "rung of the DNA ladder." The DNA molecule consists of two strands that wind around each other like a twisted ladder. Each strand has a backbone made of alternating sugar (deoxyribose) and phosphate groups. Attached to each sugar is one of four bases--adenine (A), cytosine (C), guanine (G), or thymine (T). The two strands are held together by hydrogen bonds between the bases, with adenine forming a base pair with thymine, and cytosine forming a base pair with guanine.

birth defect: An abnormality present at birth. Also called a congenital defect, it can be caused by a genetic mutation, an unfavorable environment during pregnancy, or a combination of both. The effect of a birth defect can be mild, severe, or incompatible with life.

BRCA1 and BRCA2: The first two genes found to be associated with inherited forms of breast cancer. Both genes normally act as tumor suppressors, meaning that they help regulate cell division. When these genes are rendered inactive due to mutation, uncontrolled cell growth results, leading to breast cancer. Women with mutations in either gene have a much higher risk for developing breast cancer than women without mutations in the genes.

cancer: A group of diseases characterized by uncontrolled cell growth. Cancer begins when a single cell mutates, resulting in a breakdown of the normal regulatory controls that keep cell division in check.

candidate gene: A gene whose chromosomal location is associated with a particular disease or other phenotype. Because of its location, the gene is suspected of causing the disease or other phenotype.

carrier: An individual who carries and is capable of passing on a genetic mutation associated with a disease and may or may not display disease symptoms. Carriers are associated with diseases inherited as recessive traits. In order to have the disease, an individual must have inherited mutated alleles from both parents. An individual having one normal allele and one mutated allele does not have the disease. Two carriers may produce children with the disease.

carrier screening: A type of genetic testing performed on people who display no symptoms for a genetic disorder but may be at risk for passing it on to their children. A carrier for a genetic disorder has inherited one normal and one abnormal allele for a gene associated with the disorder. A child must inherit two abnormal alleles in order for symptoms to appear. Prospective parents with a family history of a genetic disorders are candidates for carrier screening.

cell: The basic building block of living things. An adult human body is estimated to contain between 10 and 100 trillion cells.

centromere: A constricted region of a chromosome that separates it into a short arm (p) and a long arm (q).

chromatid: One of two identical halves of a replicated chromosome. During cell division, the chromosomes first replicate so that each daughter cell receives a complete set of chromosomes. Following DNA replication, the chromosome consists of two identical structures called sister chromatids, which are joined at the centromere.

chromosome: An organized package of DNA found in the nucleus of the cell. Different organisms have different numbers of chromosomes. Humans have 23 pairs of chromosomes--22 pairs of numbered chromosomes, called autosomes, and one pair of sex chromosomes, X and Y.

cloning: The process of making identical copies of an organism, cell, or DNA sequence.

codominance: A relationship between two versions of a gene. Individuals receive one version of a gene, called an allele, from each parent. If the alleles are different, the dominant allele usually will be expressed, while the effect of the other allele, called recessive, is masked. In codominance, however, neither allele is recessive and the phenotypes of both alleles are expressed.

codon: A trinucleotide sequence of DNA or RNA that corresponds to a specific amino acid. There are sixty-four different codons: sixty-one specify amino acids while the remaining three are used as stop signals.

complex disease: A disease caused by the interaction of multiple genes and environmental factors.

congenital conditions: Conditions present from birth. Birth defects are described as being congenital.

copy number variation (CNV): When the number of copies of a particular gene varies from one individual to the next. The extent to which copy number variation contributes to human disease is not yet known. It has long been recognized that some cancers are associated with elevated copy numbers of particular genes.

crossing over: The swapping of genetic material that occurs in the germ line. Crossing over results in a shuffling of genetic material and is an important cause of the genetic variation seen among offspring.

deletion: A type of mutation involving the loss of genetic material. It can be small, involving a single missing DNA base pair, or large, involving a piece of a chromosome.

diploid: A cell or organism that has paired chromosomes, one from each parent. In humans, cells other than human sex cells, are diploid and have twenty-three pairs of chromosomes. Human sex cells (egg and sperm cells) contain a single set of chromosomes and are known as haploid.

DNA (deoxyribonucleic acid): The chemical name for the molecule that carries genetic instructions in all living things. The DNA molecule consists of two strands that wind around one another to form a shape known as a double helix. Each strand has a backbone made of alternating sugar (deoxyribose) and phosphate groups. Attached to each sugar is one of four bases--adenine (A), cytosine (C), guanine (G), and thymine (T). The two strands are held together by bonds between the bases; adenine bonds with thymine, and cytosine bonds with guanine. The sequence of the bases along the backbones serves as instructions for assembling protein and RNA molecules.

DNA replication: The process by which a molecule of DNA is duplicated. When a cell divides, it must first duplicate its genome so that each daughter cell winds up with a complete set of chromosomes.

DNA sequencing: A laboratory technique used to determine the exact sequence of bases (A, C, G, and T) in a DNA molecule. The DNA base sequence carries the information a cell needs to assemble protein and RNA molecules. DNA sequence information is important to scientists investigating the functions of genes.

dominant: This refers to the relationship between two versions of a gene. Individuals receive two versions of each gene, known as alleles, from each parent. If the alleles of a gene are different, one allele will be expressed; it is the dominant gene.

double helix: The description of the structure of a DNA molecule. A DNA molecule consists of two strands that wind around each other like a twisted ladder.

duplication: A type of mutation that involves the production of one or more copies of a gene or region of a chromosome. Gene duplication is an important mechanism by which evolution occurs.

epigenetics: An emerging field of science that studies heritable changes caused by the activation and deactivation of genes without any change in the underlying DNA sequence of the organism.

epistasis: A circumstance where the expression of one gene is affected by the expression of one or more independently inherited genes. For example, if the expression of gene #2 depends on the expression of gene #1, but gene #1 becomes inactive, then the expression of gene #2 will not occur. In this example, gene #1 is said to be epistatic to gene #2.

exon: The portion of a gene that codes for amino acids.

fibroblast: The most common type of cell found in connective tissue. Fibroblasts secrete collagen proteins that are used to maintain a structural framework for many tissues. They also play an important role in healing wounds.

first-degree relative: A family member who shares about 50 percent of their genes with a particular individual in a family. This includes parents, offspring, and siblings.

fluorescence in situ hybridization (FISH): A laboratory technique for detecting and locating a specific DNA sequence on a chromosome. The technique relies on exposing chromosomes to a small DNA sequence called a probe that has a fluorescent molecule attached to it. The probe sequence binds to its corresponding sequence on the chromosome.

frameshift mutation: A type of mutation involving the insertion or deletion of a nucleotide in which the number of deleted base pairs is not divisible by three. This is important because the cell reads a gene in groups of three bases. Each group of three bases corresponds to one of 20 different amino acids used to build a protein. If a mutation disrupts this reading frame, then the entire DNA sequence following the mutation will be read incorrectly.

fraternal twins: Dizygotic twins, resulting from the fertilization of two separate eggs during the same pregnancy. They share half of their genes just like any other siblings.

gene: The basic physical unit of inheritance. Genes are passed from parents to offspring and contain the information needed to specify traits. Genes are arranged, one after another, on structures called chromosomes.

gene amplification: An increase in the number of copies of a gene sequence.

gene expression: The process by which the information encoded in a gene is used to direct the assembly of a protein molecule. The cell reads the sequence of the gene in groups of three bases. Each group of three bases (codon) corresponds to one of twenty different amino acids used to build the protein.

gene mapping: The process of establishing the locations of genes on the chromosomes.

gene pool: The total genetic diversity found within a population or a species. A large gene pool has extensive genetic diversity and is better able to withstand the challenges posed by environmental stresses. Inbreeding contributes to the creation of a small gene pool and makes populations or species more likely to go extinct when faced with some type of stress.

gene regulation: The process of turning genes on and off. Gene regulation ensures that the appropriate genes are expressed at the proper times.

gene therapy: An experimental technique for treating disease by altering the patient's genetic material. Most often, gene therapy works by introducing a healthy copy of a defective gene into the patient's cells.

genetic counseling: The professional interaction between a healthcare provider with specialized knowledge of genetics and an individual or family. The genetic counselor determines whether a condition in the family may be genetic and estimates the chances that another relative may be affected.

genetic drift: Random fluctuations in the frequencies of alleles from generation to generation due to chance events. Genetic drift can cause traits to be dominant or disappear from a population.

genetic engineering: The process of using recombinant DNA (rDNA) technology to alter the genetic makeup of an organism. Traditionally, humans have manipulated genomes indirectly by controlling breeding and selecting offspring with desired traits. Genetic engineering involves the direct manipulation of one or more genes. Most often, a gene from another species is added to an organism's genome to give it a desired phenotype.

genetic marker: A DNA sequence with a known physical location on a chromosome. Genetic markers can help link an inherited disease with the responsible gene.

genetic screening: The process of testing a population for a genetic disease in order to identify a subgroup of people that either have the disease or the potential to pass it on to their offspring.

genetic testing: The use of a laboratory test to look for genetic variations associated with a disease. The results of a genetic test can be used to confirm or rule out a suspected genetic disease or to determine the likelihood of a person passing on a mutation to their offspring.

genome: The entire set of genetic instructions found in a cell. In humans, the genome consists of 23 pairs of chromosomes, found in the nucleus, as well as a small chromosome found in the cells' mitochondria.

genome-wide association study (GWAS): An approach used in genetics research to associate specific genetic variations with particular diseases. The method involves scanning the genomes from many different people and looking for genetic markers that can be used to predict the presence of a disease. Once such genetic markers are identified, they can be used to understand how genes contribute to the disease and develop better prevention and treatment strategies.

genomics: The study of the entire genome of an organism.

genotype: An individual's collection of genes. The expression of the genotype contributes to the individual's observable traits, called the phenotype.

germ line: The sex cells (eggs and sperm) that are used by sexually reproducing organisms to pass on genes from generation to generation.

haploid: The quality of a cell or organism having a single set of chromosomes. In humans, only their egg and sperm cells are haploid.

haplotype: A set of DNA variations, or polymorphisms, that tend to be inherited together. A haplotype can refer to a combination of alleles or to a set of single nucleotide polymorphisms (SNPs) found on the same chromosome.

heterozygous: Having inherited different forms of a particular gene from each parent.

homologous recombination: A type of genetic recombination that occurs during meiosis (the formation of egg and sperm cells). Paired chromosomes from the male and female parent align so that similar DNA sequences from the paired chromosomes cross over each other. Crossing over results in a shuffling of genetic material and is an important cause of the genetic variation seen among offspring.

homozygous: A genetic condition where an individual inherits the same alleles for a particular gene from both parents.

hybridization: The process of combining two complementary single-stranded DNA or RNA molecules and allowing them to form a single double-stranded molecule through base pairing. Hybridization is a part of many important laboratory techniques such as polymerase chain reaction and Southern blotting.

identical twins: Also known as monozygotic twins. They result from the fertilization of a single egg that splits in two. Identical twins share all of their genes and are always of the same sex.

inherited trait: A trait that is genetically determined. Inherited traits are passed from parent to offspring according to the rules of Mendelian genetics.

insertion: A type of mutation involving the addition of genetic material.

intron: A portion of a gene that does not code for amino acids.

karyotype: An individual's collection of chromosomes.

knockout: An organism that has been genetically engineered to lack one or more specific genes. Scientists create knockouts (often in mice) so that they can study the impact of the missing genes and learn something about the genes' function.

linkage: The close association of genes or other DNA sequences on the same chromosome.

locus: The specific physical location of a gene or other DNA sequence on a chromosome, like a genetic street address.

mapping: The process of making a representative diagram cataloging the genes and other features of a chromosome and showing their relative locations.

marker: A DNA sequence with a known physical location on a chromosome. Markers can help link an inherited disease with the responsible genes.

Mendelian inheritance: Patterns of inheritance that are characteristic of organisms that reproduce sexually. The Austrian monk Gregor Mendel introduced the idea of dominant and recessive genes.

missense mutation: When the change of a single base pair causes the substitution of a different amino acid in the resulting protein. This amino acid substitution may have no effect, or it may render the protein nonfunctional.

mitochondrial DNA: The small circular chromosome found inside mitochondria. The mitochondria are organelles found in cells that are the sites of energy production.

mitosis: A cellular process that replicates chromosomes and produces two identical nuclei in preparation for cell division.

monosomy: The state of having a single copy of a chromosome pair instead of the usual two copies found in diploid cells. Monosomy can be partial if a portion of the second chromosome copy is present. Monosomy, or partial monosomy, is the cause of some human diseases such as Turner syndrome and cri du chat syndrome.

mutagen: A chemical or physical phenomenon, such as ionizing radiation, that promotes errors in DNA replication. Exposure to a mutagen can produce DNA mutations that cause or contribute to diseases such as cancer.

mutation: A change in a DNA sequence.

newborn screening: Testing performed on newborn babies to detect a wide variety of disorders. Typically, testing is performed on a blood sample obtained from a heel prick when the baby is two or three days old.

noncoding DNA: DNA sequences that do not code for amino acids. Most noncoding DNA lies between genes on the chromosome and has no known function. Other noncoding DNA, called introns, is found within genes. Some non-coding DNA plays a role in the regulation of gene expression.

nonsense mutation: The substitution of a single base pair that leads to the appearance of a stop codon where previously there was a codon specifying an amino acid. The presence of this premature stop codon results in the production of a shortened, and likely nonfunctional, protein.

oncogene: A mutated gene that contributes to the development of a cancer. In their normal, unmutated state, oncogenes are called proto-oncogenes, and they play roles in the regulation of cell division.

open reading frame: A portion of a DNA molecule that, when translated into amino acids, contains no stop codons. The genetic code reads DNA sequences in groups of three base pairs, which means that a double-stranded DNA molecule can read in any of six possible reading frames—three in the forward direction and three in the reverse. A long open reading frame is likely part of a gene.

personalized medicine: An emerging practice of medicine that uses an individual's genetic profile to guide decisions made in regard to the prevention, diagnosis, and treatment of disease. Knowledge of a patient's genetic profile can help doctors select the proper medication or therapy and administer it using the proper dose or regimen.

pharmacogenomics: A branch of pharmacology concerned with using DNA and amino acid sequence data to inform drug development and testing. An important application of pharmacogenomics is correlating individual genetic variation with drug responses.

phenotype: An individual's observable traits, such as height, eye color, and blood type.

point mutation: When a single base pair is altered. Point mutations can have one of three effects. First, the base substitution can be a silent mutation where the altered codon corresponds to the same amino acid. Second, the base substitution can be a missense mutation where the altered codon corresponds to a different amino acid. Or third, the base substitution can be a nonsense mutation where the altered codon corresponds to a stop signal.

polygenic trait: A trait whose phenotype is influenced by more than one gene.

polymorphism: One of two or more variants of a particular DNA sequence. The most common type of polymorphism involves variation at a single base pair. Polymorphisms can also be much larger in size and involve long stretches of DNA. Called a single nucleotide polymorphism, or SNP (pronounced snip), scientists are studying how SNPs in the human genome correlate with disease, drug response, and other phenotypes.

protein: An important class of molecules found in all living cells. A protein is composed of one or more long chains of amino acids, the sequence of which corresponds to the DNA sequence of the gene that encodes it. Proteins play a variety of roles in the cell, including structural (cytoskeleton), mechanical (muscle), biochemical (enzymes), and cell signaling (hormones).

pseudogene: A DNA sequence that resembles a gene but has been mutated into an inactive form over the course of evolution. A pseudogene shares an evolutionary history with a functional gene and can provide insight into their shared ancestry.

recessive: A quality found in the relationship between two versions of a gene. Individuals receive one version of a gene, called an allele, from each parent. If the alleles are different, the dominant allele will be expressed, while the effect of the other allele, called recessive, is masked.

recombinant DNA (rDNA): A technology that uses enzymes to cut and paste together DNA sequences of interest. The recombined DNA sequences can be placed into vehicles called vectors that ferry the DNA into a suitable host cell where it can be copied or expressed.

retrovirus: A virus that uses RNA as its genetic material. When a retrovirus infects a cell, it makes a DNA copy of its genome that is inserted into the DNA of the host cell. There are a variety of different retroviruses that cause human diseases such as some forms of cancer and acquired immunodeficiency syndrome (AIDS).

ribosome: A cellular particle made of RNA and protein that serves as the site for protein synthesis in the cell. The ribosome reads the sequence of the messenger RNA (mRNA) and, using the genetic code, translates the sequence of RNA bases into a sequence of amino acids.

RNA (ribonucleic acid): A molecule similar to DNA. Unlike DNA, RNA is single-stranded. An RNA strand has a backbone made of alternating sugar (ribose) and phosphate groups. Attached to each sugar is one of four bases—adenine (A), uracil (U), cytosine (C), or guanine

(G). Different types of RNA exist in the cell: messenger RNA (mRNA), ribosomal RNA (rRNA), and transfer RNA (tRNA).

sex chromosome: A type of chromosome that participates in sex determination. Humans and most other mammals have two sex chromosomes, the X and the Y. Females have two X chromosomes in their cells, while males have both X and a Y chromosomes in their cells.

sex linked: A trait in which a gene is located on a sex chromosome. In humans, the term generally refers to traits that are influenced by genes on the X chromosome.

single nucleotide polymorphisms (SNPs): A type of polymorphism involving variation of a single base pair.

somatic cell: Any cell of the body except sperm and egg cells. Somatic cells are diploid, meaning that they contain two sets of chromosomes, one inherited from each parent.

stem cell: A cell with the potential to form many of the different cell types found in the body. When stem cells divide, they can form more stem cells or other cells that perform specialized functions.

stop codon: A trinucleotide sequence within a messenger RNA (mRNA) molecule that signals a halt to protein synthesis. The genetic code describes the relationship between the sequence of DNA bases (A, C, G, and T) in a gene and the corresponding protein sequence that it encodes. The cell reads the sequence of the gene in groups of three bases. Of the sixty-four possible combinations of three bases, sixty-one specify an amino acid, while the remaining three combinations are stop codons.

substitution: A type of mutation where one base pair is replaced by a different base pair. The term also refers to the replacement of one amino acid in a protein with a different amino acid.

susceptibility: A condition of the body that increases the likelihood that the individual will develop a particular disease. Susceptibility is influenced by a combination of genetic and environmental factors.

syndrome: A collection of recognizable traits or abnormalities that tend to occur together and are associated with a specific disease.

tandem repeat: A sequence of two or more DNA base pairs that is repeated in such a way that the repeats lie adjacent to each other on the chromosome. Tandem repeats are generally associated with noncoding DNA. In some instances, the number of times the DNA sequence is repeated is variable. Such variable tandem repeats are used in DNA fingerprinting procedures.

telomere: The end of a chromosome. Telomeres are made of repetitive sequences of non-coding DNA that protect the chromosome from damage. Each time a cell divides, the telomeres become shorter. Eventually, the telomeres become so short that the cell can no longer divide.

trait: A specific characteristic of an organism. Traits can be determined by genes or the environment, or more commonly by interactions between them. The genetic contribution to a trait is called the genotype. The outward expression of the genotype is called the phenotype.

transcription: The process of making an RNA copy of a gene sequence. This copy, called a messenger RNA (mRNA) molecule, leaves the cell nucleus and enters the cytoplasm, where it directs the synthesis of the protein, which it encodes.

transfer RNA (tRNA): small RNA molecule that participates in protein synthesis. Each tRNA molecule has two important areas: a trinucleotide region called the anticodon and a region for attaching a specific amino acid. During translation, each time an amino acid is added to the growing chain, a tRNA molecule forms base pairs with its complementary sequence on the messenger RNA (mRNA) molecule, ensuring that the appropriate amino acid is inserted into the protein.

translation: The process of translating the sequence of a messenger RNA (mRNA) molecule to a sequence of amino acids during protein synthesis.

translocation: A type of chromosomal abnormality in which a chromosome breaks and a portion of it reattaches to a different chromosome.

X chromosome: One of two sex chromosomes.

X-linked: A trait where a gene is located on the X chromosome. Humans and other mammals have two sex chromosomes, the X and the Y. In an X-linked or sex linked disease, it is usually males that are affected because they have a single copy of the X chromosome that carries the mutation. In females, the effect of the mutation may be masked by the second healthy copy of the X chromosome.

Y chromosome: One of two sex chromosomes.

Chapter 75

Sources of Further Help and Information Related to Genetic Disorders

General

Genetics Home Reference
Website: http://ghr.nlm.nih.gov

National Digestive Diseases Information Clearinghouse
2 Information Way
Bethesda, MD 20892-3570
Toll-Free: 800-891-5389
Toll-Free TTY: 866-569-1162
Fax: 703-738-4929
Website: http://www.digestive
.niddk.nih.gov
E-mail: nddic@info.niddk.nih.gov

National Heart, Lung, and Blood Institute
National Institutes of Health
NHLBI Health
Information Center
P.O. Box 30105
Bethesda, MD 20824-0105
Phone: 301-592-8573
Fax: 301-592-8563
Website:
http://www.nhlbi.nih.gov
E-mail: nhlbiinfo@nhlbi.nih.gov

Resources in this chapter were compiled from several sources deemed reliable. All contact information was verified and updated in June 2013.

National Human Genome Research Institute
Communications and
Public Liaison Branch
National Institutes of Health
Building 31, Room 4B09
31 Center Drive, MSC 2152
9000 Rockville Pike
Bethesda, MD 20892-2152
Phone: 301-402-0911
Fax: 301-402-2218
Website: http://www.genome.gov

National Institute of Arthritis and Musculoskeletal and Skin Diseases (NIAMS)
Information Clearinghouse
National Institutes of Health
1 AMS Circle
Bethesda, MD 20892-3675
Toll-Free: 877-22-NIAMS
(877-226-4267)
Phone: 301-495-4484
TTY: 301-565-2966
Fax: 301-718-6366
Website:
http://www.niams.nih.gov
E-mail: NIAMSinfo@mail.nih.gov

National Institute of Child Health and Human Development (NICHD)
P.O. Box 3006
Rockville, MD 20847
Toll-Free: 800-370-2943
Toll-Free TTY: 888-320-6942
Toll-Free Fax: 866-760-5947
Website:
http://www.nichd.nih.gov
E-mail: NICHDInformation
ResourceCenter@mail.nih.gov

National Institute of Diabetes and Digestive and Kidney Diseases (NIDDK)
Office of Communications &
Public Liaison
Building 31, Room 9A06
31 Center Drive, MSC 2560
Bethesda, MD 20892-2560
Phone: 301-496-3583
Website:
http://www2.niddk.nih.gov

National Institute of General Medical Sciences
Office of Communications &
Public Liaison
45 Center Drive MSC 6200
Bethesda, MD 20892-6200
Phone: 301-496-7301
Website:
http://www.nigms.nih.gov
E-mail: info@nigms.nih.gov

National Institute of Neurological Disorders and Stroke
Office of Communications
National Institutes of Health
Neurological Institute
P.O. Box 5801
Bethesda, MD 20824
Toll-Free: 800-352-9424
Phone: 301-496-5751
Website:
http://www.ninds.nih.gov

Nemours Foundation
Website:
http://www.kidshealth.org

Rare Diseases Clinical Research Network
Website:
http://rarediseasesnetwork.epi
.usf.edu

Albinism

National Organization for Albinism and Hypopigmentation (NOAH)
P.O. Box 959
East Hampstead, NH 03826-0959
Toll-Free: 800-473-2310
(U.S. and Canada)
Phone: 603-887-2310
Toll-Free Fax: 800-648-2310
Website: http://www.albinism.org
E-mail: webmaster@albinism.org

Angelman Syndrome

Angelman Syndrome Association
P.O. Box 554
Sutherland, NSW Australia 2232
Website:
http://www.angelman
syndrome.org

Angelman Syndrome Foundation
4255 Westbrook Drive
Suite 219
Aurora, IL 60504
Toll-Free: 800-432-6435
Phone: 630-978-4245
Fax: 630-978-7408
Website:
http://www.angelman.org
E-mail: info@angelman.org

Canadian Angelman Syndrome Society
P.O. Box 37
Priddis,
Alberta T0L 1W0 Canada
Phone: 403-931-2415
Fax: 403-931-4237
Website:
http://www.angelmancanada.org

Blood Disorders

American Hemochromatosis Society, Inc.
4044 West Lake Mary Boulevard
Unit #104 PMB 416
Lake Mary, FL 32746-2012
Toll-Free: 888-655-IRON
(888-655-4766)
Phone: 407-829-4488
Fax: 407-333-1284
Website:
http://www.americanhs.org
E-mail: mail@americanhs.org

Canadian Fanconi Anemia Research Fund
P.O. Box 38157
Toronto, ON M5N 3A9 Canada
Phone: 416-489-6393
Fax: 416-489-6393
Website:
http://www.fanconicanada.org
E-mail:
admin@fanconicanada.org

Fanconi Anemia Research Fund, Inc.
1801 Willamette Street
Suite 200
Eugene, OR 97401
Toll-Free: 888-FANCONI
(888-326-2664)
Phone: 541-687-4658
Fax: 541-687-0548
Website: http://www.fanconi.org
E-mail: info@fanconi.org

Iron Disorders Institute
P.O. Box 675
Taylors, SC 29687
Website:
http://www.irondisorders.org
E-mail: info@irondisorders.org

National Hemophilia Foundation
116 West 32nd Street
11th Floor
New York, NY 10001
Phone: 212-328-3700
Fax: 212-328-3777
Website:
http://www.hemophilia.org

Sickle Cell Disease Association of America
231 East Baltimore Street
Suite 800
Baltimore, MD 21202
Toll-Free: 800-421-8453
Phone: 410-528-1555
Fax: 410-528-1495
Website:
http://www.sicklecelldisease.org
E-mail:
scdaa@sicklecelldisease.org

CHARGE Syndrome

CHARGE Syndrome Foundation, Inc.
141 Middle Neck Road
Sands Point, NY 11050
Toll Free: 800-442-7604
Phone: 516-684-4720
Fax: 516-883-9060
Website:
http://www.chargesyndrome.org
E-mail:
info@chargesyndrome.org

Connective Tissue Disorders

Canadian Ehlers-Danlos Association (CEDA)
183 Charlton Avenue
Thornhill, ON L4J 6E9 Canada
Phone: 905-761-7552
Fax: 905-761-7567
Website:
http://www.ehlersdanlos.ca

Canadian Marfan Association (CMA)
Centre Plaza Postal Outlet
128 Queen Street South
P.O. Box 42257
Mississauga,
ON L5M 4Z0 Canada
Toll-Free: 866-722-1722
Phone: 905-826-3223
Fax: 905-826-2125
Website: http://www.marfan.ca
E-mail: info@marfan.ca

Ehlers-Danlos National Foundation (EDNF)
1760 Old Meadow Road
Suite 500
McLean, VA 22102
Phone: 703-506-2892
Fax: 703-506-3266
Website: http://www.ednf.org
E-mail: ednfstaff@ednf.org

National Marfan Foundation (NMF)
22 Manhasset Avenue
Port Washington NY 11050
Toll-Free: 800-862-7326
Phone: 516-883-8712
Fax: 516-883-8040
Website: http://www.marfan.org
E-mail: staff@marfan.org

Osteogenesis Imperfecta Foundation
804 West Diamond Avenue
Suite 210
Gaithersburg, MD 20878
Toll-Free: 800-981-2663
Phone: 301-947-0083
Fax: 301-947-0456
Website: http://www.oif.org
E-mail: bonelink@oif.org

Cornelia de Lange Syndrome

Cornelia de Lange Syndrome Foundation
302 West Main Street, #100
Avon, CT 06001
Toll-Free: 800-753-2357
or 800-223-8355
Phone: 860-676-8166
or 860-676-8255
Fax: 860-676-8337
Website: http://www.cdlsusa.org
E-mail: info@cdlsusa.org

Cystic Fibrosis

Cystic Fibrosis Foundation
6931 Arlington Road, 2nd floor
Bethesda, MD 20814
Toll free: 800-FIGHT CF
(800-344-4823)
Phone: 301-951-4422
Fax: 301-951-6378
Website: http://www.cff.org
E-mail: info@cff.org

Fragile X Syndrome

FRAXA Research Foundation
10 Prince Place
Newburyport, MA 01950
Phone: 978-462-1866
Website: http://www.fraxa.org

National Fragile X Foundation

1615 Bonanza Street
Suite 202
Walnut Creek, CA 94596
Toll-Free: 800-688-8765
Fax: 925-938-9315
Website:
http://www.fragilex.org
E-mail: natlfx@fragilex.org

Gene Therapy

American Society of Gene & Cell Therapy

555 East Wells Street
Suite 1100
Milwaukee, WI 53202
Phone: 414-278-1341
Fax: 414-276-3349
Website: http://www.asgct.org
E-mail: info@asgct.org

Huntington Disease

Huntington's Disease Society of America

505 Eighth Avenue
Suite 902
New York, NY 10018
Toll-Free: 800-345-HDSA
(800-345-4372)
Phone: 212-242-1968
Fax: 212-239-3430
Website: http://www.hdsa.org
E-mail: hdsainfo@hdsa.org

Jewish Genetic Disorders

Center for Jewish Genetics

30 South Wells
Chicago, IL 60606
Phone: 312-357-4718
Website:
http://www.jewishgenetics.org
E-mail:
jewishgeneticsctr@juf.org

Leukodystrophy

United Leukodystrophy Foundation

224 North Second Street
Suite 2
DeKalb, IL 60115
Toll-Free: 800-728-5483
Phone: 815-748-3211
Fax: 815-748-0844
Website: http://www.ulf.org
E-mail: office@ulf.org

Lipid Storage Diseases

Batten Disease Support and Research Association

1175 Dublin Road
Columbus, OH 43215
Toll-Free: 800-448-4570
Toll-Free Fax: 866-648-8718
Website: http://www.bdsra.org
E-mail: bdsra1@bdsra.org

Canadian Fabry Association

1707 West 7th Avenue
Unit #314
Vancouver, BC V6J 5E9 Canada
Website:
http://www.fabrycanada.com

Children's Brain Disease Foundation
Parnassus Heights Medical
Building, Suite 900
San Francisco, CA 94117
Phone: 415-665-3003
Fax: 415-665-3003

Children's Gaucher Research Fund
8110 Warren Court
Granite Bay, CA 95746
Phone: 916-797-3700
Fax: 916-797-3707
Website:
http://www.childrensgaucher.org
E-mail:
research@childrensgaucher.org

Fabry Support & Information Group
108 NE 2nd Street
Suite C
P.O. Box 510
Concordia, MO 64020-0510
Phone: 660-463-1355
Fax: 660-463-1356
Website: http://www.fabry.org
E-mail: info@fabry.org

Nathan's Battle Foundation [For Batten Disease Research]
459 State Road 135 South
Greenwood, IN 46142
Phone: 317-888-7396
Fax: 317-888-0504
Website:
http://www.nathansbattle.com
E-mail: pmilto@indy.net

National Fabry Disease Foundation
4301 Connecticut Avenue NW
Suite 404
Washington, DC 20008-2369
Toll-Free: 800-651-9131
Fax: 919-932-7786
Website:
http://www.fabrydisease.org
E-mail: info@fabrydisease.org

National Gaucher Foundation
2227 Idlewood Road, Suite 6
Tucker, GA 30084
Toll-Free: 800-504-3189
Website:
http://www.gaucherdisease.org
E-mail: ngf@gaucherdisease.org

National Niemann-Pick Disease Foundation, Inc.
P.O. Box 49
401 Madison Avenue, Suite B
Fort Atkinson, WI 53538
Toll-Free: 877-CURE-NPC
(877-287-3672)
Phone: 920-563-0930
Fax: 920-563-0931
Website: http://www.nnpdf.org
E-mail: nnpdf@nnpdf.org

National Tay-Sachs and Allied Diseases Association
2001 Beacon Street, Suite 204
Boston, MA 02135
Toll-Free: 800-90-NTSAD
(800-906-8723)
Fax: 617-277-0134
Website: http://www.ntsad.org
E-mail: info@ntsad.org

Mitochondrial Diseases

Australian Mitochondrial Disease Foundation
Suite 4, Level 6
9-13 Young Street
Sydney NSW 2000 Australia
Website: http://www.amdf.org.au
E-mail: info@amdf.org.au

United Mitochondrial Disease Foundation
8085 Saltsburg Road, Suite 201
Pittsburgh, PA 15239
Toll-Free: 888-317-UMDF
(888-317-8633)
Phone: 412-793-8077
Fax: 412-793-6477
Website: http://www.umdf.org
E-mail: info@umdf.org

Neurofibromatosis

Acoustic Neuroma Association
600 Peachtree Parkway
Suite 108
Cumming, GA 30041-6899
Toll-Free: 877-200-8211
Toll-Free Fax: 877-202-0239
Phone: 770-205-8211
Fax: 770-205-0239
Website: http://www.anausa.org
E-mail: info@anausa.org

Children's Tumor Foundation
95 Pine Street, 16th Floor
New York, NY 10005-1703
Toll-Free: 800-323-7938
Phone: 212-344-6633
Fax: 212-747-0004
Website: http://www.ctf.org
E-mail: info@ctf.org

Neurofibromatosis Network
213 South Wheaton Avenue
Wheaton, IL 60187
Toll-Free: 800-942-6825
Phone: 630-510-1115
Fax: 630-510-8508
Website:
http://www.nfnetwork.org
E-mail: admin@nfnetwork.org

Neuromuscular Disorders

Charcot-Marie-Tooth Association (CMTA)
P.O. Box 105
Glenolden, PA 19036
Toll-Free: 800-606-CMTA
(800-606-2682)
Phone: 610-499-9264
Fax: 610-499-9267
Website: http://www.cmtausa.org
E-mail: info@cmtausa.org

Coalition to Cure Calpain 3 (C3)
15 Compo Parkway
Westport, CT 06880
Phone: 203-221-1611
Fax: 734-668-4755
Website:
http://www.curecalpain3.org
E-mail: info@curecalpain3.org

Cure CMD
P.O. Box 701
Olathe, KS 66051
Toll-Free: 866-400-3626
Website: http://www.curecmd.org
E-mail: info@curecmd.com

Facioscapulohumeral Muscular Dystrophy (FSH) Society
450 Bedford Street
Lexington, MA 02420
Phone: 781-301-6060
Fax: 781-862-1116
Website:
http://www.fshsociety.org
E-mail: info@fshsociety.org

Families of Spinal Muscular Atrophy
925 Busse Road
Elk Grove Village, IL 60007
Toll-Free: 800-886-1762
Phone: 847-367-7620
Fax: 847-367-7623
Website: http://www.curesma.org
E-mail: info@fsma.org

FightSMA
1321 Duke Street, Suite 304
Alexandria, VA 22134
Phone: 703-299-1144
Website: http://www.fightsma.org

Friedreich's Ataxia Research Alliance (FARA)
533 West Uwchlan Avenue
Downingtown, PA 19335
Phone: 484-879-6160
Fax: 484-872-1402
Website: http://www.CureFA.org
E-mail: info@CureFA.org

Hereditary Neuropathy Foundation, Inc.
432 Park Avenue South
4th Floor
New York, NY 10016
Toll-Free: 855-HELPCMT
(855-435-7268)
Phone: 212-722-8396
Fax: 917-591-2758
Website: http://www.hnf-cure.org
E-mail: info@hnf-cure.org

Jain Foundation
2310 130th Avenue NE
Suite B101
Bellevue, WA 98005
Phone: 425-882-1440
Fax: 425-658-1703
Website:
https://www.jain-foundation.org
E-mail:
ehwang@jain-foundation.org

Muscular Dystrophy Association (MDA)
3300 East Sunrise Drive
Tucson, AZ 85718-3208
Toll-Free: 800-572-1717
Phone: 520-529-2000
Fax: 520-529-5300
Website: http://www.mda.org
E-mail: mda@mdausa.org

Muscular Dystrophy Family Fund
1033 Third Avenue SW
Suite 108
Carmel, IN 46032
Phone: 317-249-8488
or 317-615-9140
Fax: 317-853-6743
Website: http://www.mdff.org
E-mail: info@mdff.org

Myotonic Dystrophy Foundation
P.O. Box 29543
Sunland, CA 94129
Toll-Free: 866-968-6642
Phone: 415-800-7777
Website: http://myotonic.org
E-mail: info@myotonic.org

National Ataxia Foundation (NAF)
2600 Fernbrook Lane North
Suite 119
Minneapolis, MN 55447-4752
Phone: 763-553-0020
Fax: 763-553-0167
Website:
http://www.ataxia.org
E-mail: naf@ataxia.org

Neuropathy Association
60 East 42nd Street
Suite 942
New York, NY 10165-0999
Toll-Free: 888-PN-FACTS
(888-763-2287)
Phone: 212-692-0662
Fax: 212-692-0668
Website:
http://www.neuropathy.org
E-mail: info@neuropathy.org

Parent Project Muscular Dystrophy (PPMD)
401 Hackensack Avenue
9th Floor
Hackensack, NJ 07601
Toll-Free: 800-714-KIDS
(800-714-5437)
Phone: 201-250-8440
Fax: 201-250-8435
Website:
http://www.parentprojectmd.org
E-mail:
info@parentprojectmd.org

Spastic Paraplegia Foundation
7700 Leesburg Pike
Suite 123
Falls Church, VA 22043
Toll-Free: 877-SPF-GIVE
(877-773-4483)
Fax: 877-SPF-GIVE
(877-773-4483)
Website:
http://www.sp-foundation.org
E-mail:
information@sp-foundation.org

Spinal Muscular Atrophy Foundation
888 Seventh Avenue
Suite 400
New York, NY 10019
Toll-Free: 877-FUND-SMA
(877-386-3762)
Phone: 646-253-7100
Fax: 212-247-3079
Website:
http://www.smafoundation.org
E-mail:
info@smafoundation.org

Porphyria

American Porphyria Foundation

4900 Woodway, Suite 780
Houston, TX 77056–1837
Toll-Free: 866-APF-3635
(866-273-3635)
Phone: 713-266-9617
Fax: 713-840-9552
Website: http://www
.porphyriafoundation.com
E-mail: porphyrus@aol.com

The Porphyrias Consortium

Consortium Project Coordinator
Mount Sinai School of Medicine
Department of Genetics
and Genomic Sciences
1425 Madison Avenue, 14-75A
New York, NY 10029
Toll-Free: 866-322-7968
Phone: 212-659-6779
Fax: 212-659-6780
Website:
http://rarediseasesnetwork.epi
.usf.edu/porphyrias/

Prader-Willi Syndrome

Foundation for Prader-Willi Research

5455 Wilshire Boulevard
Suite 2020
Los Angeles, CA 90036
Toll-Free: 888-322-5487
Phone: 760-536-3027
Toll-Free Fax: 888-559-4105
Website: http://www.fpwr.org

Prader-Willi Syndrome Association (USA)

8588 Potter Park Drive
Suite 500
Sarasota, FL 34238
Toll-Free: 800-926-4797
Phone: 941-312-0400
Fax: 941-312-0142
Website:
http://www.pwsausa.org

Retinoblastoma

Retinoblastoma International

18030 Brookhurst Street
Box 408
Fountain Valley, CA 92708
Website:
http://www.retinoblastoma.net
E-mail: info@retinoblastoma.net

Retinoblastoma.com

Website: http://retinoblastoma
.com/retinoblastoma/

Rett Syndrome

International Rett Syndrome Foundation

4600 Devitt Drive
Cincinnati, OH 45246
Toll-Free: 800-818-7388
Phone: 513-874-3020
Fax: 513-874-2520
Website:
http://www.rettsyndrome.org
E-mail:
admin@rettsyndrome.org

**Rett Syndrome
Research Trust**
67 Under Cliff Road
Trumbull, CT 06611
Phone: 203-445-0041
Fax: 203-445-9234
Website: http://www.rsrt.org
E-mail: monica@rsrt.org

Smith-Magenis Syndrome

**PRISMS, Inc. (Parents and
Researchers Interested in
Smith-Magenis Syndrome)**
21800 Town Center Plaza
Suite 266A-633
Sterling, VA 20164
Phone: 972-231-0035
Fax: 972-499-1832
Website: http://www.prisms.org

SMS Research Foundation
18620 SW 39th Street
Miramar, FL 33029
Phone: 203-450-9022
Website: http://www
.smsresearchfoundation.org
E-mail: info@
smsresearchfoundation.org

Trisomy Disorders

**National Association for
Down Syndrome (NADS)**
P.O. Box 206
Wilmette, IL 60091
Phone: 630-325-9112
Website: http://www.nads.org
E-mail: info@nads.org

**National Down
Syndrome Congress**
30 Mansell Court
Suite 108
Roswell, GA 30076
Toll-Free: 800-232-NDSC
(800-232-6372)
Phone: 770-604-9500
Fax: 770-604-9898
Website:
http://www.ndsccenter.org
E-mail: info@ndsccenter.org

**National Down Syndrome
Society**
666 Broadway, 8th Floor
New York, NY 10012
Toll-Free: 800-221-4602
Website: http://www.ndss.org
E-mail: info@ndss.org

Trisomy 18 Foundation
4491 Cheshire Station Plaza
Suite 157
Dale City, VA 22193
Phone: 810-867-4211
Website:
http://www.trisomy18.org
E-mail: T18info@trisomy18.org

Tuberous Sclerosis

Tuberous Sclerosis Alliance
801 Roeder Road
Suite 750
Silver Spring, MD 20910-4467
Toll-Free: 800-225-6872
Phone: 301-562-9890
Fax: 301-562-9870
Website:
http://www.tsalliance.org
E-mail: info@tsalliance.org

Tuberous Sclerosis Canada
92 Caplan Avenue, Suite 125
Barrie, ON L9N 0Z7 Canada
Toll-Free: 888-223-2410
Website: http://tscanada.ca

Urea Cycle Disorders

National Urea Cycle Disorders Foundation
Toll-Free: 800-38-NUCDF
(800-386-8233)
Website: http://www.nucdf.org
E-mail: info@nucdf.org

Vision Disorders

Childhood Glaucoma Network
Website: http://
childhoodglaucomanetwork.com

Glaucoma Associates of Texas
10740 North Central
Expressway, Suite 300
Dallas, TX 75231
Phone: 214-360-0000
Fax: 214-739-8562
Website: http://www
.glaucomaassociates.com

Glaucoma Research Foundation
251 Post Street, Suite 600
San Francisco, CA 94108
Toll-Free: 800-826-6693
Phone: 415-986-3162
Fax: 415-986-3763
Website:
http://www.glaucoma.org
E-mail: question@glaucoma.org

Williams Syndrome

Williams Syndrome Association
570 Kirts Boulevard
Suite 223
Troy, MI 48084-4156
Toll-Free: 800-806-1871
Phone: 248-244-2229
Fax: 248-244-2230
Website: http://
www.Williams-syndrome.org
E-mail: info@
williams-syndrome.org

Wilson Disease

Wilson Disease Association
5572 North Diversey Boulevard
Milwaukee, WI 53217
Toll-Free: 866-961-0533
Phone: 414-961-0533
Fax: 414-962-3886
Website:
http://www.wilsonsdisease.org
E-mail: info@wilsonsdisease.org

Index

Index

Page numbers followed by 'n' indicate a footnote. Page numbers in *italics* indicate a table or illustration.

685

K

L

Health Reference Series